Jonas and Kovner's
Health Care Delivery
in the United States

Seventh Edition

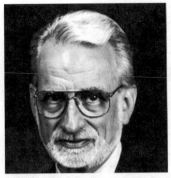

Steven Jonas, MD, MPH, earned his bachelor's degree from Columbia University, and received his master's degrees from Harvard, Yale, and New York University, respectively, with additional graduate study at the London School of Economics and the Touro College School of Law. He currently is a Professor of Preventive Medicine at the State University of New York at Stony Brook. Board-certified in preventive medicine, he is a Fellow of the American College of Preventive Medicine, the New York Academy of Medicine, and the American Public Health Association. He is a past President of the Association of Teachers of Preventive Medicine and a past member of the New York State Board for Medicine. He has authored, coauthored, and edited more than 20 books on health policy, health promotion and wellness, and national politics. He is the Founding Editor of Springer Publishing's *Series on Medical Education,* a member of the editorial boards of several other professional journals in health promotion/disease prevention, and has a regular column in the *American Medical Athletics Association Quarterly.* Jonas has also published well over 100 professional articles and book reviews in the health policy arena, and has published numerous popular articles and given many talks on sports, exercise promotion, and weight management.

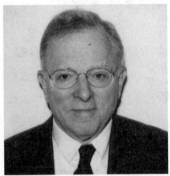

Anthony R. Kovner, PhD, is Professor of Health Policy and Management at the Robert F. Wagner Graduate School of Public Service at New York University, in New York City. He is trained in organizational behavior, health services management, and social economic development. He received bachelor's and master's degrees from Cornell University, and obtained his doctorate in public administration from the University of Pittsburgh. Kovner is an experienced health care manager, having served as CEO of a community hospital, senior health care consultant for a large union, and as manager of a group practice, a nursing home, and a large neighborhood health center. He is a board member of the Lutheran Medical Center, Augustana Nursing Home, and Health Plus, of Brooklyn, New York. He has several funded research projects, most recently focusing on better information for hospital boards and on the impact of Medicaid managed care on New York City health plans. He is the author or editor of 9 books, and the author of 43 journal articles and 24 case studies. Kovner has carried out several national demonstration programs funded by major foundations. He was the fourth recipient, in 1999, of the Gary L. Filerman prize for Educational Leadership, from the Association of University Programs in Health Administration.

Jonas and Kovner's

Health Care Delivery in the United States

Seventh Edition

Anthony R. Kovner, PhD
Steven Jonas, MD, MPH, MS, Editors

 Springer Publishing Company

Springer Publishing Company, Inc.
536 Broadway
New York, NY 10012-3955

Acquisitions Editor: Sheri W. Sussman
Production Editor: Pamela Lankas
Cover design by Susan Hauley

02 03 04 05 06 / 5 4 3 2 1

Library of Congress Cataloging-in-Publication Data

Jonas and Kovner's healthcare delivery in the United States / Anthony R.
Kovner, Steven Jonas, editors. — 7th ed.
    p. cm.
    Includes bibliographical references and index.
    ISBN 0-8261-2085-7
    1. Medical care—United States. I. Title: Healcare delivery in the U.S.
II. Title: Health care delivery in the United States. III. Kovner, Anthony R.
IV. Jonas, Steven.
    [DNLM: 1. Delivery of Health Care—United States. 2. Health
Services—United States.]
    RA395.A3 H395 2002
    362.1'0973—dc21
                                                        2002017573

Printed in the United States of America by Capital City Press.

To all those who have struggled to assure equitable insurance and access to health care for all Americans, and for all those who continue to so struggle.

Contents

III: System Performance

IV: Futures

Foreword

The health care delivery system in the United States is unique among developed nations. We spend more on health care per citizen by a factor of two. We rely on the market as a vehicle for delivering care, largely through private provision and financing. Government steps in to pay for or provide care directly to certain groups of citizens—the elderly, disabled, some of the poor—or to special beneficiaries like the military, veterans, and Native Americans. We do not have a tradition of national (federal) approaches to assuring financial access to care for all our people or to setting standards for service, quality, or performance. All of these factors make for an extremely dynamic and complex system and create a challenge to faculty and student as they explore its core institutions and track the policies and programs that cause them to change over time.

Jonas and Kovner's *Health Care Delivery in the United States* in its 7th edition meets these challenges in a number of ways. First, it provides historical perspective on the development of our health care delivery system—our basic belief in the importance of individual responsibility for health and social well-being in the United States, with government playing a role only when the private individual and community efforts fall short. It also helps us to understand that the first line of government response is that closest to the individual—at state and local levels—creating the conditions for both enormous variety and innovation in our health system as well as enormous inequities in access to and quality of care. These facts automatically ensure that any national-level change in the health system will require the management of multiple public and private stakeholders, as well as a balancing of the relationships between federal and state governmental authorities.

In this context, the book provides us with expert analyses of both the inputs to the system—the provision of human and financial resources, technology, and the institutions that pay for and provide care—and the outputs of the system in the provision of continuity of care to individuals with different levels of mental and physical health and illness and at different stages of their disease process, from primary care to hospitals to long-term care. It also examines system performance to help assess the value received for the investments.

When the book looks at future trends and influences, it does so with the recognition that in a system as complex as ours, it is critical to understand the forces acting on the system from outside and inside and to be aware that aligning these forces to make desired changes will be a real challenge. It will depend on public understanding, professional standards and, most of all, political will to balance the multiple interests at stake. We also see that assuring the health of our nation involves actions outside the health care delivery system to influence personal risk behaviors, physical environmental conditions, and critical social environmental factors such as socioeconomic status and education.

Finally, and very important, this book has a point of view about health policy. First, it must include factors beyond personal health care to take on the critical challenges of population education and prevention. Second, the critical challenge facing us in our personal health care system is ensuring access to health care of acceptable quality at reasonable cost for all our people. Achieving this goal is still the major unsolved health policy issue of our time and one that all future health professionals must understand and be willing to tackle. Students using this book as a resource will be well on their way to understanding and playing an effective role in addressing the policy and management challenges of our health care system now and for the future.

JO IVEY BOUFFORD, MD
Dean, Robert F. Wagner Graduate
School of Public Service
New York University

Organization of This Book

This book, *Health Care Delivery in the United States,* 7th edition, is organized into four parts: I—"Perspectives," II—"Settings," III—"System Performance," and IV—"Futures" (see Figure 1). The titles of these four parts can be formulated as answers to the following questions. How do we assess and also understand the health care sector of our economy? Where is health care provided and what are the characteristics of those institutions that provide health care? What are some of the determinants of how well the system performs? Over the short term, where is the health care sector going in terms of the health of the people, the cost or care, access, and quality?

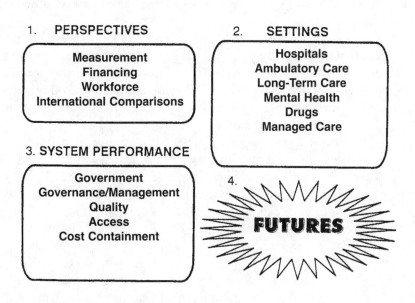

FIGURE 1   Health care delivery in the United States.

Part I, "Perspectives," is divided into an introduction and chapters on measurement, financing, workforce, and international comparisons. The introductory chapter on the state of health care delivery in the United States focuses on what we as a nation, in the estimation of the authors, are doing "right" and what we are doing "wrong." Next Jonas and Chiasson present the basics on how health and health care are measured in the United States. Then Thorpe and Knickman analyze where the money to pay for health services comes from and on what the money is spent. Chris Kovner and Salsberg describe the health care workforce and focus on issues of supply and demand for doctors and nurses. Rodwin then compares health care systems in several developed countries and asks how the United States can learn from others in evaluating and proposing changes in our system of health care delivery.

Part II, "Settings," contains six chapters, on hospitals and health systems, ambulatory care, long-term care, mental health, pharmaceuticals, and managed care. Tony Kovner describes how hospitals are organized and financed, and how they are forming themselves into health systems in response to the pressures from managed care. Mezey examines the different ways of providing ambulatory care, and how primary care is changing. Feldman then describes how long-term care is organized and financed, and how nursing home and home care too are changing in the managed care environment. Continuing Part II, Sharfstein, Stoline, and Koran examine how mental health services have evolved and how they are organized and financed. In a chapter that is new to this 7th edition of our textbook, Strongin describes the pharmaceutical sector of our nation's economy and how rapidly increasing drug expenditures are influencing health care delivery. Smits and Tony Kovner conclude Part II by examining managed care and how well it meets the expectations that purchasers and other stakeholders have for it.

Part III, "System Performance," is divided into five chapters, on government, governance and management, quality, access, and cost containment. Sparer describes the major role that government plays in the purchasing, regulating, and delivery of health care, focusing on the Medicare and Medicaid programs and how these are evolving. Tony Kovner examines what health institution governance is, and who owns health care organizations and how they are managed. Horn analyzes indicators of health care quality including the structure, process, and outcomes of care, and specifies key factors in designing quality improvement programs. Billings and Cantor review the levels of access various groups of Americans have to health care, and they make suggestions for improving access. Thorpe, in reviewing cost containment strategies, explains the trends in the growth of health care expenditures and the history of efforts to contain costs.

Finally, in Part IV, "Futures," Knickman attempts to specify what health care in the United States will look like over the near term. What are the key drivers for change? What do customers and taxpayers want from the system? Knickman forecasts the following areas where change may be most significant: innovation in serving the elderly and the chronically ill; advances in molecular genetics and a range of technological innovation; larger and more complex health systems; and changes in Medicare, the use of information technology, and health promotion.

Each of these 17 chapters contains learning objectives, a topical outline, a list of key words, questions, and a case study for further analysis and discussion. Following the primary text are a glossary, a guide to sources of data, a guide to using the World Wide Web, and an index by subject.

Contributors

John Billings, JD, is currently an associate professor at the Robert F. Wagner Graduate School of Public Service at New York University, and he is the director of the school's Health Research Program. Mr. Billings's recent work has involved analysis of patterns of hospital admission rates and emergency department utilization as tools to evaluate access barriers to outpatient care and to assess the performance of the ambulatory care delivery system. Mr. Billings is currently the principal investigator on a project funded by the Robert Wood Johnson Foundation to assess models for delivering primary care to low-income populations and is coprincipal investigator with Columbia University and the United Hospital Fund of New York to evaluate the impact of Medicaid managed care in New York City. Previously, Mr. Billings headed the Ambulatory Care Access Project, a 4-year effort to evaluate access barriers in New York City and urban areas in five other states. He has also worked extensively analyzing the problems of the medically indigent and developing solutions for coverage and provision of care for the uninsured in Florida, Virginia, North Carolina, Pennsylvania, Utah, and the District of Columbia. Mr. Billings's other health policy work has focused on issues related to quality of care, the management of quality in the inpatient and outpatient setting, and the physician decision-making process. Mr. Billings holds a law degree from the University of California at Berkeley.

Joel C. Cantor, ScD, is the Director of the Center for State Health Policy and Professor of Public Policy at Rutgers, The State University of New Jersey. Dr. Cantor's research focuses on issues of health care financing and delivery at the state and local levels. His recent work includes studies of the effect of health care market competition on access to care, the organization of the health care safety net for the uninsured, and the role of minority physicians in improving access to care of underserved populations. Dr. Cantor has published widely on health policy topics, and serves on the editorial board of the policy journal *Inquiry.* Prior to joining the faculty at Rutgers, Dr. Cantor served as Director of Research at the United Hospital Fund of New York and Director of Evaluation Research at the Robert Wood Johnson Foundation.

Mary Ann Chiasson, MPH, DrPH, is Vice President for Research and Evaluation at the Medical and Health Research Association of New York City, Inc. (MHRA). Before joining MHRA, she served as Assistant Commissioner for Disease Intervention Research at the New York City Department of Health for 9 years with scientific and administrative responsibility for AIDS surveillance, AIDS Research, and Vital Statistics and Epidemiology. Dr. Chiasson is an epidemiologist and her research focuses on disease surveillance, the epidemiology of HIV (particularly risk factors for heterosexual transmission and gynecologic manifestations of HIV), women's reproductive health, and infant mortality. Dr. Chiasson received her MPH and DrPH in epidemiology from the School of Public Health, Columbia University, and is an Associate Professor of Clinical Public Health (Epidemiology) at the Joseph L. Mailman School of Public Health, Columbia University.

Penny Hollander Feldman, PhD, is Vice President for Research and Evaluation and Director of the Center for Home Care Policy and Research at the Visiting Nurse Service of New York (VNSNY). Prior to joining VNSNY, Dr. Feldman served on the faculties of Harvard University's Kennedy School of Government and the Department of Health Policy and Management at the Harvard School of Public Health, where she continues as a member of the faculty. At the Center for Home Care Policy and Research, she directs research projects focused on improving the quality, outcomes and cost-effectiveness of home-based care; supporting informed policy-making by federal, state, and local decision makers; promoting equitable access and outcomes for older persons, especially those who are disadvantaged; and strengthening methods for home care research. Dr. Feldman is the program director of the Home Care Research Initiative, a national research program established by the Robert Wood Johnson Foundation in 1995. She also directs the AdvantAge Initiative, a project designed to develop indicators of "elder friendliness" for communities that seek to improve their capacity to meet the needs of a rapidly growing older population. Dr. Feldman served as a member of the Institute of Medicine's Committee on Improving Quality in Long-Term Care, which issued its final report in the winter of 2001. She earned her PhD in Political Science from Harvard University.

Michal D. Gursen, MPH, MS, is a Research Analyst at the Center for Home Care Policy and Research at the Visiting Nurse Service of New York. At the Center, she is involved in multiple projects, including the Home Care Research Initiative of the Robert Wood Johnson Foundation, and the AdvantAge Initiative, a project designed to develop indicators of "elder friendliness" for communities that seek to improve their capacity to meet the needs of older persons. Before coming to the Center, Ms. Gursen worked at New York State Psychiatric Institute where she investigated psychoeducational interventions for people with mental illness. Prior to that, she worked at Mount Sinai School of Medicine where she researched psychosocial pathways leading to drug use. Ms. Gursen earned her MPH in Health Policy and Management with a concentration in Effectiveness and Outcomes Research, and her MS in Social Work, from Columbia University.

Susan D. Horn, PhD, is senior scientist for the Institute for Clinical Outcomes Research (ICOR), and Vice President of Research for International Severity Information Systems, Inc. (ISIS), both located in Salt Lake City, Utah. In addition, she is a Research Professor at the University of Texas–Houston, School of Nursing and a professor in the Department of Medical Informatics at the University of Utah School of Medicine in Salt Lake City. From 1991 to 1995, she was Senior Scientist at Intermountain Health Care in Salt Lake City. In 1982, Dr. Horn and her colleagues began developing the Comprehensive Severity Index (CSI®), with inpatient, outpatient, hospice, rehabilitation, and long-term care components for adult and pediatric patients. The CSI software system is used to collect disease-specific, physiologic severity data for clinical practice improvement and risk-adjusted outcomes. She has authored over 115 publications on statistical methods, health services research, severity of illness measurement, clinical practice improvement, and quality of care. Dr. Horn is coeditor of *Clinical Practice Improvement: A New Technology for Developing Cost Effective, Quality Health Care,* Faulkner & Gray, Washington, D.C., 1994, and editor of *Clinical Practice Improvement Methodology: Implementation and Evaluation,* Faulkner & Gray, 1997. She earned a BA in mathematics at Cornell University in 1964, and a PhD in statistics at Stanford University in 1968.

James R. Knickman, PhD, is Vice President for Research and Evaluation at The Robert Wood Johnson Foundation. Prior to joining the Foundation in October 1992, Dr. Knickman was a Professor of Health Administration at New York University's Robert Wagner Graduate School of Public Service. Dr. Knickman has published extensively on a range of health care issues. He has done research on insurance markets and health care reimbursement systems with particular attention to long-term care services. He also has written about methods for improving health services for urban, vulnerable populations such as the homeless, the frail elderly, and individuals with HIV illness. Dr. Knickman has served on a range of state government, local government, and health care sector advisory committees, and has offered consultation to a range of health sector organizations. Currently, he serves on the Board of Trustees of Robert Wood Johnson

University Hospital. Dr. Knickman received his PhD in Public Policy Analysis from the University of Pennsylvania and did undergraduate work at Fordham University.

Lorrin M. Koran, MD, Professor of Psychiatry at Stanford University Medical Center, is the Director of the Obsessive Compulsive Disorders Clinic and Chief of the Psychiatric Consultation Service. His research interests include new drug treatments for obsessive-compulsive and depressive disorders, and characteristics of the mental health services delivery system. Dr. Koran has served as Special Assistant to the Director of the National Institute of Mental Health. He received his MD from Harvard Medical School.

Christine T. Kovner, RN, PhD, is a Senior Fellow, Hartford Institute for Geriatric Nursing, and Professor in the Division of Nursing, Steinhardt School of Education, New York University. Dr. Kovner is the editor of *Nursing Counts,* a newsletter about the nursing workforce. She has worked as a public health nurse, home care coordinator, and as a director of staff development in a small acute care hospital. Her research interests are nursing resource use and the cost of nursing care.

Andrew P. Mezey, MD, MS, is Vice Chair for Research and Director of the Division of General Pediatrics in the Department of Pediatrics at Maimonides Medical Center in Brooklyn, New York. He was formerly Associate Dean of Graduated Medical Education and Affiliations at the Albert Einstein College of Medicine. From 1989–1994 he was Medical Director of the Jacobi Medical Center, a member hospital of the New York City Health and Hospitals Corporation. He received his MD degree from New York University in 1960 and an MS degree in management in 1992, also from NYU. He was coeditor of *Primary Care Pediatrics: A Symptomatic Approach,* is on the editorial board of the American Academy of Pediatrics book *Caring for Your Baby and Young Child: Birth to Age 5,* and the former coeditor of the journal *Emergency and Office Pediatrics.* He is a member of the New York State Board of Midwifery and the New York State Council on Graduate Medical Education. He has recently been recognized by *New York Magazine* as being among the best doctors in New York in primary care pediatrics.

Pamela Nadash, BPhil, is a Research Associate at the Center for Home CAre Policy and Research, Visiting Nurse Service of New York (VNSNY). She is also working toward her PhD at Columbia University, earning a joint degree between the Mailman School of Public Health and the Political Science department. She contributes to the work of the Home Care Research Initiative of the Robert Wood Johnson Foundation and is currently conducting research on VNSNY's managed long-term care program, VNS CHOICE. Before embarking on her doctorate, she worked at the National Council on the Aging as Director of the National Institute on Consumer-Directed Long-Term Services, sitting on the management team of the Cash and Counseling Demonstration and Evaluation program and also supporting the National Program Office of The Robert Wood Johnson-funded Independent Choices grants program. Ms. Nadash has also conducted research on the experience of children with special health care needs in managed care. While working at the Policy Studies Institute in London, she acted as coinvestigator for a major study of cash payments for personal care services in the UK. Ms. Nadash earned her BA from Bryn Mawr College and a BPhil (a master's degree) in political theory from Oxford University.

Jennifer A. Nelson, MPH, is a Research Associate in the Research and Evaluation Unit at Medical and Health Research Association of New York City, Inc. Her research interests include reproductive health and maternal and child health. Recent work has focused on childhood obesity and family planning and STD service provision. She has also worked in a reproductive health clinic and was a Peace Corps Volunteer at a rural health clinic in Niger, West Africa, providing growth monitoring services, nutritional counseling, and family planning education. She received an MPH from the Center for Population and Family Health at the Joseph L. Mailman School of Public Health of Columbia University.

Lesley Reis graduated *magna cum laude* from Boston University with a Bachelor of Arts in International Relations. She is pursuing her Masters of Public Administration in Health Policy and Management at New York University. Ms. Reis has worked on a variety of public health research projects at the Massachusetts Department of Public Health, the Harvard School of Public Health, and the Boston University School of Medicine. She currently works at the Memorial Sloan-Kettering Cancer Center in New York City and served as an Administrative Resident at the State University of New York School of Optometry in August 2001.

Victor G. Rodwin, PhD, is director of the World Cities Project, a joint venture of the International Longevity Center (ILC-USA) and the Robert F. Wagner Graduate School of Public Service, New York University (NYU), where he is Professor of Health Policy and Management. He is a recipient of the 1999 Robert Wood Johnson Investigator Awards in Health Policy for his research project, "Health and Megacities: New York, London, Paris and Tokyo." At NYU since 1985, Dr. Rodwin teaches courses on health policy, comparative analysis of health systems, and community health and medical care. He has served successively as Director of the Advanced Management Program for Clinicians (AMPC) and of the International Initiative, both in the Wagner School. Professor Rodwin is author and editor of several books including *Japan's Universal and Affordable Health Care* (Japan Society, 1994), *Public Hospital Systems in*

New York City and Paris (with D. Jolly, C. Brecher, and R. Banter, New York University Press, 1992), *The Health Planning Predicament: France, Quebec, England and the United States* (University of California Press, 1984) and several others published in English and French. He is also author of numerous articles, book chapters, reports, and essays.

Edward S. Salsberg, MPA, is the Executive Director of the Center for Health Workforce Studies at the School of Public Health at the University at Albany of the State University of New York (SUNY). Mr. Salsberg established the Center in 1996. The Center, which conducts dozens of health workforce studies each year, is a national leader in the field. It is one of four organizations nationally to receive a federal cooperative agreement to support state level health workforce data analysis. Mr. Salsberg has also authored and co-authored numerous reports and papers on the health workforce. Mr. Salsberg is a member of the U.S. delegation to the International Physician Workforce Conference; a member of the steering committee of the National Academy for State Health Policy, and a member of the American Hospital Association's Commission on Workforce for Hospitals and Health Systems. Mr. Salsberg received his Masters in Public Administration from the New York University Wagner School.

Steven S. Sharfstein, MD, is President, Medical Director, and Chief Executive Officer of Sheppard Pratt, a nonprofit behavioral health system in Baltimore; Clinical Professor of Psychiatry at the University of Maryland; and a practicing clinician for over 20 years. He specializes in psychotherapy and psychopharmacology for patients with long-term mental illness. He spent 13 years with the National Institute of Mental Health, where he was Director of Mental Health Service Programs and also held positions in consultation/liaison psychiatry and research in behavioral medicine on the campus of the National Institutes of Health. He has written on a wide variety of clinical and economic topics and has published more than 140 articles, 40 book chapters, and 10 books, including (as coauthor) *Madness and Government: Who Cares for the Mentally Ill?*, a history of the federal community mental health centers program. A graduate of Dartmouth College and the Albert Einstein College of Medicine, he trained in psychiatry at the Massachusetts Mental Health Center in Boston from 1969 to 1972. Dr. Sharfstein also received a master's degree in public administration from the Kennedy School of Government in 1973 and a certificate from the Advanced Management Program at the Harvard Business School in 1991. He was Secretary of the American Psychiatric Association from 1991 to 1995. Dr. Sharfstein is also a member of the Presidential Advisory Commission on Consumer Protection and Quality in the Health Care Industry.

Helen L. Smits, MD, MACP, is currently a Visiting Professor at the Robert F. Wagner Graduate School of Public Service and Visiting Scholar at the Institute for Medicare Practice at New York University Mount Sinai.

Her major area of research has been the oversight and regulation of the quality of medical care across a broad range of settings. Dr. Smits served from 1993 to 1996 as the Deputy Administrator of the Health Care Financing Administration. From 1996 to 1999 she was President and Medical Director of Health Right, Inc., a Medicaid-only managed care plan in Connecticut. She was the Director of the John Dempsey Hospital at the University of Connecticut from 1986 through 1993. She is a member of the Institute of Medicine and serves on their Robert Wood Johnson Health Policy Fellowships Board and the Committee on Federal Quality Oversight. She served from 1996 to 2000 as a member of the Board of Governors of the Clinical Center at the National Institutes of Health. She is cochairperson of the Strategic Framework Board of the National Quality Forum. She is a former member and former Chair of the Board of Commissioners of the Joint Commission on the Accreditation of Health Care Organizations as well as a former member of the Board of Regents of the American College of Physicians (now ACP-ASIM).

Michael S. Sparer, MD, is an associate professor at the Joseph L. Mailman School of Public Health at Columbia University. He has doctoral degrees in political science from Brandeis University and in law from Rutgers School of Law (Newark). Sparer studies and writes about the politics of health care with an emphasis on the state and local role in the American health care system. Among his current projects are an evaluation of the organizational and financial issues affecting managed care plans formed by safety net providers, a study of the politics of Medicaid managed care in New York City, and an examination of state efforts to provide long-term care services through managed care delivery systems. He is the author of *Medicaid and the Limits of State Health Reform* (Temple University Press, 1996) as well as numerous articles and book chapters.

Anne M. Stoline, MD, obtained her undergraduate degree from Kalamazoo College. She attended medical school and psychiatry residency at The Johns Hopkins School of Medicine, where she coauthored *The New Medical Marketplace.* During several years as staff psychiatrist at the Sheppard and Enoch Pratt Hospital under the mentorship of Dr. Steven Sharfstein, she coauthored several chapters and articles about managed mental health care. She currently serves as Director of Women's Mental Health at Mercy Medical Center in Baltimore, Maryland.

Robin J. Strongin, MPA, is a principal with Polidais LLC, a Washington, D.C.-based health care consulting firm. Prior to consulting, Ms. Strongin was a senior research associate with the National Health Policy Forum at George Washington University where she specialized in issues related to bioterrorism and medical technology, including devices, pharmaceutical, and biotechnology concerns. Ms. Strongin was formerly Acting Executive Director and Director of Research Programs for the Health Care Technology

Institute, a privately funded organization dedicated to the support of public policy research and analysis of issues related to health care technology. Ms. Strongin has served as staff to the National Leadership Coalition on Health Care and the Prospective Payment Assessment Commission (now the Medicare Payment Advisory Commission), and as a Presidential Management Intern in the Health Care Financing Administration as well as in the Office of Congressman James J. Florio (D-NJ). Ms. Strongin holds a bachelor's degree in psychology and a master's degree in public administration, with a concentration in health administration.

Kenneth E. Thorpe, PhD, is currently Robert W. Woodruff Professor and Chair of the Department of Health Policy and Management, Rollins School of Public Health at Emory University. He was formerly Visiting Professor of Health Policy and Tropical Medicine, Tulane University. Prior to that, he was Deputy Assistant Secretary for Health Policy in the Department of Health and Human Services. He has served as consultant to the Rand Corporation and the Subcommittee on Health Insurance for the New York State Council on Health Care Financing, where he aided in the development of New York's new hospital payment system. His primary research interests include evaluations of the impact of public policies on hospital and nursing home behavior. Recent projects include an evaluation of the cost and access implications of alternative hospital payment methodologies in New York's (Medicare) waiver program and the impact of DRG payment on hospital readmission rates, as well as his ongoing research evaluating the RUG-II nursing home payment system in New York. Most recently, his research has focused on the effects of proposed employer health insurance mandates and expansions of Medicaid. He received his MA in public policy analysis from Duke University and his PhD from the Rand Graduate School.

I

Perspectives

The first part of the book, "Perspectives," has five chapters: Introduction: The State of Health Care Delivery in the United States, Measurement, Financing for Health Care, The Health Care Workforce, and Comparative Health Systems. In chapter 1, Kovner and Jonas present issues and concerns with health care delivery and the constraints and opportunities facing those who wish to improve the system. To those who say, "We don't have a health care *system* in the United States," Kovner and Jonas say, "Well, try and change something important—such as Medicare, how specialist physicians get paid, or how hospital information systems could be standardized—and see how hard it is to change it." The authors argue that it is right for Americans to have a national (not a wholly public) system, that the United States can afford national health insurance, and that we can ill afford not to have such a plan. Currently, there are "winners" among those groups that have an interest in health care delivery (those who have adequate health insurance and employers who don't pay for health insurance benefits for their workers), and "losers" (the uninsured, and employers who pay "too much" for their employees' health benefits). Kovner and Jonas suggest that more attention should be paid to "winners" and "losers" under the present system, and that the United States as a nation should reduce some of the inequalities. Kovner and Jonas indicate what they see as "right" and "wrong" with American health care delivery, and invite readers to join in discussions and initiatives to improve the health of the nation's population.

In chapter 2, Jonas and Chiasson discuss how health and health care are measured and quantified. Among other things, they review the data that are available, such as statistics on morbidity, health status, health-related

1

behaviors, and utilization. In chapter 3, Thorpe and Knickman explain how the money spent on health care is spent, where the money comes from to pay for health services, how clinicians and hospitals are paid, and why expenditures have been increasing at a rate significantly above the rate of inflation.

Chris Kovner and Salsberg, in chapter 4, describe the types of health care workers in the United States and the impact of the changing health care system on the health workforce. They discuss the following issues: the accountability of the professions, duplication and coordination among the professions, and assuring an adequate supply of doctors and nurses. In chapter 5, Rodwin presents key features of health care systems in France, Canada, and Great Britain and what might be learned from them that could be helpful for making changes in the health care delivery system in the United States.

1

Introduction: The State of Health Care Delivery in the United States

Anthony R. Kovner and Steven Jonas

LEARNING OBJECTIVES

- ☐ Understand defining characteristics of the American health care delivery system.
- ☐ Identify issues and concerns with the current delivery system.
- ☐ Understand the causes of current issues and concerns.
- ☐ Analyze stakeholder interests in health care delivery.
- ☐ Identify goals for health care delivery that are realistic and politically feasible.

TOPICAL OUTLINE

Defining characteristics of the American health care delivery system
Issues and concerns
Stakeholder interests in health care delivery
Goals for health care delivery

KEY WORDS

health care delivery, life expectancy, infant mortality, quality of care, chronic care, health care providers, Medicare, national health insurance, stakeholders, comprehensive coverage, universal health insurance, access

This introduction shall give a brief overview of some of the distinguishing characteristics of the American *health care delivery* system, review issues and concerns, and make recommendations for change in health care delivery. As long ago as 1932, a presidential commission studied the American system and pointed out that the United States had the economic resources to provide satisfactory medical service to all the people at costs that they can meet (Committee on the Costs of Medical Care, 1932/1970, p. 2). It still does. We wish to address the question of why we still have a system that doesn't do better for all Americans. If we do not come up with our own satisfactory answers to why we have the system that we do, it is likely that we can only devise unrealistic recommendations for change, that will not be implemented by the powers that be. Of course, the powers that be could fall, as did the Berlin Wall (and the powers that were in the USSR). That, however, is an alternative way of looking at things that we choose not, at this time, to consider.

DEFINING CHARACTERISTICS OF THE AMERICAN HEALTH CARE DELIVERY SYSTEM

Americans spend a lot of money on health care, over $4,300 per capita, much more than any developed country. At the same time, over 44 million Americans lack financial coverage for basic health services, again a much higher percentage than is found in any developed country. We have the most highly developed medical technology, the most expensive hospitals, and the most highly paid doctors in the world, so that Americans who can afford it have access to the best that medical treatment can offer.

ISSUES AND CONCERNS

But what value do we, as a population, get for the money that we spend? Is the health of Americans overall better than that of people in other developed countries? No. For example, among the world's developed countries the United States is not among the leaders in *life expectancy* from birth (U.S. Census Bureau [USCB], 1999, Table 1352). Nor are we among the leaders in low *infant mortality* rates. We lead the rest of the world in only one health statistic, life expectancy after the age of 80. There are several possible causes for this occurrence. It might be due to the better underlying health status of the survivors. It might be due to the better access to high technology for those who can afford care.

There are other distressing aspects of our health care delivery system beyond excessive cost and less than the best population health outcomes. The *quality of care* is uneven. Too much money is spent on administration, in major part because the financing of care is so extraordinarily complex. Too little money is spent on *chronic care*. There is fragmentation and discontinuity of care. In part because of the complexity of the financing system, there is overregulation of *health care providers* by government and insurers. Millions of Americans follow poor health practices: smoking too much tobacco and drinking too much alcohol, for example. There are also those who engage in acts of violence, with easy access to firearms. And there are those who eat too much of the wrong foods. In addition, millions of Americans are poor and cannot read—these characteristics create health problems such as the lack of knowledge about good health practices and how to gain access to services.

Part of the problem is that millions of Americans are ambivalent about a healthy lifestyle, what it consists of, and how to implement it. Americans want to look and feel terrific—but to what extent are we Americans willing to change our behaviors so that we get enough sleep and proper exercise, eat the proper amount of the right foods, and do not use tobacco or abuse alcohol?

What Most of Us Can Agree On

Of the leading priorities, national health care system reform was not a top voting issue in the 1998 congressional elections, ranking well below where it did in 1992. More narrowly focused issues such as *Medicare* reform, coverage for the uninsured and dealing with managed care are seen as the highest health care priorities by voters (Blendon, Benson, Brodie, Altman, James, & Hugick, 1999). We think that most Americans in principle agree upon the following: (1) all Americans should have access to basic health services, (2) the country can afford to provide all Americans with such access, and (3) we need to improve the effectiveness of the government in holding the private health sector accountable for providing better value for the dollars that we spend. But in the legislative arena, health care is never dealt with in principle. With regard to specifics, those whose interests benefit from the status quo simply don't want to make changes, or if they do the changes they support are designed to support their interests rather than those of the consumer and taxpayer. Americans don't agree about how we should pay for providing all Americans with access to basic health services. Nor do we agree upon what "basic health services" are; for example, to what extent are nonmedical services to the frail elderly a health service, to be afforded all Americans?

WHY DO WE HAVE THE SYSTEM THAT WE HAVE?

Readers of this text are primarily students in the various health care professions, who have their own opinions on many of these issues and concerns. Some would argue that the answer to "not getting enough value for the dollars we spend and for insuring all Americans" is the creation of a *national health insurance* system that assures basic health benefits to all, and that will contain health care costs by government regulation. Before reaching conclusions as to what "treatments" are indicated for what diagnoses, however, it is useful to understand the reasons that many of the various *stakeholders* in the health care delivery system prefer the system for the most part the way that it is now, to be changed only in certain ways that would be more favorable to their interests. Stakeholders are groups who can affect or who are affected by the current system. For the purposes of this book, we shall divide health care stakeholders into the six groups listed in Table 1.1.

Table 1.1, of course, drastically oversimplifies a complex political economy. For example, patients who require chronic care have different interests than those who are basically healthy; nurses have interests that are different from physicians, as do generalist from specialist physicians; whereas the interests of insurance plans, educators, consultants, researchers, and unions and trade organizations (all included above as vendors and suppliers) are often very different from each other. Note also that in this Table, "the people" appear in two different categories, "taxpayer" and "patient." This is because, of course, most of the time most people are not sick and don't think about what it's like to be sick and lacking insurance. We must not forget that health expenditures equal health incomes, that every dollar spent on someone in health care is also revenue or income for someone else. Provider interests narrowly focus on bottom-line issues much of the time. They are usually more effective in influencing the kinds of governmental legislation they desire than are more broadly focused consumer interests.

What we learn from Table 1.1 is that there are groups of stakeholders who favor *comprehensive coverage* (patients, vendors and suppliers, and providers), and other stakeholder groups who favor limits on payments to providers (taxpayers, and employers and payers). Of course, the same individuals in these stakeholder groups can belong to different interest groups depending on, for example, whether the individual or the provider is healthy or sick.

We are not saying that both expressed preferences for comprehensive—but not unlimited—insurance coverage, and adequate—but limited—payments to providers cannot be solved by one solution, such as national health insurance. We are saying that typically no one stakeholder group favors policies that include *both* comprehensive coverage *and* limited payments to providers. And given the risk of losing what a stakeholder group has, whether this is adequate health insurance at work or an adequate income as a health care provider, the major provider/payment system interest groups have demonstrated no interest in even a compromise solution, such as to provide full basic coverage for everyone at some reasonable cost.

WHAT IS TO BE DONE?

Let us assume that we could agree on the desirability of achieving the three goals we have highlighted: (a) access to basic health care for all Americans,

TABLE 1.1   Stakeholder Interests in Health Care Delivery

Stakeholder groups	Policies they favor	Policies they oppose
Taxpayers	Limits on provider payment	Higher taxes
Patients	Comprehensive coverage Quality of care Lower out-of-pocket costs	Limited access to care Increased patient payments
Providers	Income maintenance Autonomy Comprehensive coverage	Limits on provider payment
Vendors and suppliers	Comprehensive coverage Research funding	Limits on provider payment
Employers and payers	Cost containment Administrative simplification Elimination of cost shifting	Governmental regulation
Regulators (government)	Disclosure and reporting by providers Cost containment Access to care Quality of care	Provider autonomy

(b) *universal health insurance* coverage for all Americans, and (c) more effective governmental regulation of private providers, in a system that would be financed at a reasonable level. What must we do to make attainment of these goals a reality? First, we have to define in measurable terms what we mean by these statements of purpose. For example, how should *basic* health care and *necessary* primary care services be defined? We could define basic health care as what is covered in a typical employer's benefit plan, or in a typical plan for governmental employees. But there is a lot of disagreement even here. For example, to what extent should nursing home and home care be covered? But we have to start somewhere and cost it out. We can have whatever specific coverages are politically preferable but we can't have everything covered at a price American voters are willing to pay.

Second, we have to measure how well the system is performing now with regard to the three issues. For example, who doesn't have *access* to basic health care, and what are the consequences to how many of those involved, and for the rest of us, in paying for subsequent care?

Third, we have to have an acceptable plan to implement the recommendations. For example, to finance the additional coverages, either we have to provide narrower coverages or lower payments to providers, or raise additional revenues from other sources. This is not the place to discuss these implementation issues. You will find them discussed in greater depth in the chapters that follow (for example, those on financing, cost containment, access, and futures).

IT'S UP TO YOU

Every reader of this text is a stakeholder in the American health care delivery system. We believe that after you have read this book, you will wish the American health care delivery system to move, faster, in the direction of greater access, universal insurance, and more effective (not more) governmental regulation.

We hope our text will provide you with data and perspectives so that you can form your own conclusions and develop future lines of inquiry so that you can get answers to your own questions about these issues. We have been fascinated in our own teaching, learning, and undertaking of research over the years, by the difficulty in finding satisfactory solutions. We have been humbled by the tremendous pace of change in the delivery of health care in terms of new technologies and therapies, new demands and consumer preferences, and new ways of organizing services and training the health care workforce. At the same time, the underlying problems of lack of coverage, fragmentation of services, and grossly uneven access remain virtually unchanged. The journey to understanding and changing the world's most complicated, expensive and often dysfunctional, or at least wasteful, health care delivery system is both exhilarating and exhausting. We hope that you will enjoy it.

CASE STUDY

Politicians have suggested extending Medicare to the rest of the American population. They intend to pay for increasing the population eligible for these benefits by increasing payroll taxes and premiums. Discuss which groups or interests in American society are likely to favor or oppose such legislation, and for what reasons.

DISCUSSION QUESTIONS

1. What are the characteristics of the American health care delivery system?
2. What are the problems and issues resulting from these characteristics?
3. What are the reasons for these problems and issues?

4. What are some suggestions to overcome the opposition of certain interest groups to national health insurance for all Americans?
5. What is likely to be the response from these interests to your suggestions?

REFERENCES

Blendon, R. J., Benson, J. M., Brodie, M., Altman, D. E., James, M., & Hugick, L. (1999). Voters and health care in the 1998 election. *Journal of the American Medical Association, 282,* 189–194.

Committee on the Costs of Medical Care. (1970). *Medical care for the American people.* Washington, DC: USDHEW. (Original work published 1932)

U.S. Census Bureau. (1999). *Statistical abstract of the United States: 1999* (119th edition). Washington, DC: Author.

2

Measurement

Steven Jonas and Mary Ann Chiasson

LEARNING OBJECTIVES

☐ List and characterize the major categories of data used to describe the people served *and not served* by the health care delivery system.
☐ List and characterize the major categories of data used to describe the health care delivery system and its activities.
☐ Describe the principal sources of health and health services data and state how and where to find them (using Appendix B as well as this chapter).
☐ Define the "Key Words" listed.

TOPICAL OUTLINE

Quantitative perspectives
Census data
Vital statistics
Morbidity
Health status and health-related behaviors
Utilization of health care services
Conclusions

KEY WORDS

data, census, vital statistics, surveillance, demographic characteristics, rates, numerator, denominator, morbidity, mortality, natality, infant mortality, crude and specific rates, age-adjusted and age-standardized rates, incidence, prevalence, health status, provider- and patient-perspective utilization, ambulatory services, hospitalization, health services utilization, program planning

Quantitative description and analysis provide the basic means for understanding both the nature and health status of the population the health care delivery system is meant to serve, and how the system operates. Data are used to describe the population and its health, to plan for and target services and interventions and to measure the delivery of services and the outcomes of interventions. Commonly used data can be divided into five broad categories: census data; vital statistics data (births, deaths, marriages, and divorces); surveillance data; administrative data; and survey research data.

Data useful in describing the health of a community can be obtained from a variety of sources collected for a variety of different purposes. Data collected through surveillance, defined as the ongoing, systematic collection of information by established, often legally mandated reporting systems, directly monitor the health of the public (communicable diseases, cancer registries). Health-related data also may be collected as an adjunct to a civil registration procedure (births and deaths), or may be collected by health care providers (health services utilization) and governmental and nongovernmental insurers, or they may be collected through population-based health and behavior interview surveys.

Given the nature of most data gathering and reporting on the one hand, and book-writing and publishing on the other, by the time this book is published virtually none of the data presented in this chapter will be current. Thus, the utility of the numbers presented is not to be found in their description of current reality at the time this book is being read. Rather, the data presented are to be viewed as examples of *how* numbers can be and are used to better understand the health care delivery system, those it serves, and those outside the system.

The explosion in information technology has revolutionized our access to data. Virtually all the numbers presented in this chapter are from national surveys and data collection systems; summaries of these data are available on the Internet, in addition to being published on a regular, usually annual, basis. (See Appendix B for descriptions of the principal data sources.) Thus, the most recent numbers available for many data categories of interest can be found at the time they are needed with a few clicks of a computer mouse. It is important to note, however, that because data collection and analysis are lengthy processes, the most recent available data are usually several years old.

Despite this technological revolution, not all important data categories are regularly *(or ever)* collected or reported. Most routinely used population and health data come from data collection systems that monitor conditions of public health importance as mandated by federal, state, or local law. Publicly supported data systems are traditionally under-funded, and health care financing must balance the need for these systems and the information they provide on the part of public officials, health care providers, health planners, researchers, and the public with the need for treatment and prevention programs.

Mortality data serve as one example of how public health officials have attempted to maximize data collection while minimizing cost. Cause of death by diagnosis (e.g., heart disease, cancer, diabetes) is usually easily determined and regularly reported on the death certificate, while underlying risk factors (e.g., lifestyle, obesity, cigarette smoking) are not. As an inexpensive way of increasing the collection of this important information, some jurisdictions have added items to the death certificate related to the decedent's history of smoking and alcohol use. These efforts, however, have had limited success because this information is difficult to obtain. Therefore, one often must look beyond the traditional vital statistics reports to gain an understanding of the causes of morbidity and mortality.

Population-based surveys can provide this additional data. Such surveys are routinely used to collect more detailed, risk-related information from a relatively small sample of individuals chosen to be representative of the population. Data from interview surveys have been invaluable in linking behaviors to health outcomes and in describing the underlying prevalence of these behaviors at the national level.

Unfortunately, findings from national surveys usually cannot be extrapolated to the state or local level since neither health-related behaviors nor illnesses are randomly distributed in the population and the number of individuals in any single sociodemographic subgroup is likely to be too small to provide reliable information at the state or local level. In recent years, statewide surveys have become more common but, again, the findings usually cannot be generalized to the local level. Thus, although many characteristics of the population of a given geographic area can be described using readily accessible sources like census and vital statistics data, all too often health officials, health planners, and researchers can obtain only imprecise estimates of the incidence and prevalence of chronic diseases and health-related behaviors in the specific populations of interest to them.

This chapter focuses primarily on national data. The principal sources of the data presented are the *National Vital Statistics Reports*,[1] *Vital Statistics of the United States*, and special studies published in the National Center for Health Statistics (NCHS) publication *Vital and Health Statistics*, Series 20. Some of these data are also published regularly in the *Statistical Abstract of the United States* and the recurrent publication *Health, United States*. Detailed state and local vital statistics data are available from each

---

[1] Until the appearance of Vol. 47, No. 1 in 1988, this publication was known as the *Monthly Vital Statistics Report*. With the change of name came some changes in the ways that and frequency with which the relevant data are reported, but it is still the primary frequently published source for vital statistics data for the United States.

state's health department. Data from the many surveys and data collection systems of the Department of Health and Human Services including those from the NCHS and the National Center for Chronic Disease Prevention and Health Promotion are also included. Some of these surveys, particularly the Behavioral Risk Factor Surveillance System, collect state-specific data. (See Appendix B for descriptions of each of these sources as well as the website addresses where they can be accessed.)

QUANTITATIVE PERSPECTIVES

Purposes

There are three major purposes for characterizing a population's health and health care status quantitatively: description, program planning and evaluation, and performance measurement.

Description

There are three quantitative perspectives that can be used for description: the size and demographic characteristics of the population, direct measures of health and health status, and utilization of health services. First, quantification *describes* the population being served using simply the *numbers* of people and what are called their *demographic* (from the Greek "describing the people") characteristics. Among the important demographic indices are: age, sex, race, birthplace, geographic location, and such social characteristics as marital status, income, educational attainment, and employment. Demographic characteristics such as geographic location (do many people live near standing water inhabited by mosquitoes carrying West Nile virus?) and age distribution (are there many infants and/or people older than 65?) by themselves may well provide some indication of the population's relative disease risks.

Second are the *direct measures of health and ill health* in a population. Given the current level of sophistication of data gathering and analysis, it is much easier to characterize the latter than the former. The ill-health status of the population is described by measures of mortality (death) and morbidity (sickness). Mortality and morbidity may be counted for the population as a whole—referred to as crude rates, or mortality and morbidity may be counted by cause, or by demographic characteristics used to describe segments of the population (e.g., age, sex)—called specific rates.

Disease-specific mortality and morbidity rates highlight the major clinically apparent health and illness problems in the population. The infant mortality rate gives some indication both of general health levels and the availability of medical care. The distribution of crude and disease-specific mortality and morbidity rates by place, age, sex, ethnic group, and social class shows which population subgroups are being affected by what diseases. The prevalence of behavioral risk factors like smoking, sedentary lifestyle, and sun exposure in the population suggests the level and kinds of interventions needed and provides a window into future health care needs.

The third quantitative perspective for viewing a population in terms of health and ill health is the *utilization and quality of its health services:* what kinds of services are offered, who uses how many of what kinds of services, when, and where, and what the patient outcome is. Utilization can be measured quantitatively and qualitatively from three points of view: that of the consumer, that of the provider, and that of an accrediting organization. For example, physician-patient encounters can be reported in terms of how many visits the average patient makes to the physician each year. The same set of events can be reported in terms of how many patient visits the average physician provides each year. The type and frequency of the visits themselves and the outcomes of medical procedures can also be compared to national standards.

Patient-perspective utilization data can provide some idea about the possible differential (over- or under-) utilization of health services by social class, ethnicity, and geography. It is also important to include measures of health status when examining utilization rates since older, sicker patients would obviously use more services than healthier patients. Provider-perspective utilization data can tell us, for example, about physician and hospital workloads, in terms of provider characteristics (size, location, services offered, etc.). Taken together, these two perspectives can identify barriers to health care access at the individual and institutional level, while the findings of accrediting organizations provide a picture of the types and quality of services being provided.

In summary, health status and services quantification describes how many of what kind of people are at risk, what kinds of diseases and ill health conditions they have, how those problems are distributed in the population, who goes where for how many of what kinds of health services, delivered by which types of providers, and, in some cases, what the outcome is of these services. These descriptive data can also be used for the following purposes.

Program Planning and Evaluation

The second purpose of quantification in health care delivery is program planning and evaluation. It may be done, for example, by a private physician, a hospital, a health services network, a city or state health services administration, or a federal government agency. Descriptive data can reveal the existence of health or health services problems and can be used to help design solutions to identified problems or unmet needs. Since not everyone who is in need of a specific service will use it, data-based utilization projections are essential for estimating costs as well as service needs. Once new programs are under way, having data on them is necessary if they are to be evaluated. It is essential to know whether the program, once it is operational, is being used by those for whom it was intended.

It must be remembered, however, that data alone are not sufficient for effective and useful planning. Before data can have any real meaning for planning, the agencies and institutions in charge must first make a policy decision to actually engage in the process. They must also agree to make their planning data-based. (Too often in the real world, program planning, even if it is done, is not data-based.) Further, to make the planning process work, the policy makers who have authorized it must also have decided that once arrived at, a suitable plan will be implemented. Some of the data-based questions to be asked in any health services planning exercise are listed in Table 2.1.

Performance Measures

With the advent of managed care and the increasing need to control health care costs, interest in what health care does and how well it does it has intensified, as has competition among providers and plans. The NCQA (National Committee for Quality Assurance) HEDIS (Health Plan Employer Data and Information Set) clinical measures have been developed to assess managed care quality and the HEDIS CAHPS (Consumer Assessment of Health Plans) composite measures, which include patient satisfaction measures as well as health care and health care provider ratings, serve as important indicators of the industry's overall performance (National Committee for Quality Assurance [NCQA], 2000).

Numerous forms of health plan report cards have been developed to help consumers (formerly patients) and health care purchasers compare health plans and make informed choices. NCQA includes information about a health plan's performance in five key areas: access and service, qualified providers, staying healthy (e.g., immunization and screening programs), getting better, and living with illness (see Figure 2.1). While interpreting report cards can sometimes be a difficult task for consumers, there are likely to be many benefits beyond choosing the appropriate health plan. Never have the practice patterns of providers been under such public scrutiny, and the overall level of care is likely to improve as a result of this monitoring and feedback.

Numbers and Rates

Population, health status, and utilization data all can be presented in two forms: numbers and rates. A *number* is simply a count of conditions, individuals, or events. A *rate* has two parts: a numerator and a denominator. The numerator is the number of conditions, individuals, or events counted. The denominator is (usually) a larger group of persons, conditions, or

TABLE 2.1   Major Classes of Data Used for Health Services Planning

1. How many people live in the proposed service area, where are they located, and what forms of transportation are available?

2. What are the age, sex, and marital status distributions?

3. What are the education levels, income, ethnicity, languages spoken?

4. What is the sickness and health profile?

5. How is the population size and composition changing over time?

6. What are the financial resources of the target population and what sorts of health insurance coverage do they have?

7. What are the existing health care resources, where are they, and how are they used?

8. What do existing providers see as their needs? How do they view the new facility, and how will they relate to it?

events from among which the subset described by the numerator data is drawn. For example, for 1997, the crude death rate for the United States was 8.6 per 1000 population (U.S. Bureau of the Census [USBOC], Table 130).

It is customary to present a rate as applying during a particular time period. For example, one could determine that 1,000 deaths occurred in a particular population during a year. This number of deaths can become the numerator of a rate. Let's say that the whole population in which those deaths occurred numbers 100,000. Then the mortality rate for that population is 1,000/100,000, per year. This can be expressed as the rate per thousand (in this case, 10) or any other formulation that is useful, per year.

The magnitude of the denominator is usually chosen to make the rate a number of reasonable size with a numerator of one or higher. Thus, the less frequent the event being counted by the numerator, the larger the denominator needs to be. For example, crude death rates for a whole population, all causes, are usually given as per thousand population. Cause-specific mortality rates are usually presented as per 100,000 or even as per 1,000,000 population, depending upon the frequency of the event to which the rate refers.

Both denominators and numerators can be quite specific, as can their units. For example, in describing deaths from lung cancer that are caused by cigarette smoking, an age-/cause-specific rate could be the number of deaths per year from lung cancer in males over age 45 who have smoked two or more packs of cigarettes per day for 20 years or more (the numerator), divided by the number of *all* males over 45 who have smoked two or more packs of cigarettes per day for 20 years or more (the denominator). The units of the numerator and the denominator in health indices can also be different. For example, in cause-specific mortality rates, the unit for the numerator is deaths by cause, while the unit for the denominator is the total number of persons in the population being served.

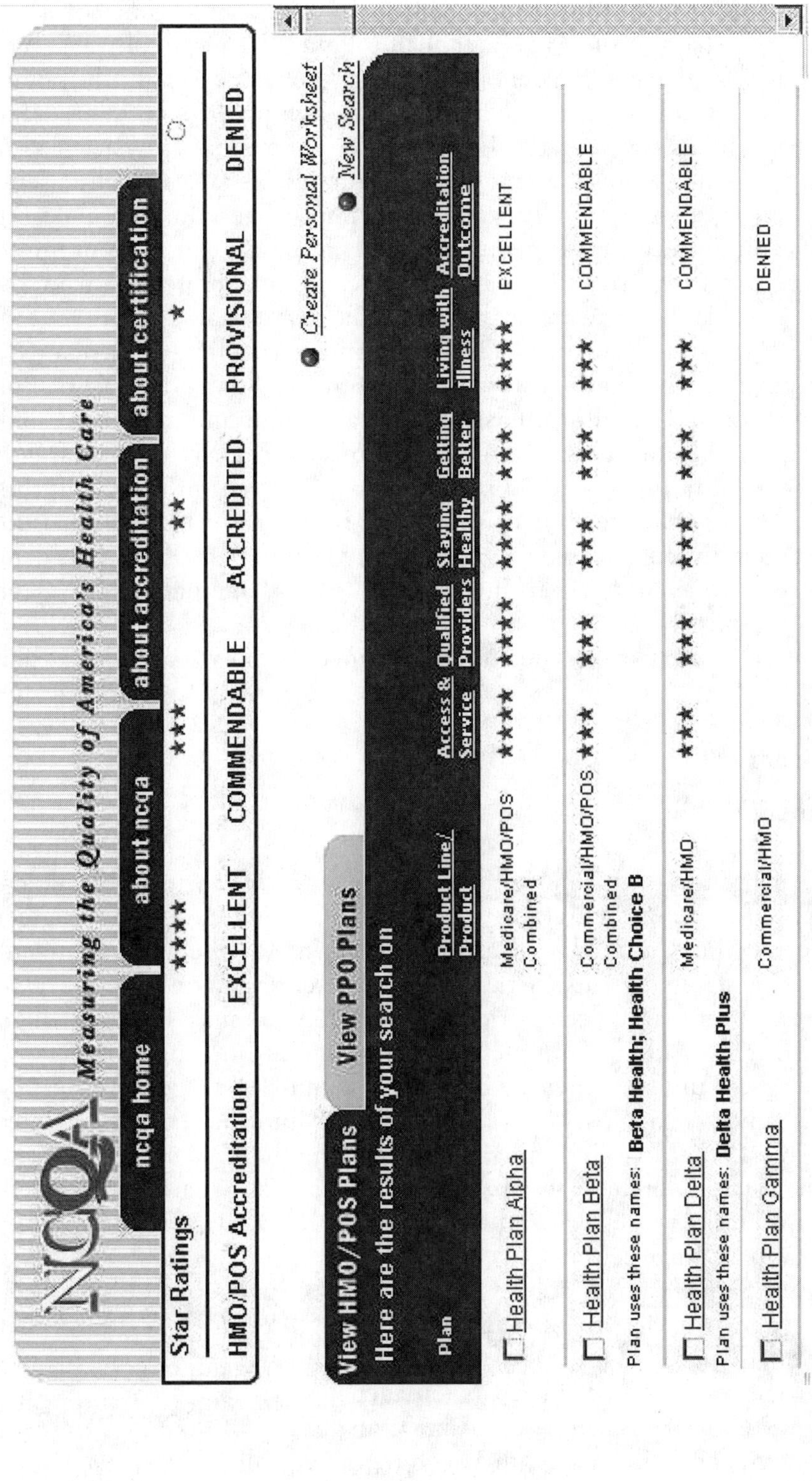

NCQA — Measuring the Quality of America's Health Care

ncqa home | about ncqa | about accreditation | about certification

Star Ratings

HMO/POS Accreditation				
★★★★	★★★	★★	★	○
EXCELLENT	COMMENDABLE	ACCREDITED	PROVISIONAL	DENIED

View HMO/POS Plans | View PPO Plans

Here are the results of your search on

Plan	Product Line/Product	Access & Service	Qualified Providers	Staying Healthy	Getting Better	Living with Illness	Accreditation Outcome
☐ Health Plan Alpha	Medicare/HMO/POS Combined	★★★★	★★★★	★★★★★	★★★	★★★★	EXCELLENT
☐ Health Plan Beta	Commercial/HMO/POS Combined	★★★	★★★	★★★	★★★	★★★	COMMENDABLE
Plan uses these names: **Beta Health; Health Choice B**							
☐ Health Plan Delta	Medicare/HMO	★★★	★★★	★★★	★★★	★★★	COMMENDABLE
Plan uses these names: **Delta Health Plus**							
☐ Health Plan Gamma	Commercial/HMO						DENIED

● Create Personal Worksheet
● New Search

FIGURE 2.1 NCQA's health plan report card.
Provided by NCQA.

Although rates are usually fractions (as in a crude death rate of 8.6 per 1000) occasionally they will be whole numbers. For example, in measuring total morbidity in a population, one may find that the number of diagnosed disease conditions is greater than the number of people. The rate then is usually given with a denominator of 1. For example: "In the population of a central African city there are 2.5 diseases per person." This usage also occurs in utilization rates. For example: "The annual physician-visit rate in the United States is about 6 per person." Rates are especially useful for measuring and describing changes over time, in everything from deaths to per capita health care expenditures. It is important to keep in mind, however, that there are no hard and fast rules for data presentation, and it is always crucial to be aware of the size of the denominator.

Health service utilization rates constitute a special group of rates. Usually they do not have customary numerators and denominators. For example, hospital-specific admission rates are commonly presented simply as a number per unit of time, as follows: "In 1997, the admission rate for hospital Y was 1,000 per month." One reason for using this formulation is that the sizes of the populations served by both institutional and individual providers are generally not known. These data generally refer to events, not to individuals, that is, one patient can have multiple admissions.

Now let us turn to a consideration of certain classes of data in some detail.

CENSUS DATA

Numbers

The Constitution of the United States requires that a census of the nation be taken at least once every 10 years (USBOC, 1999, p. 1). The original purpose of the census was to provide the basis for the apportionment among the states of seats in the House of Representatives of the U.S. Congress. A census has been carried out every 10 years since 1790. Although every effort is made for completeness, the Census Bureau has estimated that in 1990 it undercounted by between 1% and 2%, ranging from 5.0% for Hispanics, through 4.4% for blacks, to 0.7% for nonHispanic whites (USBOC, 1999, p. 1). Preliminary estimates for the 2000 census indicate that the total undercount was reduced to under 1%, whereas the undercount for blacks was 0.78% and for Hispanics 1.25% (U.S. Census Public Information Office, 2001).

The primary reasons for undercounting are thought to be fear of authority in general on the part of members of those population segments that are undercounted, and fear in particular by certain persons of being reported for one reason or another to such agencies as those responsible for immigration, social services, or criminal justice, even though guarantees are made by the census takers that such reporting will not occur.

In addition to carrying out the decennial censuses, the Census Bureau makes interim population estimates on various parameters, based on information gathered from samples and a variety of other sources. The estimated U.S. resident population as of July 1, 1998 was 270,299,000 (USBOC, 1999, Table 2). In addition, there were about 262,000 U.S. citizens (including members of the military) living abroad.

Births, deaths, immigration, and emigration are the four factors producing change in population size. During the 1970s and 1980s, the population growth rate in the U.S. averaged about 1.0% per year (USBOC, 1999, Tables 2 and 4). During the 1960s the population had grown at the rate of about 1.3% per year. The decline in rate of growth resulted primarily from a decrease in the birth rate. It is projected that population growth will likely decline further, to 0.6% per year by 2050.

Nevertheless, the "mid-range" U.S. population size projection for that year is still about 393 million, an increase of about 33% over the 1995 population. Even without taking into account the accompanying changes in the age composition of a population growing ever older as well as growing in size, the bearing of such factors as simple population size and growth rate on health services need and utilization is obvious.

Demographic Characteristics

In 1996, 79.9% of the U.S. population lived in what are called metropolitan statistical areas (MSAs, variously also referred to, with slightly different definitions, as standard metropolitan statistical areas [SMSAs], and consolidated metropolitan statistical areas [CMSAs]) (USBOC, 1999, Table 40). The figures for 1960 and 1980 were 63% and 78%, respectively, suggesting an increasingly urban population. (The definitions of "metropolitan statistical area" and its variants have varied over time. See the current edition of the *Statistical Abstract of the United States* for the current definitions.)

As of 1998, it was estimated that the U.S. population was 48.9% male, 87.3% nonblack, and had a median age of 35.2 (34.1 for males, 36.3 for females) (USBOC, 1999, Tables 13 and 14; see Table 202), up considerably from 28 in 1970. In 1998, 12.7% of the population was age 65 and over, an increase from 9.8% in 1970. In 1998, about 62% of males and 58% of females 18 and over were married, contrasting with 69% and 63%, respectively, in 1980 (USBOC, 1999, Table 62). In 1995, over 1.5 million Americans were imprisoned (USBOC, 1999, Tables 380 and 381).

During the next 50 years, the population is expected to age dramatically and this is likely to have a profound impact, not only on health and health care delivery in the United States, but on society itself. In 1995, there were 34 million people ages 65 and older, representing 13% of the population. Mid-range projections for 2050 indicate that there will be 79 million people ages 65 and older, representing 20% (one fifth!) of the population. Within this group of older Americans, the proportion of those 85 and over is growing the fastest and it is projected to more than double from nearly 4 million (1.4% of the population) in 1995 to over 8 million (2.4%) in 2030, then to more than double again in size from 2030 to 2050 to 18 million (4.6%). The effects on the need for health care and social services are likely to be staggering (USBOC, 1997).

Other realized and anticipated changes in the demographic composition of the United States are likely to have important but less dramatic effects. Educational attainment continues to rise and in March of 1995, 82% of adults ages 25 and over had completed at least high school, and 23% had earned a bachelor's degree. Attainment varied by race/ethnicity, however, with 83% of whites, 74% of blacks, and 53% of Hispanics having at least a high school degree (USBOC, 1997).

Another change that will affect the U.S. linguistically, culturally, and socially is the increase in the number and proportion of foreign born in the population. Foreign born persons declined from a high of 14.7% in 1910 to a low of 4.8% in 1970 and increased steadily to 9.7% of the total population in 1999—nearly one in ten. The majority were born in Latin America (50.7%), Asia (27.1%), and Europe (16.1%) (USBOC, 1997). Since the foreign born tend to live in central cities within a metropolitan area, cultural competence within health care delivery systems in these areas is essential in the 21st century.

In addition to sources cited, the information presented so far in this chapter comes primarily from the "Population" section of the *Statistical Abstract of the United States: 1999* (USBOC, 1999). Additional information necessary to develop a comprehensive profile of the population is contained in the "Vital Statistics," "Education," "Social Insurance and Human Services," "Labor Force, Employment, and Earnings," and "Income Expenditures, and Wealth" sections of the same publication and on the Bureau of the Census website.

VITAL STATISTICS

What Are They and How Are They Collected

In public health, "vital statistics" include data on births, deaths, fetal deaths, marriages, and divorces (National Center for Health Statistics [NCHS], 2001). Birth and death data, in particular, are probably the most widely studied and reported on indicators of the health status of a community. In the United States, primary responsibility for collecting these data lies with the state. In addition to the 50 states, the District of Columbia and New York City are independent vital registration areas. Vital registration systems are operated by the state government (or local for New York City and the District of Columbia), and are usually a function of the state department of health or its equivalent. These agencies in turn frequently delegate power to county or local health departments or local registrars to receive and process birth and death certificates. Not all states collect all categories of data although all states have collected birth and death data since 1933.

The first vital statistic to be collected in the United States on an annual basis was mortality. While there is no constitutional requirement for states to participate, in 1900, 10 states and the District of Columbia voluntarily became the first "death registration states," carrying out that task and forwarding the results to the federal government (USBOC, 1999, p. 73). Beginning in 1915, 10 states and the District of Columbia formed a "birth registration area," collecting birth data on an annual basis. Fetal deaths have been counted annually since 1922. Since 1933, the birth and death registration area has included all of the states and the District of Columbia. A "marriage registration area" was first formed in 1957. By 1999 it included 42 states and the District of Columbia. The "divorce registration area" was established in 1958. By 1999 it covered 31 states and the Virgin Islands.

Until 1946, the Census Bureau assembled and reported on vital statistics at the national level. From 1946 to 1960, the work was performed by the Bureau of State Services of the U.S. Public Health Service, and since 1960, the National Center for Health Statistics (NCHS), Centers for Disease Control and Prevention, USDHHS, has carried out this function. NCHS shares the costs incurred by the states in providing vital statistics data for national use. Through cooperative activities of the states and NCHS, standard forms for data collection and model procedures for the uniform registration of vital events are developed and recommended for state use. All states model their birth and death certificates after the U.S. standard certificates of live birth and death. Certified copies of birth and death certificates are legal documents: the original certificates remain on file with the state.

Although the process varies slightly from state to state, in general, the birth certificate is used to legally register births occurring in that state by collecting information on the newborn's name, date, time and place of birth, and name, address, and date and place of birth for the mother and father. This information is included on the copy of the birth certificate the state provides to the mother. A confidential portion of the original certificate filed by the hospital of birth contains extensive demographic and medical information on the mother and newborn that may include a chronology of the birth, maternal medical (e.g., gestational diabetes), and behavioral risk factors in the pregnancy (e.g., smoking), birth weight, abnormal conditions, and congenital anomalies of the newborn. The hospital or other facility where the birth occurs is required to complete and file the birth certificate with the state. Thus, the health care system bears the actual responsibility for collecting and reporting birth data.

In a similar manner, death certificates are used to register every death in the state where it occurs. Although there is variation from state to state, the certificate collects extensive information about the decedent including date, time, and place of death; name; age; sex; race/ethnicity; birthplace; usual occupation; and marital status. The certificate also provides a format for reporting causes of death. Generally, a licensed physician must pronounce death and certify the cause. The conditions reported on the certificate are coded by the state health department through the use of a classification structure and selection and modification rules contained in the applicable revision of the International Classification of Diseases (ICD) published by the World Health Organization (as discussed below). These coding rules provide a template for the international standardization of mortality data and improve its usefulness by systematically selecting a single cause of death from the reported sequence of conditions. The single cause selected through this procedure is called the underlying cause of death while the combination of the underlying cause of death and all other causes listed on the certificate constitutes the multiple causes of death. Unless otherwise specified, mortality statistics refer to the underlying cause of death. See Figure 2.2 (pp. 24–27) for a copy of the U.S. standard certificate of death.

NCHS calculates the national vital statistics rates. The population denominators, both total and by numerous demographic subgroups, are based upon the actual number of persons counted by the Census Bureau on April 1 of each decennial year, as well as the midyear estimates made for other years. As discussed previously, cause of death is classified according to the *International Classification of Diseases, Ninth Revision, Adapted for Use in the United States* (ICDA[2]; NCHS, 1979a).

Natality

Natality data refer only to live births. In 1998, about 3.94 million babies were born in the United States, an increase of 2% from 1997 and the first increase since 1990 (Ventura, Martin, Curtin, Matthews, & Park, 2000). As in 1997, the live birth rate was 14.6 per 1,000 population, the lowest rate recorded since 1975–1976 and 12.6% below the highest rate recorded in recent years, 16.7% in 1993. Until the earlier turnaround that occurred in 1975–1976, the birth rate had been steadily dropping from a post-World War II high of 25, reached in 1955, the peak of the so-called "baby boom."

The "fertility rate" is defined as the number of births per 1,000 women aged 15–44 (women of childbearing age). For 1998 compared to 1997, it increased 1% to 65.6. That was down from the post-World War II high of 123 reached in 1957 (USBOC, 1999, Table 93), down 7.5% from the 1990 rate, and slightly above the low of 65 recorded in 1976.

---

[2] ICD classification is also used in other coding schemes. The ICD-9-Clinical Modification (ICD-9-CM) is an extension of the ICD-9 that is used to code and classify morbidity data from inpatient and outpatient records, physician offices, and most NCHS surveys. All hospitals in the U.S. receiving federal funds are required to use this classification system. ICD is revised periodically to incorporate changes in medicine: ICD-10 was implemented by NCHS on January 1, 1999 but ICD-10-CM is still under development. The most important effect of ICD revisions is a discontinuity of trends in causes of death. See footnote 3.

Mortality

Crude Death Rates

Mortality data are reported rather neatly. Death is a well-defined event. As noted, there is one primary reporting authority for deaths, usually the local health department or registrar. Since both hospitals and funeral directors are legally required to report all deaths, we can assume that almost all deaths are reported.

For 1998 the crude death rate (total deaths per 100,000 population) in the United States was 864.7 (Murphy, 2000). This compares with a rate of 878.3 for 1980, and 852.9 for 1992. Mortality is relatively high during the first year of life, drops by increasing age group to a relatively low level until the mid-40s, and then begins to climb again (USBOC, 1999, Tables 129 and 131). Males have a higher mortality rate than females, at all ages. Data on differential death rates by the basic demographic variables of age, ethnicity, and sex can be found in the *National Vital Statistics Reports, Vital Statistics of the United States,* special studies published in the NCHS publication *Vital and Health Statistics,* Series 20, as well as the *Statistical Abstract* (refer to Appendix B).

Age-Adjusted Death Rates

In addition to crude death rates, age-adjusted (standardized) death rates are also commonly used to compare relative mortality risk across groups over time. These constructed rates eliminate variability due to differences in the age composition of various populations. Differences in age composition may have a large impact on the crude rate because of the widely different mortality rates experienced by different age groups. Statistically, an age-adjusted death rate is a weighted average of the age-specific death rates in which the weights are fixed population proportions by age. For the past 50 years the existing standard has been based on the 1940 U.S. population, but beginning with the 1999 death data, a new standard will be based on the 2000 population (Anderson & Rosenberg, 1998). This change is being made because the age composition of the 1940 population no longer reflects the increasing proportion of the U.S. population in the older age groups with higher death rates.

Although the discussion of crude versus age-adjusted death rates may appear to be of interest only to statisticians, the following example will help to illustrate the kinds of interpretation errors that can be made when mortality data are viewed by only one measure. The crude death rate for the U.S. *rose* 3.2% from 852.2 per 100,000 population in 1979 to 880.0 in 1995. In contrast, during this time period, the age-adjusted death rate *dropped* 12.7% from 577.0 per 100,000 U.S. standard population (1940) to 503.9, showing that the increase in the crude rate was due to the increasing proportion of the population in older age groups with higher death rate, not to a higher death rate by age group (Anderson & Rosenberg, 1998).

TYPE/PRINT IN PERMANENT BLACK INK FOR INSTRUCTIONS SEE OTHER SIDE AND HANDBOOK

U.S. STANDARD CERTIFICATE OF DEATH

LOCAL FILE NUMBER

STATE FILE NUMBER

DECEDENT

1. DECEDENT'S NAME (First, Middle, Last)

2. SEX

3. DATE OF DEATH (Month, Day, Year)

4. SOCIAL SECURITY NUMBER

5a. AGE—Last Birthday (Years)

5b. UNDER 1 YEAR — Months / Days

5c. UNDER 1 DAY — Hours / Minutes

6. DATE OF BIRTH (Month, Day, Year)

7. BIRTHPLACE (City and State or Foreign Country)

8. WAS DECEDENT EVER IN U.S. ARMED FORCES? (Yes or no)

9a. PLACE OF DEATH (Check only one; see instructions on other side)
HOSPITAL: ☐ Inpatient ☐ ER/Outpatient ☐ DOA
OTHER: ☐ Nursing Home ☐ Residence ☐ Other (Specify)

9b. FACILITY NAME (If not institution, give street and number)

9c. CITY, TOWN, OR LOCATION OF DEATH

9d. COUNTY OF DEATH

10. MARITAL STATUS—Married, Never Married, Widowed, Divorced (Specify)

11. SURVIVING SPOUSE (If wife, give maiden name)

12a. DECEDENT'S USUAL OCCUPATION (Give kind of work done during most of working life. Do not use retired.)

12b. KIND OF BUSINESS/INDUSTRY

13a. RESIDENCE—STATE

13b. COUNTY

13c. CITY, TOWN, OR LOCATION

13d. STREET AND NUMBER

13e. INSIDE CITY LIMITS? (Yes or no)

13f. ZIP CODE

14. WAS DECEDENT OF HISPANIC ORIGIN? (Specify No or Yes—If yes, specify Cuban, Mexican, Puerto Rican, etc.) ☐ No ☐ Yes Specify:

15. RACE—American Indian, Black, White, etc. (Specify)

16. DECEDENT'S EDUCATION (Specify only highest grade completed) Elementary/Secondary (0-12) | College (1-4 or 5+)

SEE INSTRUCTIONS ON OTHER SIDE

PARENTS

17. FATHER'S NAME (First, Middle, Last)

18. MOTHER'S NAME (First, Middle, Maiden Surname)

INFORMANT

19a. INFORMANT'S NAME (Type/Print)

19b. MAILING ADDRESS (Street and Number or Rural Route Number, City or Town, State, Zip Code)

DISPOSITION

20a. METHOD OF DISPOSITION ☐ Burial ☐ Cremation ☐ Removal from State ☐ Donation ☐ Other (Specify)

20b. PLACE OF DISPOSITION (Name of cemetery, crematory, or other place)

20c. LOCATION—City or Town, State

21a. SIGNATURE OF FUNERAL SERVICE LICENSEE OR PERSON ACTING AS SUCH

21b. LICENSE NUMBER (of Licensee)

22. NAME AND ADDRESS OF FACILITY

SEE DEFINITION ON OTHER SIDE

Complete items 23a-c only when certifying physician is not available at time of death to certify cause of death.

23a. To the best of my knowledge, death occurred at the time, date, and place stated.
Signature and Title ▲

23b. LICENSE NUMBER

23c. DATE SIGNED (Month, Day, Year)

PRONOUNCING PHYSICIAN ONLY

ITEMS 24-26 MUST BE COMPLETED BY PERSON WHO PRONOUNCES DEATH

24. TIME OF DEATH   M

25. DATE PRONOUNCED DEAD (Month, Day, Year)

26. WAS CASE REFERRED TO MEDICAL EXAMINER/CORONER? (Yes or no)

NAME OF DECEDENT: _____
For use by physician or institution

CENTER FOR HEALTH STATISTICS — 1989 REVISION

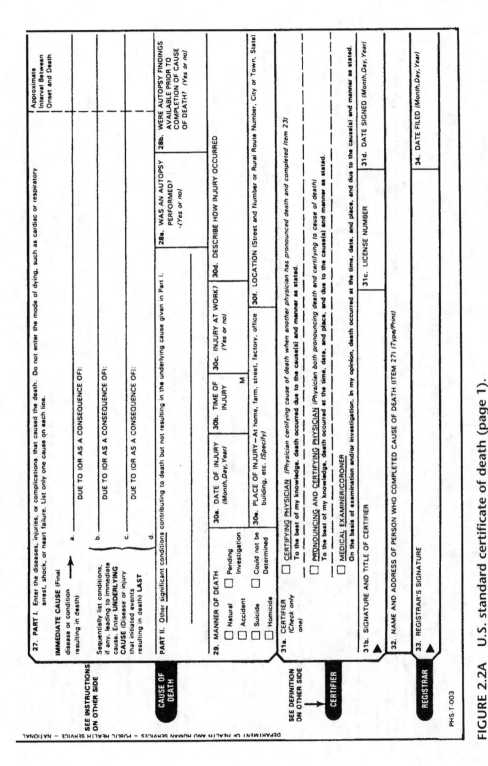

FIGURE 2.2A   U.S. standard certificate of death (page 1).

From The Centers for Disease Control, National Center for Health Statistics, 1989. Hyattsville, MD: National Center for Health Statistics.

INSTRUCTIONS FOR SELECTED ITEMS

Item 9.-- Place of Death

If the death was pronounced in a hospital, check the box indicating the decedent's status at the institution (inpatient, emergency room/outpatient, or dead on arrival (DOA)). If death was pronounced elsewhere, check the box indicating whether pronouncement occurred at a nursing home, residence, or other location. If other is checked, specify where death was legally pronounced, such as a physician's office, the place where the accident occurred, or at work.

Items 13-a-f. -- Residence of Decedent

Residence of the decedent is the place where he or she actually resided. This is not necessarily the same as "home State," or "legal residence." Never enter a temporary residence such as one used during a visit, business trip, or a vacation. Place of residence during a tour of military duty or during attendance at college is not considered as temporary and should be considered as the place of residence.

If a decedent had been living in a facility where an individual usually resides for a long period of time, such as a group home, mental institution, nursing home, penitentiary, or hospital for the chronically ill, report the location of that facility in items 13a through 13f.

If the decedent was an infant who never resided at home, the place of residence is that of the parent(s) or legal guardian. Do not use an acute care hospital's location as the place of residence for any infant.

Items 23 and 31 -- Medical Certification

The PRONOUNCING PHYSICIAN is the person who determines that the decedent is legally dead but who was not in charge of the patient's care for the illness or condition which resulted in death. Items 23a through 23c are to be completed only when the physician responsible for completing the medical certification of cause of death (Item 27) is not available at time of death to certify cause of death. The pronouncing physician is responsible for completing only items 23 through 26.

The CERTIFYING PHYSICIAN is the person who determines the cause of death (Item 27). This box should be checked only in those cases when the person who is completing the medical certification of cause of death is not the person who pronounced death (Item 23). The certifying physician is responsible for completing items 27 through 32.

The PRONOUNCING AND CERTIFYING PHYSICIAN box should be checked when the same person is responsible for completing items 24 through 32, that is, when the same physician has both pronounced death and certified the cause of death. If this box is checked, items 23a through 23c should be left blank.

The MEDICAL EXAMINER/CORONER box should be checked when investigation is required by the Post Mortem Examination Act and the cause of death is completed by a medical examiner or coroner. The Medical Examiner/Coroner is responsible for completing items 24 through 32.

Item 27. -- Cause of Death

The cause of death means the disease, abnormality, injury, or poisoning that caused the death, not the mode of dying, such as cardiac or respiratory arrest, shock, or heart failure.

In Part I, the immediate cause of death is reported on line (a), which gave rise to the cause are reported on lines (b), (c), and (d). The underlying cause, should be reported on the last line used in Part I. No entry is necessary on lines (b), (c), and (d) if the immediate cause of death on line (a) describes completely the train of events. ONLY ONE CAUSE SHOULD BE ENTERED ON A LINE. Additional lines may be added if necessary. Provide the best estimate of the interval between the onset of each condition and death. Do not leave the interval blank; if unknown, so specify.

In Part II, enter other important diseases or conditions that may have contributed to death but did not result in the underlying cause of death given in Part I.

See examples below.

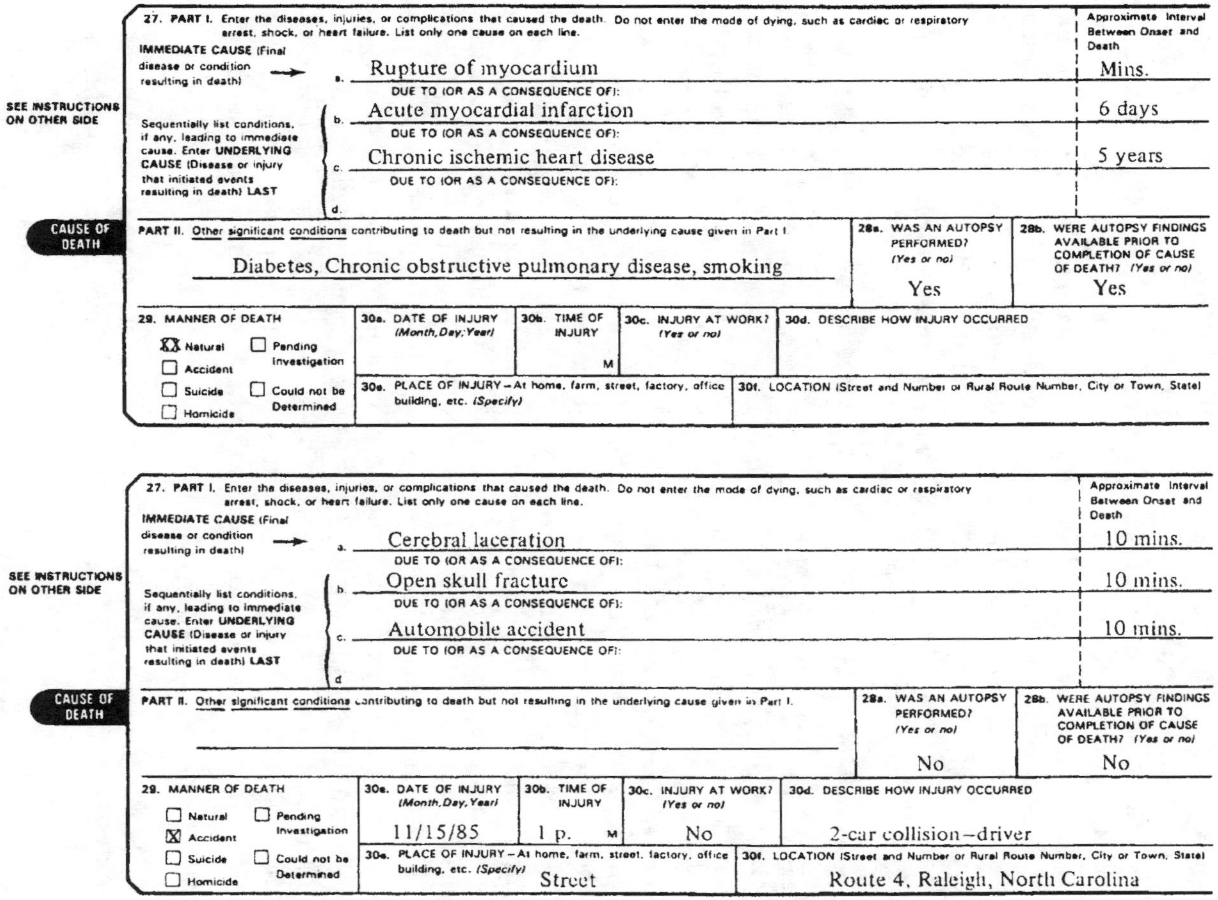

SEE INSTRUCTIONS ON OTHER SIDE

CAUSE OF DEATH

27. PART I. Enter the diseases, injuries, or complications that caused the death. Do not enter the mode of dying, such as cardiac or respiratory arrest, shock, or heart failure. List only one cause on each line.

IMMEDIATE CAUSE (Final disease or condition resulting in death) →

a. Rupture of myocardium — Mins.

DUE TO (OR AS A CONSEQUENCE OF):

b. Acute myocardial infarction — 6 days

DUE TO (OR AS A CONSEQUENCE OF):

c. Chronic ischemic heart disease — 5 years

DUE TO (OR AS A CONSEQUENCE OF):

d.

Sequentially list conditions, if any, leading to immediate cause. Enter UNDERLYING CAUSE (Disease or injury that initiated events resulting in death) LAST

Approximate Interval Between Onset and Death

PART II. Other significant conditions contributing to death but not resulting in the underlying cause given in Part I: Diabetes, Chronic obstructive pulmonary disease, smoking

28a. WAS AN AUTOPSY PERFORMED? (Yes or no) Yes

28b. WERE AUTOPSY FINDINGS AVAILABLE PRIOR TO COMPLETION OF CAUSE OF DEATH? (Yes or no) Yes

29. MANNER OF DEATH: [X] Natural [ ] Pending Investigation [ ] Accident [ ] Suicide [ ] Could not be Determined [ ] Homicide

30a. DATE OF INJURY (Month, Day, Year)

30b. TIME OF INJURY M

30c. INJURY AT WORK? (Yes or no)

30d. DESCRIBE HOW INJURY OCCURRED

30e. PLACE OF INJURY—At home, farm, street, factory, office building, etc. (Specify)

30f. LOCATION (Street and Number or Rural Route Number, City or Town, State)

SEE INSTRUCTIONS ON OTHER SIDE

CAUSE OF DEATH

27. PART I. Enter the diseases, injuries, or complications that caused the death. Do not enter the mode of dying, such as cardiac or respiratory arrest, shock, or heart failure. List only one cause on each line.

IMMEDIATE CAUSE (Final disease or condition resulting in death) →

a. Cerebral laceration — 10 mins.

DUE TO (OR AS A CONSEQUENCE OF):

b. Open skull fracture — 10 mins.

DUE TO (OR AS A CONSEQUENCE OF):

c. Automobile accident — 10 mins.

DUE TO (OR AS A CONSEQUENCE OF):

d

Sequentially list conditions, if any, leading to immediate cause. Enter UNDERLYING CAUSE (Disease or injury that initiated events resulting in death) LAST

Approximate Interval Between Onset and Death

PART II. Other significant conditions contributing to death but not resulting in the underlying cause given in Part I.

28a. WAS AN AUTOPSY PERFORMED? (Yes or no) No

28b. WERE AUTOPSY FINDINGS AVAILABLE PRIOR TO COMPLETION OF CAUSE OF DEATH? (Yes or no) No

29. MANNER OF DEATH: [ ] Natural [ ] Pending Investigation [X] Accident [ ] Suicide [ ] Could not be Determined [ ] Homicide

30a. DATE OF INJURY (Month, Day, Year) 11/15/85

30b. TIME OF INJURY 1 p. M

30c. INJURY AT WORK? (Yes or no) No

30d. DESCRIBE HOW INJURY OCCURRED 2-car collision—driver

30e. PLACE OF INJURY—At home, farm, street, factory, office building, etc. (Specify) Street

30f. LOCATION (Street and Number or Rural Route Number, City or Town, State) Route 4, Raleigh, North Carolina

FIGURE 2.2B U.S. standard certificate of death (page 2).

From The Centers for Disease Control, National Center for Health Statistics, 1989. Hyattsville, MD: National Center for Health Statistics.

Disease-Specific Mortality

Disease-specific causes of death are used to monitor prevention and treat-ment practices and programs. Determination of the disease-specific cause of death in a given case can present some problems. In most cases it is the responsibility of a physician to certify that a patient is dead and to deter-mine any underlying causes of death. Physicians have varying diagnostic styles, perspectives, and abilities, however, and may have little or no first-hand knowledge of the patient's medical history. Furthermore, there have been changes in the medical understanding and technical definitions of causes of death over time.[3] As an example of the potential difficulty, con-sider the following question: In a patient who dies from a heart attack that resulted from the complications of diabetes, is the cause of death diabetes or coronary artery disease? It is up to the physician to determine the imme-diate cause of death (most would say heart attack) and then to sequentially list conditions leading to the immediate cause entering the underlying cause (disease or injury) that initiated the chain of events leading to death last. Ultimately, physicians are responsible for cause of death coding: most physicians follow NCHS coding instructions but some do not.

In 1998 the 10 leading causes of death by disease-specific diagnostic cat-egory (excluding "symptoms and ill-defined conditions" and "all other dis-eases") were heart disease, cancer, stroke, chronic obstructive pulmonary disease, pneumonia and influenza (primarily pneumonia), "accidents and adverse effects" (all leading to personal injury as the cause of death), dia-betes mellitus, suicide, kidney disease, and liver disease (*National Vittal Statistics Reports* [NVSR], 1999, Table E).

With a few notable exceptions, the leading causes were similar in 1990: the top three, heart disease, cancer, and stroke, remained the same, fol-lowed by personal injury, chronic obstructive pulmonary disease, pneu-monia and influenza, diabetes mellitus, suicide, liver disease, and "other infectious and parasitic diseases" (predominantly human immunodeficiency virus and AIDS) (USBOC, 1999, Table 137). The rates for heart disease, cancer, and personal injury were somewhat higher in 1990 while the rates for stroke and chronic obstructive pulmonary disease were somewhat lower. In certain categories we are making progress, including the dramatic decline in deaths due to AIDS, which followed the introduction of effective therapy in 1996. Figure 2.3 illustrates the changing causes of death since 1900. Heart disease is the only cause that has been in the top five since 1900.

Risk Factor-Specific Mortality

In the modern United States, most deaths are caused by chronic diseases or conditions (such as personal injury) in which environmental and personal

---

[3] For a detailed discussion of this problem, see "Estimates of Selected Comparability Ratios Based on Dual Coding of 1976 Death Certificates by the Eighth and Ninth Revisions of the International Classification of Diseases," *Monthly Vital Statistics Report, 28*(11, Suppl.), February 1980.

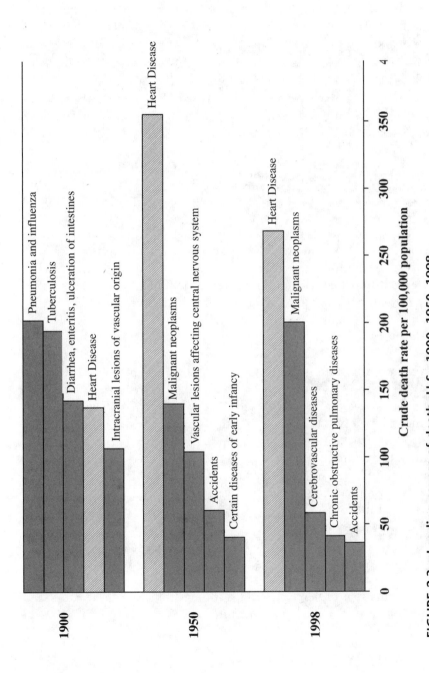

FIGURE 2.3 Leading causes of death, U.S., 1900, 1950, 1998.

Sources: Murphy, S. L. (2000). Deaths: Final Data for 1998. *National Vital Statistics Reports* (Vol. 48, No. 11). Hyattsville, MD: National Center for Health Statistics; Centers for Disease Control and Prevention (accessed 10/18/01. *Historical Data: Leading Causes of Death, 1900–1978* [on-line]. Available: www.cdc.gov/nchs/data/lead0078.pdf.

risk factors play a major causative role. To make the mortality data picture more useful for understanding what is truly going on in matters of health status and for program planning, in 1993 McGinnis and Foege (1993) took a different approach to characterizing the causes of death in the United States.

They went beyond the classic lists of death-associated disease-specific diagnoses to the identification of the major external (nongenetic) factors known to be causally associated with death. After an exhaustive review of the literature covering the period of 1977–1993 McGinnis and Foege were able to attribute approximately half of all deaths occurring in 1990 to the following ten risk factors: tobacco use (400,000 deaths annually), diet and activity patterns (300,000), alcohol use (100,000), microbial agents (90,000), toxic agents (60,000), firearms (35,000), sexual behaviors (30,000), motor vehicle use (25,000), and use of the "illicit drugs," primarily heroin and cocaine (20,000).

The picture arising from the McGinnis and Foege analysis is particularly helpful in planning public health programs to prolong life, especially healthy life. Using it, one can focus on changeable/modifiable human behaviors, for example, cigarette smoking, eating patterns, physical activity, and exercise, rather than classical, diagnostically related disease-specific prevention for such conditions as heart disease, cancer, and stroke. The former, focusing on the here and now, have much more relevance to the otherwise healthy patient than do the latter, concerning as they do an event that may or may not happen to any one individual, in the future.

Infant Mortality

The infant mortality rate is the number of deaths under the age of 1 year among children born alive, divided by the number of live births in that year. A nation's infant mortality rate is related to a variety of socioeconomic, environmental, and health care factors and is considered a fairly sensitive indicator of general health levels in a population. In 1998, the infant mortality rate in the United States was 7.2 per 1,000 live births, the lowest ever recorded in the United States (Matthews, Curtin, & MacDorman, 2000). The rate has been declining steadily since 1940, when it was 47 (Grove & Hetzel, 1968, Table 38). In fact, the infant mortality rate has been falling since it was first recorded in this country at 99.9 in 1915.

The most striking feature of the U.S. infant mortality rate is that while it has consistently declined over the years, the rate for blacks has just as consistently remained about double the white rate (USBOC, 1999, Table 133). Detailed examinations of the relationships among ethnicity, other factors, and infant mortality are contained in *Vital and Health Statistics* (NCHS, 1992).

Marriage and Divorce

In 1997 the marriage rate stood at 8.9 per 1,000 population (USBOC, 1999, Table 155), down from 10.6 in 1970. The divorce rate, that had stood at 5.2

per 1,000 population in 1980 (USBOC, 1999, Table 155), was 4.3 in 1997, significantly less than half of the marriage rate for the first time in some years. Both the marriage and divorce rates have dropped over time (phenomena that may be related). Detailed analyses of birth, marriage, and divorce statistics can be found in the *Vital and Health Statistics*, Series 21, "Data on Natality, Marriage and Divorce," as well as in the *National Vital Statistics Reports.*

MORBIDITY

Definitions

Morbidity refers to sickness and disease. Like mortality, morbidity data can be expressed in both numbers and rates. Like other data, morbidity data can be cross-tabulated with the broad range of demographic characteristics. Morbidity data are extremely important in characterizing the health status of a population. Since many widely prevalent diseases and conditions of ill health do not appear in mortality figures, by themselves the latter are not adequate for health status characterization. This is particularly so in a country like the United States, in which communicable diseases, with a few notable exceptions such as AIDS, pneumonia, and influenza, are major causes of morbidity but not mortality.

Morbidity data can be reported in terms of both incidence and prevalence. Incidence is the number of new cases of the disease in question occurring during a particular time period, usually a year. For example: "In 1997, there were about 58,000 new cases of AIDS reported in the United States" (NCHS, 1999b, Table 54). Prevalence is the total number of cases existing in a population during a time period, or at one point in time (in which case it is known as point-prevalence). For example, in 1999, the estimated total number of cases of AIDS (both living and dead) reported in the United States since the first known case report was made, was 620,000, of whom about 300,000 had died (NCHS, 1999b, Table 54). The prevalence of living AIDS cases in 1999 was 320,000.

The list of significant nonfatal causes of ill health in the United States includes arthritis, low-back pain, the common cold, influenza, nonfatal injuries, dermatitis, and mild emotional and sexual problems (NCHS, 1999a, p. 5). There are other diseases that may kill but do so rarely in relation to their prevalence. Included in this category are sexually transmitted diseases (STD) other than AIDS, duodenal ulcer, and gall bladder disease. Morbidity data highlight not only the important diseases and the patterns of their distribution in the population; the data also illustrate disease-related limitations of activity.

Counting and reporting morbidity are not nearly as simple as reporting mortality, however; consider the following questions: What is meant by the term "sickness," and just when is a person "sick"? Who decides? The physician? The patient? Furthermore, while state law requires that all deaths be reported, only one category of sickness, the infectious diseases, are reportable in every state.

Until the advent of antibiotics and vaccines, death and disability caused by infectious diseases posed the greatest risk to the U.S. population. After several decades of complacency, the emergence of new threats (e.g., AIDS, hantavirus, *E. coli* 0157:H7, hepatitis C) and the resurgence of old threats (tuberculosis) together with concerns about antibiotic resistance and the risk of bioterrorism have reignited interest in and funding for infectious disease surveillance.

As of January 1, 1998, a total of 52 infectious diseases were designated as notifiable at the national level. "A notifiable disease is one for which regular, frequent, and timely information regarding individual cases is considered necessary for the prevention and control of the disease" (Centers for Disease Control and Prevention [CDC], 1998, p. iii). States voluntarily report cases, and the incidence of infectious diseases appears in a weekly publication of the Centers for Disease Control and Prevention of the United States Public Health Service called *Morbidity and Mortality Weekly Report*. An annual summary of notifiable diseases in the U.S., and individual disease (AIDS) and disease category summaries (sexually transmitted diseases) are also published by the CDC.

Surveillance for infectious diseases relies on physicians and it is well known that some physicians fail to report certain diseases, even when legally required to do so. There are many reasons why physicians fail to report, including the time it takes to complete the required paperwork. Some physicians will not report sexually transmitted diseases in private patients, on the grounds of "avoiding embarrassment." Physicians may not report tuberculosis because of possible economic consequences for the patient in terms of maintaining employment. Many physicians fail to report cases of common childhood viral infections because these infections are considered "inconsequential," even though they may have serious sequelae and may signal incomplete coverage by immunization programs.

Surveillance for several classes of infectious diseases (tuberculosis, sexually transmitted diseases, and AIDS), which involves reporting individual cases by name to local and state health departments, generated considerable controversy during the 20th century. An intense debate surrounding named reporting of HIV infection continues today, fueled by fear of discrimination and the potential for breaches of confidentiality (Bayer & Fairchild, 2000). This debate highlights the importance of privacy and confidentiality protections for all surveillance systems, in particular, and medical records in general. Although most surveillance systems are protected by state law and the names of individuals with infectious diseases are retained by the state and not included in reports sent to federal agencies, many people support federal regulation of surveillance systems.

Other diseases, events, and conditions of public health significance are reportable in at least some states including, among others, cancer, injuries, lead poisoning, childhood asthma, and congenital malformations. In recognition of cancer's place as the second leading cause of death in the United States, Congress responded to the need for cancer surveillance by establishing the National Program of Cancer Registries in 1992 (Cancer Registries Amendment Act, 1992), which provides support to either enhance existing registries or implement them in 45 states, 3 territories, and the District of Columbia. There are, however, no mandatory reporting requirements for many disease categories that are equally important, such as heart disease, diabetes, and stroke, to say nothing of very common, sometimes crippling but usually nonfatal conditions like arthritis and osteoporosis, as well as such negative health conditions as sedentary lifestyle, obesity, and cigarette smoking.

Data

Turning to the data itself, for mortality there is only one possible source—and it isn't the patient. For morbidity, it is obvious that both providers and patients can be data sources and, as a result, quite different pictures of the same reality can be obtained. Providers can report morbidity by diagnostic categories and also by patients' chief complaints—that is, what the patient reports to the physician as being the problem.

Patients don't usually come to a physician saying "I think I've got diabetes mellitus, Doc," however, but rather something like, "Doc, I've been feeling kind of weak, I'm drinking a great deal of water and urinating a lot. Do you think maybe something's wrong?" It is up to the physician to characterize the problem and make a diagnosis, that he or she can then report. Patients can also report their chief complaints directly to data gatherers, as in a population survey.

From a chief complaint profile for a population, obtained from either source, a partial picture of morbidity patterns can be drawn. One advantage of deriving information directly from a population sample as opposed to deriving information only from people seeking medical care is that certain people with certain types of illnesses will never come to medical attention. Thus morbidity surveys that gather information only from providers will not give a complete picture.

In the United States, morbidity data are published on a regular basis by the National Center for Health Statistics (NCHS) and as noted, for the reportable communicable diseases by the Centers for Disease Control and Prevention (in the *Morbidity and Mortality Weekly Report*). From the NCHS, the data sources include the National Health and Nutrition Examination Survey (NHANES), the National Health Interview Survey (NHIS), the National Hospital Discharge Survey (NHDS), the National Ambulatory Medical Care Survey (NAMCS), and the National Hospital Ambulatory Medical Care Survey.

The results of these surveys are published periodically in both *Vital and Health Statistics* and *Advance Data*. Series 1 of *Vital and Health Statistics* contains the general methodological and historical accounts of the whole endeavour. Detailed descriptions of all the surveys can be found in Appendix I of *Health, United States 1999* (NCHS, 1999b).

Considering some examples of morbidity data, in 1996 the incidence of acute conditions was 164 per 100 persons per year, down a bit from 174 per 100 in 1995 (NCHS, 1999a, p. 3). Most common were respiratory conditions (including the common cold and influenza) (79 per 100), injuries (22 per 100), infective and parasitic diseases (21 per 100), and digestive system conditions (6.7 per 100).

Persons sought medical attention for these conditions about two thirds of the time. Acute conditions were associated with about 624 days of restricted activity per 100 persons per year, leading to about 272 days in bed due to illness and 297 school-loss days per 100 persons 5–17 years of age, and for persons 18 and over, about 284 work-loss days per 100.

About 14.4% of the population experienced limitation in all activity due to chronic conditions (NCHS, 1999a, p. 5). The major chronic conditions causing limitations in activity in 1996 (in descending order of frequency) were arthritis, sinusitis, deformity or orthopedic impairment, hypertension, hay fever or allergic rhinitis without rhinitis, hearing impairment, and heart disease (NCHS, 1999a, p. 4).

An example of provider-perspective data, the National Hospital Discharge Survey (NHDS) reports on hospital utilization by age and sex of patients, their lengths of stay, and their diagnoses and surgical and non-surgical procedures. It affords a rather accurate illness profile of hospitalized patients. It must be remembered, however, that the overwhelming majority of ill persons do not require hospitalization. Thus, the morbidity profile of the population as a whole does not match that seen in hospitals. The results of the NHDS are published in *Vital and Health Statistics,* Series 13, and in *Advance Data from Vital and Health Statistics,* published on an irregular basis. Selected results are also published periodically in *Health, United States.*

The National Ambulatory Medical Care Survey (NAMCS; NCHS, 1974a, 1974b) was developed in the 1970s as a component of the National Health Survey. It is a continuing survey of private, nonfederally employed office-based physicians practicing in the United States (Woodwell, 2000). The data are collected using a stratified random sample of all office-based physicians (both allopathic and osteopathic) in the contiguous United States, excluding anesthesiologists, pathologists, radiologists, and physicians engaged primarily in teaching, research, and administration. In the early 1990s, the data were being reported primarily by physician specialty.

In the NAMCS, morbidity data are collected from both the patient's and the physician's perspectives. For example, in 1998 the five leading groups of symptoms causing patients to come to a physician's office were referable to the respiratory system; musculoskeletal system; eyes and ears; skin, hair, and nails; and digestive system (Woodwell, 2000, Table 8). The seven leading physician's diagnoses were acute upper respiratory infections, excluding pharyngitis; essential hypertension; arthropathies (joint problems); diabetes mellitus; otitis media and Eustachian tube disorders (both ear problems), rheumatism, excluding back; and cancer (Woodwell, 2000, Table 5).

HEALTH STATUS AND HEALTH-RELATED BEHAVIORS

In 1979, the Office of the Assistant Secretary for Health (OASH) of the U.S. Department of Health and Human Services published the first national health status report, *Healthy People: The Surgeon General's Report on Health Promotion and Disease Prevention* (OASH). Subsequently, the Office of Disease Prevention and Health Promotion (ODPHP), part of OASH, published *Promoting Health and Preventing Disease: Objectives for the Nation* (ODPHP, 1980, 1986). Two hundred sixteen objectives were established for dealing with 15 major diseases and conditions that can be prevented using existing knowledge and techniques.

The 15 major diseases and conditions were grouped into three sets of five; conditions were grouped according to the appropriate prevention strategy. For example, high blood pressure and sexually transmitted diseases were grouped in "Preventive Health Services"; such problems as toxic agent control and occupational safety and health were in "Health Protective Services"; and such conditions as cigarette smoking and sedentary lifestyle were grouped in "Health Promotion Programs."

In 1991, the U.S. Public Health Service published the next comprehensive update for the program, *Healthy People 2000*, in which three broad goals were identified that focus on increasing the span of healthy life, reducing health disparities, and achieving access to preventive services for everyone (USPHS). In 1995, *Healthy People 2000: Midcourse Review* was published (USDHHS). The project had expanded its scope to set National Health Promotion and Disease Prevention Objectives for dealing with 22 diseases, conditions, and health-related behaviors (and the means for tracking them), including: physical activity and fitness, nutrition, tobacco use, substance abuse (alcohol and other drugs), family planning, mental health and mental disorders, violent and abusive behavior, unintentional injuries, occupational safety and health, environmental health, food and drug safety, oral health, maternal and infant health, heart disease and stroke, cancer, diabetes and chronic disabling conditions, HIV infection, sexually transmitted diseases, and immunization and infectious diseases. Objectives were also established for educational and community-based programs, clinical preventive services, and surveillance and data systems. For the 22 designated areas a total of 520 objectives and sub-objectives were established (USDHHS, 1995, Appendix A).

Then in 2000, the next decennial iteration, *Healthy People 2010* (USDHHS, 2000) appeared, which is designed to achieve two overarching goals: increase the quality and years of healthy life; and eliminate health disparities by gender, race/ethnicity, income and education, disability, geography, and sexual orientation. The 2010 objectives were consolidated from 520 to 467 and they are being tracked by 190 data sources (USDHHS, 2000).

In support of the "Healthy People" efforts, beginning in 1985 the National Center for Health Statistics carried out a Health Promotion/ Disease Prevention (HP/DP) Survey as part of the ongoing National Health Interview Survey (NHIS; NCHS, 1988). The HPDP Survey was repeated in 1990 and 1995 and subsequently questions have been incorporated into the NHIS and other surveys. Results are published in *Vital and Health Statistics,* Series 10; *Advance Data;* and *Morbidity and Mortality Weekly Report* (reporting data from the related Behavioral Risk Factor Surveillance System).

Key findings include (NCHS, 1999b, Tables 61–71); as of 1995, 24.7% of persons 18 or older regularly smoked cigarettes, about 19% of persons between 20 and 74 years of age had an elevated serum cholesterol, about 23% of persons had hypertension, close to 35% of the population between 20 an 74 could be classified as overweight, and (as of 1990) of the 72% of men and 51% of women who drank alcohol, 13.6% of the men and 3.4% of the women could be classified as "heavier" drinkers. Note that this "risk factor" approach to morbidity has much in common with the McGinnis-Foege approach to classification of causes of death.

Since data from national surveys generally cannot be analyzed by state, all states and the District of Columbia began participating in the Behavioral Risk Factor Surveillance System (BRFSS) in 1994. These telephone surveys monitor the state-level prevalence of personal health behaviors like smoking that play a major role in premature morbidity and mortality. Data from BRFSS and the Youth Risk Behavior Surveillance System (YRBS), which samples high school students, complement the data from the NHIS. The National Center for Chronic Disease Prevention and Health Promotion at the CDC is responsible for the BRFSS and YRBS. (See *Healthy People 2010,* Volume II, for a complete discussion of data sources used for tracking progress.)

UTILIZATION OF HEALTH CARE SERVICES

Introduction

We come now to the third quantitative perspective for viewing a population in terms of health and ill health: how the population utilizes the health care delivery system. We have pointed out that in quantifying the utilization of health services, the same series of events can be counted from either the patient's or the provider's perspective. The results of the two types of counts are not always the same. Thus, when discussing utilization one has to be careful to distinguish between the two approaches.

It should be noted that reliable utilization data is regularly reported primarily for services provided by licensed MDs and DOs (Doctors of

Osteopathic Medicine) in licensed allopathic (MD-staffed) and osteopathic hospitals, and by licensed dentists. In the United States there is an unknown amount of "alternative therapy" provided by such healing disciplines as chiropractic, naturopathy, homeopathy, acupuncture/acupressure therapy and its variants, and "holistic health practitioners," among many others. These practitioners do not report utilization, they are not surveyed, and payment for much of their service is only sporadically reimbursed by insurance companies.

While regular utilization statistics are not collected, however, a one-time sampling survey estimated that over 40% of all adults use at least one alternative therapy, with an average annual visit rate among users of 7.6 (Eisenberg et al., 1998). In 1997, as in 1990, there were more visits made to alternative therapists (629 million) than to primary care physicians (485 million).

Ambulatory Services

As we have noted, the NHIS provides patient-perspective data for the utilization of ambulatory services. According to the NHIS, in 1996 there were about 5.9 physician contacts per person (NCHS, 1999a, Table 71). Of these, about 54% took place in a physician's office, 12% in a hospital (primarily in the outpatient department including the emergency department), 12% on the telephone, with the balance at home and in other locations. Females averaged 6.9 visits per year, whereas males averaged 5.2. Whites averaged 6.1 visits, while blacks averaged 5.4. Persons in families with an annual income of $10,000 or less averaged 8.4 visits per year, while persons in families with an annual income of $35,000 or more averaged 5.4 visits per year. Persons in the southern geographic region of the U.S. averaged the most visits, 6.3. All of these numbers were down somewhat from 1994.

There are several sources of provider data on the utilization of ambulatory services. The most comprehensive one is the National Ambulatory Medical Care Survey (NAMCS), described briefly above, reported upon most commonly in *Advance Data*. In addition to morbidity data, the NAMCS provides data on visits by age, race, sex, geographic region, metropolitan/nonmetropolitan living area, type of physician, and duration of visit. The other major source of provider-perspective ambulatory service utilization data is the American Hospital Association's (AHA) annual publication *Hospital Statistics*, published each summer. It reports hospital clinic and emergency department visits by such variables as number of beds, ownership, type, geographical region, and medical school affiliation.

Utilization of Hospital Inpatient Services

Turning to utilization of hospital inpatient services, from the patient perspective the National Health Interview Survey reported that in 1996 there were about 26.8 million discharges from short-stay hospitals, including about 3.5 million deliveries (down from 31.1 million discharges in 1991). These patients used about 142 million inpatient days of care with an average length of stay of 5.9 days (down from 199 million days in 1991) (NCHS, 1999a, Table 77). Other classes of data provided by the NHIS are utilization according to various hospital characteristics, morbidity (discussed previously), and an analysis of surgery.

The NCHS also provides provider-perspective hospital utilization data through the National Hospital Discharge Survey (Hall & Popovic, 2000). The NCHS points out that because of "differences in collection procedures, population sampled, and definitions" the results from the NHIS and the NHDS are not entirely consistent (NCHS, 1979b, p. 1 and footnotes; 1999b, Tables 89 and 90). For example, for 1996 the NHIS reported significantly fewer discharges from short-stay hospitals than did the NHDS: 82.4 per thousand population for the former compared with 102.3 per thousand for the latter (NCHS, 1999b, Tables 8 and 90).

Hospital utilization data are also published in the AHA's *Hospital Statistics.* For AHA-registered hospitals, the publication presents much data on bed size, admissions, occupancy rate, average daily census, and fiscal parameters, according to hospital type, size, ownership, and geographical location (see also chapter 6, "Hospitals and Health Systems"). Certain provider-perspective hospital utilization data also appear in *Health, United States.*

Data are also available on the quality of health care utilization events. The most widely used measures are the NCQA HEDIS clinical measures that focus on some of the nation's most serious and prevalent diseases and conditions. In addition, patient outcomes including survival can be measured for specific medical procedures. For example, New York State has taken a leadership role in setting standards for cardiac surgery services, monitoring outcomes, and sharing performance data with patients, hospitals, and physicians (New York State Department of Health, 2000). Mortality rates have plummeted since the publication of the first survey.

CONCLUSIONS

As we have seen in this chapter, an abundance of data concerning the U.S. population, its health, and how it uses the health care delivery system are collected and published in print and available on the Internet. Such ready access to data from multiple sources should not lull the reader into a less critical approach to using and interpreting these data. The reliability of the source of the data together with data collection methods must always be assessed. Additionally, although data sources may be reliable, not all data are consistent with one another as noted just above in the discussion of the differing hospital utilization rates obtained by NHIS and NHDS. This lack of consistency results in part from a lack of coordination of data collection efforts: even such seemingly standard information as race/ethnicity is recorded in different ways on different surveys and administrative data bases. Furthermore, there is the obvious gap between the provider-perspective and the patient-perspective on the counts, content, and quality of events.

There have been criticisms of the federal statistical collection, reporting, and analysis systems over a period of many years. A 1979 study by the Office of Technology Assessment found "federal data collection activities . . . to be overlapping, fragmented, and often duplicative" (1979, p. iii).[4] In brief, the report recommended that a "strengthened coordinating and planning unit within HHS" be established that "would embody three basic characteristics: sufficient authority to impose decisions on agencies; the necessary statistical and analytical capabilities to conduct activities requiring technical expertise and judgement; and adequate resources to build a viable core effort" (Office of Technology Assessment, 1979, p. 55).

The Department of Health and Human Services (DHHS) Data Council (http://aspe.hhs.gov/datacncl/index.htm), established in 1995, is the current iteration of a department-wide information systems committee. Not only does its charge embody the recommendations of the 1979 OTA report, but it has been expanded to encompass electronic information policy, including data standards, privacy, telemedicine, and enhanced health information for consumers.

Near universal access to the Internet and the widespread availability of high-speed computing capabilities have made the Council's tasks more difficult in some areas and easier in others. The electronic information advances of the 1990s have greatly improved communication at all levels and expanded access to databases and the capacity to link multiple databases. This has been a boon to health planners and researchers, but has raised serious public concerns about protecting the privacy of health-related information. In response to these concerns, Congress passed the Health Insurance Portability and Accountability Act of 1996 (HIPAA), the Administrative Simplification provisions of which will ultimately reshape the way the health care industry collects, processes, stores, protects, and exchanges patient records. For the first time, national standards are mandated to protect the privacy of personal health records, and common standards are set for electronic transmission of patient information within the health care industry. Implementation by the DHHS Data Council is expected in 2001.

Privacy concerns are likely to hold center stage among the many policy issues related to data collection and use, but other issues of importance include the following: the utility and application of clinical trials methodology to the study of health outcomes; health services malpractice and malpractice litigation; technological and ethical matters arising from the use of

---

[4] This report will still be valuable to students of the federal data system and its users. It not only described data collection activities and the way they were organized and supervised, but also presented and analyzed all of the statutory authorities that establish those existing at the time (that happen to be almost all still in use).

electronic data collection and analysis; the relationship between data collected and data actually used; the decision-making process governing what is counted and what data are disseminated; cost/benefit analysis of health services interventions; government data collection requirements, utilization, and costs; the impact of the Internet on health data requirements and availability; what to do when we have too much or too little data; and what is changing and will change about health care data collection, publication, and analysis.

There will always be gaps in our data collection systems. Nevertheless, we know a great deal about health, disease, and illness in the United States, and about the functioning of the U.S. health care delivery system. Further, given whatever problems there may or may not be with the available health and health care data, we need to remember above all that data mean little unless they are put to proper use.

CASE STUDY

As Director of Human Resources for a large private university, you would like to tell the President what the university is getting for the money it spends on health services for its employees and their dependents. Right now you receive only the total dollar amount spent on claims each month. What other kinds of information about these claims would you ask the health insurance companies to provide you, and why do you suppose the university doesn't get such information now?

DISCUSSION QUESTIONS

1. What are the uses of health data?
2. What are the uses of health services data?
3. How do health and health services data relate to each other?
4. How should data be used in the health and health services planning process?
5. What are the similarities and differences between disease-specific and risk-factor-specific health and illness data?
6. What impact has the Internet had on health and health services data utilization and dissemination in the United States?

REFERENCES

Advance Data (1997, May 20). National Ambulatory Medical Care Survey: 1997 summary. *Advance Data* (No. 305).

Anderson, R. N., & Rosenberg, H. M. (1998). Age standardization of death rates: Implementation of the year 2000 standard. In *National Vital Statistics Reports* (Vol. 47, No. 3). Hyattsville, MD: National Center for Health Statistics.

Bayer, R., & Fairchild, A. L. (2000). Surveillance and privacy. *Science, 290,* 1898–1899.

Cancer Registries Amendment Act, Pub. L. No. 102-515 (1992).

Centers for Disease Control and Prevention. (1998). Summary of notifiable diseases, United States, 1998. *Morbidity and Mortality Weekly Report, 47*(53), 1–92.

Eisenberg, D. M., Davis, R. B., Ettner, S. L., Appel, S., Wilkey, S., Van Rompay, M., & Kessler, R. C. (1998). Trends in alternative medicine use in the United States, 1990–1997. *Journal of the American Medical Association, 280,* 1569–1575.

Grove, R. D., & Hetzel, A. M. (1968). *Vital statistics rates for the United States: 1940–1960.* Washington, DC: National Center for Health Statistics.

Hall, M. J., & Popovic, J. R. (2000). *1998 summary: National Hospital Discharge Survey.* Advance data from *Vital and Health Statistics,* No. 316. Hyattsville, MD: National Center for Health Statistics.

Health Insurance Portability and Accountability Act of 1996, Pub. L. No. 104-191, Title II, Subtitle F, 261–264 (1996).

Matthews, T. J., Curtin, S. C., & MacDorman, M. F. (2000). Infant mortality statistics from the 1998 period linked birth/infant death data set. In *National Vital Statistics Reports* (Vol. 48, No. 12). Hyattsville, MD: National Center for Health Statistics.

McGinnis, J. M., & Foege, W. H. (1993). Actual causes of death in the United States. *Journal of the American Medical Association, 270,* 2207–2212.

Murphy, S. L. (2000). Deaths: Final data for 1998. In *National Vital Statistics Reports* (Vol. 48, No. 11.) Hyattsville, MD: National Center for Health Statistics.

National Center for Health Statistics. (1974a). National Ambulatory Medical Care Survey: Background and methodology: United States, 1967–1972. *Vital and Health Statistics,* Series 2, No. 61.

National Center for Health Statistics. (1974b). The National Ambulatory Medical Care Survey: Symptom classification. In *Vital and Health Statistics*, Series 2, No. 63.

National Center for Health Statistics. (1979a). *International classification of diseases, ninth revision, adapted for use in the United States.* Hyattsville, MD: U.S. Government Printing Office.

National Center for Health Statistics. (1979b). *Health resources statistics: Health manpower and health facilities, 1976–1977* (DHEW Pub. No. [PHS] 79-1509). Hyattsville, MD: U.S. Government Printing Office.

National Center for Health Statistics. (1988). Health promotion and dsease prevention, U.S., 1985. *Vital and Health Statistics,* Series 10, No. 163.

National Center for Health Statistics. (1992). Infant mortality rates: Socioeconomic factors. *Vital and Health Statistics,* Series 22, No. 14.

National Center for Health Statistics. (1999a). Current estimates from the National Health Survey, 1994. *Vital and Health Statistics,* Series 10, No. 200.

National Center for Health Statistics. (1999b, September). *Health United States 1999, health and aging chartbook* (DHHS Pub. No. [PHS] 99-1232). Hyattsville, MD: Centers for Disease Control and Prevention.

National Committee for Quality Assurance. (2000). *The state of managed care quality, 2000.* Washington, DC: Author.

New York State Department of Health. (2000, September). *Coronary artery bypass surgery in New York State 1995–1997.* Albany, NY: New York State Health Department.

National Vital Statistics Reports. (1999). Births and deaths: Preliminary data for 1998. In *National Vital Statistics Reports* (Vol. 47, No. 25). Hyattsville, MD: National Center for Health Statistics.

Office of the Assistant Secretary for Health. (1979). *Healthy people: The surgeon general's report on health promotion and disease prevention* (DHEW Pub. No. [PHS] 70-55071). Washington, DC: U.S. Government Printing Office.

Office of Disease Prevention and Health Promotion. (1980). *Promoting health/ preventing disease: Objectives for the nation.* Washington, DC: U.S. Government Printing Office.

Office of Disease Prevention and Health Promotion. (1986). *The 1990 health objectives for the nation.* Washington, DC: U.S. Government Printing Office.

Office of Technology Assessment. (1979). *Selected topics in federal health statistics.* Washington, DC: U.S. Government Printing Office.

U.S. Bureau of the Census. (1997, March). *How we're changing. Demographic state of the nation: 1997* (Current Population Reports Special Studies, Series P23-193). Washington, DC: U.S. Government Printing Office.

U.S. Bureau of the Census. (1999). *Statistical abstract of the United States: 1999.* (119th edition). Washington, DC: U.S. Government Printing Office.

U.S. Department of Health and Human Services. (1995). *Healthy people 2000: Midcourse review and 1995 revisions.* Washington, DC: U.S. Government Printing Office.

U.S. Public Health Service. (1991). *Healthy people 2000: National health promotion and disease prevention objectives* (DHHS Pub. No. [PHS] 91-50213). Washington, DC: U.S. Government Printing Office.

Ventura, S. J., Martin, J. A., Curtin, S. C., Matthews, T. J., & Park, M. M. (2000). Births: Final data for 1998. In *National Vital Statistics Reports* (Vol 48, No. 3). Hyattsville, MD: National Center for Health Statistics.

Woodwell, D. A. (2000). *National Ambulatory Care Survey: 1998 summary.* Advance data from *Vital and Health Statistics,* no. 315. Hyattsville, MD: National Center for Health Statistics.

3

Financing for Health Care

Kenneth E. Thorpe and James R. Knickman

LEARNING OBJECTIVES

- ☐ Quantify health care spending in the United States over time.
- ☐ Describe the major sources of health care spending.
- ☐ List and tabulate the major categories of services purchased.
- ☐ Differentiate between public and private health care spending.
- ☐ Demonstrate an understanding of the extent to which health care spending is rising and the factors that contribute to such growth.

TOPICAL OUTLINE

What the money buys
Where the money comes from
How the money is paid out
The rising costs of health care
Conclusions

KEY WORDS

prospective payment, capitation, managed care, uninsured, sources and uses of funds

Central to the design and functioning of the U.S. health care delivery system is its ever-evolving system for paying for services provided to patients. The types of services delivered and the organizational approaches to delivering

44

them are heavily influenced by how health care is paid for and the aggregate resources available for buying health care services.

The financing system that has evolved over the past 35 years in the
United States rests upon a complex blend of public and private activities
and responsibilities. It is quite different from the largely public financing
systems that exist in many other advanced, industrialized countries. An
understanding of how health care is paid for is essential to developing an
understanding of the general organization of health care in America.

The way health services are paid for has been undergoing tremendous
change since the early 1980s. The rate of change has intensified during the
1990s. The basic system for reimbursing hospital care has been completely
restructured by many payers for care. The way physicians and long-term
care are being paid is being restructured. As highlighted in the text that
follows, even within the several broad categories for raising the money and
then spending, variations can be found among providers and payers alike.
It can be predicted with confidence that the financing system will continue
to evolve over time. Thus, this chapter attempts to explain not only the
current structure of financing approaches but also the principles behind
the financing system.

In explaining how the American health care financing system operates,
this chapter focuses on (a) what the money devoted to health care buys,
(b) where the money comes from, (c) how health care providers are paid,
and (d) why health care expenditures have been increasing rapidly for several decades.

As displayed in Table 3.1, $1228.5 billion, or 13.9% of the gross domes-
tic product (GDP), was spent for health services in 1999. These expenditures represent $4,340 per year for each person. The health care sector is
clearly a major element of the American economy. Health care expenditures have been increasing at a rapid rate over the past 35 years, though
growth slowed substantially during the latter half of the 1990s. Health care
expenditures totaled only $43 billion in 1965, or 5.8% of the GDP. From
1965 onward, health care outlays rose, on the average, 11.7% each year,
reaching a peak inflation rate of 15.3%. While growth in health care expenditures continues to exceed by a wide margin the overall inflation rates
prevalent in the American economy, since 1991, health care expenditures
have risen at an average rate of only 6.7% per year. This was still well above
the overall inflation rate, however. Important elements of the study of
health care finance, therefore, are the analysis of the dynamics of that
spending in the United States, and describing what is being achieved by
the ever-increasing health care expenditure levels.

WHAT THE MONEY BUYS

National health care expenditures, as measured by the federal Health
Care Financing Administration (HCFA), are grouped into two categories:

TABLE 3.1 Aggregate and Per Capita National Health Expenditures, by Source of Funds and Percentage of Gross National Product, Selected Calendar Years, 1929–2000

Calendar year	Total GNP[a]	Total health expenditures			Private health expenditures			Public health expenditures		
		Amount[a]	Per capita	Percentage of GNP	Amount[a]	Per capita	Percentage of Total	Amount[a]	Per capita	Percentage of GNP
1929	$103.3	$3.6	$29	3.5	$3.2	$25	86.4	$0.5	$4	13.6
1935	72.2	2.9	23	4.0	2.4	18	80.8	0.6	4	19.2
1940	99.7	4.0	30	4.0	3.2	24	79.7	0.8	6	20.3
1960	503.7	26.9	146	5.3	20.3	110	75.3	6.6	36	24.7
1970	982.4	74.7	359	7.6	47.5	228	63.5	27.3	131	36.5
1980	2,631.7	248.0	1,049	9.4	142.2	601	57.3	105.8	448	42.7
1990	5,542.9	675.0	2,601	12.2	390.0	1,502	57.8	285.1	1,098	42.2
1991	5,917	761.7	2,901	12.9	441.4	1,681	58	320.3	1,220	42.0
1992	6,244[b]	834.2	3,145	13.4[c]	478.8	1,805	57.4	355.4	1,340	42.6
1993	6,553[b]	892.1	3,330	13.6[c]	505.5	1,887	56.7	386.5	1,443	43.3
1995	7,254[b]	988.5	3,621	13.6[c]	532.1	1,949	53.8	456.4	1,673	46.2
1997	8,111[b]	1092.4	3,927	13.5[c]	586.0	2,107	53.8	502.2	1,806	46.2
1999*	8,845[b]	1228.5	4,340	13.9[c]	669.2	2,364	54.5	559.3	1,976	45.5
2000*	9,194[b]	1316.2	4,611	14.3[c]	722.6	2,531	54.9	593.6	2,079	45.1

* projected
[a] In billions of dollars
[b] Gross domestic product
[c] Percentage of gross domestic product

Adapted from: Levit, K., et al. (1996). National Health Expenditures, 1995. *Health Care Financing Review, 18*(1), 175–214; Gibson, R. M. et al. (1984). National Health Expenditures, 1983. *Health Care Financing Review, 6*(2), 1–29; Gibson, R. M. (1979). National Health Expenditures, 1978. *Health Care Financing Review, 1*(1), 14, 19; Health Care Financing Administration, Office of the Actuary: National Health Statistics Group; accessed July 15, 2000 at www.hcfa.gov.

(a) research and medical facility construction and (b) payments for health services and supplies (see Table 3.2). Personal health care expenses constituted the bulk of the latter—$879 billion in 1995. It was projected that total expenditures would have increased to $1,150 billion for the year 2000. In 2000, it was projected that five types of personal health care expenditures would account for over 85% of the total: 36.8% to hospitals, 22.5% to physicians, 8.2% to nursing home care, 12.6% for drugs and drug sundries, and 5.2% for dentists' services. Projections in other categories of expenditures include "other professional services," such as podiatry and speech therapy, 6.8%; "other health services," 3.4%; administrative expenses, 5.7%; government public health activities, 3.8%; and construction, 1.5%. The costs of medical education are not included in these HCFA figures except insofar as they are inseparable from hospital expenditures and the cost of biomedical research.

WHERE THE MONEY COMES FROM

Ultimately, the people pay all health care costs. Thus, when we say health care monies come from different sources, we really mean that dollars take different routes on their way from consumers to providers: through government, private insurance companies, and independent plans, in addition to personal out-of-pocket payments. For 2000, it was projected that close to 20% of personal health care expenditures would be out-of-pocket ($199.5 billion). At the same time, the government share was nearly 44% (about $500 billion), with the federal government bearing over three fourths of that. Approximately 33% was paid through insurance companies ($337 billion) (Levit, Lazenby, Braden, Cowan, McDonnell, & Sivarajan, 1996).

Public Sources

It was projected that 44% of personal health care expenditures would be transferred by the public sector in 2000 ($500 billion), compared with 44% in 1995, 40% in 1980, 22% in 1965, 22% in 1950, and 9% in 1929. The increase, especially since 1965, is largely a result of greater federal expenditures. Proportionately, state and local government outlays have remained rather constant over time, in the 10%–13% range. The significant rise in federal spending is accounted for by the Medicare and Medicaid programs, Titles XVIII and XIX, respectively, of the Social Security Act.

Medicare

Medicare was inaugurated on July 1, 1966. It originally provided a range of medical care benefits for persons age 65 and over who were covered by the Social Security system. The 1972 amendments to the Social Security

TABLE 3.2 Aggregate and Per Capita Amount and Percentage Distribution of National Health Expenditures, Selected Calendar Years 1960–2000

Type of expenditure	Aggregate amount ($Billions)				
	1960	1980	1990	1995	2000*
Total	27.1	250.1	697.5	988.5	1316.2
Health Services and Supplies	25.4	238.9	672.9	957.8	1275.5
Personal Health Care	23.9	219.4	614.7	878.8	1150.9
Hospital Care	9.3	102.4	256.4	350.1	424.0
Physicians' Services	5.3	41.9	146.3	201.6	258.7
Dentists' Services	2.0	14.4	31.6	45.8	60.2
Other Professional Services	0.6	8.7	34.7	52.6	77.9
Home Health Care	0.0	1.3	13.1	28.6	36.0
Drugs and Drug Sundries	4.2	21.6	59.9	83.4	145.5
Eyeglasses and Appliances	0.8	4.6	10.5	13.8	15.0
Nursing Home Care	1.0	20.0	50.9	77.9	94.1
Other Health Services	0.7	4.6	11.2	25.0	39.5
Expenses for Repayment and Administration	1.2	12.2	38.6	47.7	74.5
Government Public Health Activities	0.4	7.2	19.6	31.4	50.2
Research and Medical Facility Construction	1.7	11.3	24.5	30.7	40.7
Research	0.7	5.4	12.2	16.6	20.6
Construction	1.0	5.8	12.3	14.0	20.1

Type of expenditure	Per capita amount ($)				
	1960	1980	1990	1995	2000*
Total	142.56	1063.80	2,683	3,621	4,611
Health Services and Supplies	133.61	1016.16	2,589	3,508	4,468
Personal Health Care	125.72	933.22	2,364	3,219	4,032
Hospital Care	48.92	435.56	986	1,282	1,485
Physicians' Services	27.88	178.22	563	738	906
Dentists' Services	10.52	61.25	122	168	211
Other Professional Services	3.16	37.01	133	193	273
Home Health Care	0.0	5.53	50	105	126
Drugs and Drug Sundries	22.09	91.88	230	306	510

* Projected.
Source: Health Care Financing Administration, Office of the Actuary, Data from the Office of National Health Statistics, available: www.hcfa.gov

Act extended benefits to persons age 65 and older who do not meet the criteria for the regular Social Security program but who are willing to pay a premium for coverage. In July 1973 benefits were further extended to the disabled and their dependents, and those suffering from chronic kidney disease (Russell et al., 1974).

In the Omnibus Budget Reconciliation Act of 1989 (OBRA 1989), Medicare changed the way physicians are paid. Previously, Medicare payment rates for a service were based on the amounts physicians charged. The new payment system is a national fee schedule that assigns relative values to services based on the time, skill, and intensity it takes to provide them. The relative values are then adjusted for geographic variations of payment. This system went into effect on January 1, 1992.

The Balanced Budget Act of 1997 included several further changes in the Medicare program. The act increased substantially the variety of health plans that may receive Medicare payments and enrollees. For example, Medicare beneficiaries can now choose among several types of managed care, if such plans chose to participate. In addition, the act added several new services to the Medicare benefit package, including preventive screening for prostate cancer, mammography, and colorectal screening, among other preventive benefits. As part of Congress's larger effort to balance the budget by the year 2002, the act produced $116 billion in Medicare savings between federal fiscal years 1998 and 2002.

Medicaid

Unlike Medicare, Medicaid is a program run jointly by federal and state governments; the name is more or less a blanket label for 50 different state programs designed specifically to serve the poor. Beginning in January 1967, Medicaid provided federal funds to states on a cost-sharing basis (according to each state's per capita income) so that welfare recipients could be guaranteed payments for medical services. Payment in full was to be afforded to the aged poor, the blind, the disabled, and families with dependent children if one parent was absent, unemployed, or unable to work. Four types of care were required to be covered: (a) inpatient and outpatient hospital care, (b) other laboratory and X-ray services, (c) physician services, and (d) nursing facility care for persons over age 21. Legislation enacted in subsequent years added coverage of home health services for those entitled to nursing facility services and early and periodic screening, as well as diagnostic and treatment services for persons under age 21.

The 1972 Social Security Act amendments added family planning to the list of "musts." States must also now cover the services of rural health clinics, community and migrant health centers, health centers for the homeless, and similar qualified centers, as well as nurse-midwives and nurse practitioners. Currently, the law specifies another 31 optional services that states may elect to cover, including prescription drugs, intermediate care facilities for the mentally retarded, optometrists' services, dental services, and eyeglasses. States may place certain limits on the extent to which services are covered. For example, they may limit the number of covered prescriptions or hospital days.

Eligibility for Medicaid is determined by the states within federal guidelines. By and large, Medicaid is available only to very low-income persons.

The program also has categorical restrictions; that is, only families with children, pregnant women, and those who are aged, blind, or disabled can qualify.

State Children's Health Insurance Program

As of 1998, over 11.6 million children were uninsured for health services (that is, they were covered neither by Medicaid or a parent's private health insurance policy). To address this issue, the Congress passed the State Children's Health Insurance Program (SCHIP) as part of the Balanced Budget Act of 1997. The SCHIP has some similarities with the Medicaid program. It is financed both by the federal government and states. However, the federal government pays a higher percentage of the cost of this program compared to Medicaid: on average, 70% of the cost of SCHIP, compared with 56% for Medicaid. The SCHIP is also voluntary; states may choose to participate or not. Moreover, if they do participate, they have some flexibility in the health insurance package offered, and the number of children eligible for the program. Under federal law, the states may enroll children in families with incomes up to 200% of the (federally determined) "poverty" level or they may enroll children in families with incomes up to 50 percentage points above that level currently determinative of Medicaid eligibility. Also, in contrast to Medicaid, only otherwise uninsured children are eligible for coverage under SCHIP. While some states have been rather slow to implement the program, approximately 3 million uninsured children have been enrolled as of 2000.

Other Public Expenditures

In 1997, Medicare and Medicaid accounted for 83.5% of public outlays for personal health care services. In 1997, state and local government outlays accounted for 22.0% of the $432.4 billion spent on public programs. It is projected that all government public health activities will cost $50.2 billion in 2000, accounting for less than 4% of national health care spending. It must be noted, however, that while federal prevention and disease control operations are included in this figure, excluded are funds expended at the state and local levels by departments other than health for air and water pollution control, sanitation, and sewage treatment (Letsch, Levit, & Waldo, 1988). The relatively low level of government funding for public health activities relative to health insurance payments deserves special attention, in view of the growing recognition of the relationship between the environment and health and the importance of preventive care and health promotion.

Worker's compensation is an insurance system operated by the states, each with its own law and program, that provides covered workers with some protection against the costs of medical care and loss of income resulting from work-related injury and, in some cases, sickness (Congressional Research Service, 1976; Price, 1979a, 1979b; U.S. National Commission on

State Workmen's Compensation Laws, 1973). The first worker's compensation law was enacted in New York in 1910; by 1948 all states had enacted such laws. The theory underlying worker's compensation is that all accidents, irrespective of fault, must be regarded as the result of the risks of working in industry, and that the employer and employee shall share the burden of loss.

Private Sources

The bulk of private health care expenditures come from two sources: individuals receiving treatment and private insurers making payments on the behalf of patients. In 1998, private expenditures totaled $584 billion, 56.4% of all personal health care expenditures. In 1965, prior to the advent of Medicare and Medicaid, private expenditures accounted for 76.9% of all personal health care expenditures; in 1935, 82.4%; in 1929, 88.4% (Gibson, 1979). This recent decline in the private share of total expenditures is due to the sharp drop in out-of-pocket payments associated with increased federal spending, as well as the slower growth in private health insurance payments. In 1965, 53% of personal health care expenditures was paid directly by the patient; in 1998, it was 20%. Yet because of inflation and other factors, the per capita dollar amount paid directly in 1995 was over eight times what it was in 1970 (Levit et al., 1996). Since 1965, private insurers have paid between 20% and 35% of personal health care costs. Their share was $45.3 billion in 1978, 27% of the total; in 1998, it was $118 billion, or 35% of the total.

Before considering the private health insurance in any depth, the manner in which the term *insurance* is used in the health care industry should be clarified. Insurance originally meant and still usually refers to the contribution by individuals to a fund for the purpose of providing protection against financial losses following relatively unlikely but damaging events. Thus, there is insurance against fire, theft, and death at an early age. All of those events occur within a group of people at a predictable rate but are rare occurrences for any one individual in the group.

Health care utilization, on the other hand, is not a rare occurrence. On average, each person in the United States visits a physician five times a year. One of every six Americans is admitted to a hospital at least once a year. Other than coverage for catastrophic illness, a fairly rare event, health insurance has become a mechanism for offsetting expected rather than unexpected costs. The experience of the many is pooled in an effort to reduce outlays for any one individual to a manageable prepayment size. Perhaps the term *assurance* more appropriately describes the health care payment system that has evolved. In Britain, assurance is used to denote coverage for contingencies that must eventually happen (e.g., life assurance), whereas insurance is reserved for coverage of those contingencies, like fire and theft, that may never occur in the life of a given individual.

Structure of the Private Insurance Industry

The organization of private insurance in the United States is undergoing dramatic changes. The most notable one, described below, is the growth in "managed care" and the rapid consolidation of managed care health plans of one sort or another. As of 1998, nearly 86% of all workers were enrolled in some form of managed care. This represents a dramatic change: only 55% of workers were enrolled in managed care plans just 2 years earlier. Before 1980 virtually all private insurance was provided by either the national system of Blue Cross and Blue Shield plans or by commercial insurance companies, which offered health care insurance as one of many types of insurance products available to employers. These insurance companies charged employers or individuals annual premiums and generally paid health care providers on what is termed a fee-for-service basis. A set amount, often prescribed by the insurance plan, is negotiated between the insurer and the provider, and is paid by the insurance company to a provider each time a beneficiary uses a covered service.

Starting in the early 1980s, however, a range of new insurance approaches and a range of new relationships between insurers and providers have emerged. Health maintenance organizations (HMOs), which deliver services on a "capitated" basis—paying the provider a flat rate for each person/year covered rather than on a fee-for-service basis—have been expanding rapidly. Between 1995 and 1999, the number of Americans enrolled in HMOs increased by 16 million persons, to 79.3 million. Preferred provider organizations (PPOs), which either limit beneficiaries to the use of a set list of physicians and other providers, or provide economic incentives to use physicians who have offered discounts to the insurer, are also expanding rapidly. They accounted for 25% of all private health insurance coverage in 1996 (see Table 3.3). In 1999, this number increased to 38% of all private insurance. "Point of service" plans, which generally require members to go to providers within their networks for certain services but which give them the option to go to nonnetwork providers for other services, generally at a much higher cost, accounted for 16% in 1996. In 1999, the proportion increased to 25%.

A second major change in the structure of the insurance industry is the growth of "self-insured" or self-funded health plans. Self-insurance is the assumption of claim risk by an employer, union, or other group, whereas self-funding refers to the payment of insurance claims from an established bank or trust account (Arnett & Trapnell, 1984). Self-insurance offers potential advantages to employers: they are exempt from most premium taxes and are able to retain interest on reserves (Arnett & Trapnell, 1984).

Blue Cross and Blue Shield

The establishment of payment mechanisms to defray the costs of illness by a third party on behalf of patients was established during the Great

TABLE 3.3   Enrollment in Managed and Unmanaged Group Health Plans, 1996

Plan type	Percentage of enrollment	
	1996[a]	1999[b]
Conventional FFS	26	9
HMO	33	28
PPO	25	38
POS	16	25

Sources: [a]KPMG Peat Marwick, *Health Benefits in 1996,* Table 9; [b]Kaiser Family Foundation and Health Research Education Trust Employer Health Benefits, 1999 annual survey (1999).

Depression. Previously, private hospitals had sought to assure reimbursement for their services through public education campaigns directed at encouraging their users, primarily middle-income Americans, to put money aside to pay for unpredictable medical expenses (Law, 1974). When hard times undermined the savings approach, the hospitals' attention turned to the development of a stable income mechanism. A model was at hand in the independent "prepayment" plan pioneered in 1929 at Baylor University Hospital in Texas to assure certain area schoolteachers of some hospital coverage. Under the plan, 1,250 teachers prepaid 50 cents a month to provide themselves with up to 21 days of semiprivate hospitalization annually.

In the early 1930s, nonprofit prepayment programs offering care at a number of hospitals were organized in several cities. The American Hospital Association (AHA) vigorously supported the growth and development of these plans, soon to be named Blue Cross, and the special insurance legislation that was required for their establishment in each state (Law, 1974). The AHA set standards for plans and then offered its seal of approval to plans meeting the standards. A provider-insurer partnership was firmly established. Indeed, not until 1972 did national Blue Cross formally separate from the AHA.

While Blue Cross developed as a hospital insurance system, a system called Blue Shield developed independently, beginning in 1939, as an insurer for certain physician services. These two insurers originally tended to be financially and organizationally distinct. They have many similarities, however, and for many years have worked together to provide hospital and physician payments on behalf of their beneficiaries.

Commercial Insurance

Commercial insurance companies (Aetna, Metropolitan Life, etc.) entered the general health insurance market cautiously. They had realized losses on income replacement policies during the Depression and were leery of the Blue Cross/Blue Shield's initial emphasis on providing a comprehensive benefits package. However, a Supreme Court decision recognizing that fringe benefits could legally be subject to the collective bargaining process, following as it did the freezing of industrial wages during World War II, proved too much of a temptation. While employers could not raise wages, they could improve fringe benefits packages. Thus a new market was born.

In the main, Blue Cross offered hospitalization insurance; Blue Shield covered in-hospital physician services and a limited amount of office-based care. The commercial companies offered both. As in the case of the Blues, commercial insurance is primarily provided to groups of persons through employee fringe benefit packages negotiated through collective bargaining. Individual policies can be purchased, but they are usually quite expensive and/or have limited coverage.

The commercials also sell major medical and cash payment policies. The former, directed primarily at catastrophic illness, pay all or part of the treatment costs beyond those covered by basic plans. They are sold on both a group and an individual basis. Cash payment policies pay the insured a flat sum of money per day of hospitalization and are usually sold directly to individuals, often through mass advertising campaigns. Although the daily cash payment sum is usually small, it can help defray costs left uncovered by other insurance.

Like the Blues, the commercials are subject to supervision by state insurance commissioners, although such supervision does not include rate regulation. One general requirement is that commercials establish premium rates high enough to cover claims made under the insurance they provide. Solvency of the insurer is the principal aim of insurance commission surveillance in this instance (Krizay & Wilson, 1974).

During the 1990s, the distinction between many of the commercial and Blue Cross plans blurred. To enhance their competitive pricing position vis-à-vis their commercial counterparts, several Blue Cross plans converted to for-profit status, or planned to. This shift was accompanied by the establishment of companion foundations designed to continue the provision of "community- benefits/functions" performed previously. In addition, the range of products offered through commercial and Blue Cross/Blue Shield plans has become virtually identical. Both of these trends were precipitated by the increasing demands placed on the industry to deliver cost containment.

HMOs

The form of health insurance that is reshaping the way many Americans relate to the health sector is the HMO (Health Maintenance Organization; see also chapter 11). HMOs integrate the delivery of health care and the provision of insurance for health care, being both the "fiscal agent" (money-raiser and spender) and the health care provider. Although there are many different types of HMOs, the central concept is that an annual payment is made by or for beneficiaries to a group of providers which then, for this capitated flat payment, delivers all covered services to those enrolled. The HMO concept fundamentally changes the traditional approach of paying physicians and other providers on a fee-for-service, "piece-work" basis. Both commercial insurers and Blue Cross plans have actively entered the managed care market place.

There are four distinct types of HMOs (Group Health Association of America, 1986). The traditional type is the "staff" model, in which the fiscal agent employs salaried physicians who generally spend all their time delivering services to the HMO's enrollees. The "group" model is a slight variant of this, in that the physicians as a single group contract with the fiscal agent to deliver services. In a "network" type of HMO the fiscal agent has contracts with a number of multi-specialty physician groups to provide services to enrollees. Often, these physician groups also deliver services to non-HMO patients. The fourth HMO type is the "independent practice association" (IPA) model, in which the fiscal agent contracts with a range of private, office-based physicians, solo and in specialty group practices, to provide services to HMO enrollees. Again, IPA physicians generally provide services to both HMO enrollees and patients with other forms of insurance.

HMOs vary in how they relate to hospitals. Some HMOs own their own hospitals. Others relate to community hospitals through a variety of fiscal arrangements. These include some version of a capitation payment and some form of discounted per diem or per case reimbursement mechanism.

The reason for increased enrollment in HMOs in recent years (see Table 3.4), driven primarily by employers, is principally the expectation and claim that HMOs can reduce health care costs while providing coverage that has fewer co-payment features and uncovered services than is the case under traditional health insurance forms. Many earlier studies found that HMOs, particularly group and staff models, reduce hospital use and total costs (Amould, Debruck, & Pollard, 1984; Congressional Budget Office, 1995; Luft, 1978, 1981; Manning, 1984; Roemer & Shonick, 1973; Wolinsky, 1980). Physicians working in HMOs generally have a strong incentive to use resources efficiently because of the capitated payment approach. Most important, HMO providers have strong incentives to avoid hospitalizations. Studies consistently indicate that even after adjusting for demographic differences, HMO patients are hospitalized 15%–40% less often than fee-for-service patients (Luft, 1981). At issue is whether HMOs produce one-time, or continued reductions in use and spending. While most agree that HMOs do indeed generate lower use rates, the most recent data suggest that the yearly growth in HMO premiums relative to other forms of managed care and traditional fee-for-service plans rises at similar rates (Kaiser Family Foundation, 2000). If true, this would indicate that HMOs appear to generate an important one-time reduction in utilization and spending.

PPOs

The other significantly expanding form of insurance coverage is that which uses what are called Preferred Provider Organizations (PPOs). As is the case

TABLE 3.4   Number of HMO Members (in Millions), 1976–1999

Year	As of June	As of December
1976	6.0	NA*
1977	6.3	NA
1978	7.6	NA
1979	8.2	NA
1980	9.1	NA
1981	10.2	NA
1982	10.8	NA
1983	12.5	NA
1984	15.1	NA
1985	18.9	NA
1986	23.7	25.7
1987	28.6	29.3
1988	NA	32.7
1989	NA	34.7
1990	NA	36.5
1991	NA	38.6
1992	NA	41.4
1996	NA	63.3
1999	NA	80.8

* NA: data not available

Adapted from Gruber, R., Shadle, M., & Polich, C. L. (1988). From Movement to Industry: The Growth of HMOs. *Health Affairs, 7*(3), p. 197. Group Health Association of America. (1988). National Directory of HMOs Database. *Health Affairs,* Summer. *Interstudy,* Competitive Edge. (1997). *HMO Directory 7.1,* Excelsior, MN: Author; *Interstudy,* Competitive Edge. (1999). *HMO Directory 10.1.* Minneapolis, MN: Author.

with HMOs, there are many different types of PPOs. Broadly, the concept means that beneficiaries use physicians who have agreed to give price discounts to their insurer, the PPO. The beneficiary usually is provided some incentive to use a provider from the "preferred" list, in the form of either lower insurance premiums or waiver of cost-sharing requirements.

As indicated in Table 3.3, PPOs accounted for 25% of the private insurance market in 1995. In 1999, PPOs accounted for 38% of the market. The PPO sector has been growing steadily, especially in areas where there is significant competition for patients among physicians and other health care providers. In competitive markets, insurers are more likely to be able to persuade providers to offer price discounts in return for a chance to increase patient volume. Increasingly, PPOs are being established not by insurers but by groups of non-HMO physicians interested in maintaining patient visit volume in the face of competition from HMOs.

Extent of Private Health Insurance Coverage in the United States

Private health insurance coverage for Americans is extensive but far from complete. As of 1999, all but 44 million had some form of health insurance. These latest figures indicate that, despite the recent strong growth in the economy experienced through the year 2000, the percentage of uninsured continues to rise. For instance, during 1993, at the start of the economic recovery, 15.2 % of Americans were uninsured (tabulations from March 1994 and March 1997 *Current Population Survey,* available: www.bls.census.gov/cps/cpsmain.htm). The percentage uninsured had risen to about 16.1% in 1999. The rising proportion of Americans without health care insurance (which did, while still substantial, decline slightly in 1999), even as the economy has improved, is a cause for ongoing policy concern.

A further problem is that while large numbers of individuals have some health insurance coverage, the breadth of their coverage is uneven. An examination of the proportion of total consumer expenditures met by private insurance for various types of care indicates variations in coverage (see Table 3.5). As noted earlier, in 1998 expenditures made through private health insurance amounted to about 33.1% of the total. Table 3.5 shows percentages for 1995 and prior years as the proportions of total expenditures met, for the several categories of health care covered by such insurance. Many individuals do have some coverage for drugs, physicians' office visits, and dental care. In practice, thought, that coverage often does not go very far.

One type of service that has a very low level of insurance coverage is custodial long-term care (see also chapter 8). As noted above, Medicare coverage for long-term care that involves rehabilitation has recently been expanded. Very few long-term care services are for rehabilitation, however; most are custodial, involving chronic care of the frail elderly. As of the late 1990s, Medicare paid less than 7% of all home care costs, and private insurance paid less than 1%. The current system of financing long-term care relies on out-of-pocket expenditures by the elderly who can afford them. In most states, for elderly persons who become impoverished by the costs of such services, the state Medicaid program will then pick up the cost.

Although private insurance has played a very small role in providing coverage for long-term care services, in recent years a market for private long-term care insurance has been emerging, and the types of policies available has been expanding. In addition, numerous proposals have been made for developing an integrated public-private insurance system for financing long-term care services that would combine private insurance and some public resources now devoted to Medicaid long-term care services (Knickman, 1988; White House Domestic Policy Council, 1993).

How the Money Is Paid Out

Paying Physicians

As indicated in Table 3.2, physician services account for approximately 20% of all health care expenditures. The method used to pay physicians influences not only this 20% of the health care bill, however, but also that major share of total health care costs that are controlled largely by

TABLE 3.5   Percentage of Consumer Health Expenditures Met by Private Health Insurance, 1950–1991, Selected Years

Year	Total	Hospital care	Physician's services	Prescribed drugs (out of hospital)	Dental care
1950	12.2	37.1	12.0	a*	a
1960	27.8	64.7	30.0	a	a
1965	30.5	70.1	34.0	2.4	1.6
1966	30.4	71.0	34.0	2.7	2.0
1967	32.8	76.7	36.7	3.5	2.5
1968	34.5	78.8	40.5	3.6	3.1
1969	35.5	77.7	41.1	4.0	3.9
1970	37.2	77.7	43.7	3.9	5.3
1971	39.1	80.9	43.7	4.9	6.3
1972	39.0	76.5	45.8	5.0	7.2
1973	39.0	75.4	46.0	5.6	8.1
1974	41.4	77.3	49.8	6.2	11.0
1975	45.0	82.6	51.3	6.7	15.8
1976	47.0	84.6	53.1	7.9	19.6
1977	45.5	79.3	52.9	7.9	20.2
1981	54.5	82.9	58.9	13.4	34.9
1982	56.2	83.2	60.4	14.6	34.4
1983	56.5	83.5	60.6	14.8	34.9
1984	56.0	80.0	62.6	14.6	35.7
1985	55.5	79.4	62.2	14.8	36.5
1986	55.8	79.4	62.9	15.1	37.4
1987	56.2	79.5	62.9	15.6	37.6
1988	59.4	87.1	70.1	15.6	43.2
1989	61.0	88.6	70.5	15.2	43.7
1990	61.9	90.1	71.6	15.9	44.0
1991	62.9	91.1	72.2	16.9	44.7
1995	62.5	91.6	73.2	NA**	50.2
1998	62.8	90.1	76.5	NA	49.7

* coverage insignificant
** NA: data not available

Adapted from Carroll, M.S., & Arnett II, R.H. (1979). Private health insurance plans in 1977: Coverage, enrollment and financial experience, *Health Care Financing Reviews, 1*(3), p. 14; Gibson, R. M., Levitt, K. R., Lazenby, H., & Waldo, D. (1984). National Health Expenditures, 1983, *Health Care Financing Review, 6*(2), 1–29, Table 3; Letsch, S., et al., National Health Expenditures, 1987. *Health Care Financing Review, 10*(Winter), 109–129, Table 1; Sonnerfeld, S., Waldo, P. Lemieux, J., & Makvsick, D. (1991). Projections of nation's health expenditures through the year 2000. *Heath Care Financing Review, 13*(1), 1–27; Levit, K., et al. (1996). National Health Expenditures 1995. *Health Care Financing Review, 18*(1), Table 16.

physicians' decisions. It is important to emphasize the role of physicians in determining the use of hospital resources by patients, in prescribing drugs, and in ordering medical tests.

As already mentioned, methods used by insurers to reimburse physicians are undergoing substantial change. The growth of HMOs and PPOs is changing the ability of physicians to set prices freely. Increased regulation of fees by Medicare is also affecting the way physicians are reimbursed.

Fee-for-Service

The dominant mechanism for paying physicians continues to be some variation of the fee-for-service system, though this is rapidly giving ground to various capitation arrangements. Traditionally, under fee-for-service a physician simply sets a price for each type of service delivered, and then the patient or his/her insurer pays this price.

The Medicare program's system for paying physicians is based on fee-for-service. However, over the years the physician payment mechanism has been modified. Prior to 1992, the system was based in part on a comparison of the fee each doctor set for a given type of service and that set by the other physicians in a community. This was the basis of the so-called "usual and customary fee" system. Medicare never paid an individual physician an amount that exceeded the 75th percentile of charges by all physicians in a community (this was termed the "prevailing" fee).

Resource-Based Relative-Value Scale

Under OBRA 1989, the system for paying physicians under Medicare was substantially changed. Under the new payment system, each physician service is assigned a "relative value" based on a calculation of the time, skill, and intensity it takes to provide it. The relative values are then adjusted for geographic variations and multiplied by a national conversion factor to determine the dollar amount of payment. This fee schedule, called the resource-based relative value scale (RBRVS), went into effect on January 1, 1992.

This approach was intended to lead to a relative increase in payment for cognitive services (i.e., physical examinations and diagnostic visits) and relative decreases for services that involve procedures. This rebalancing would occur because the previous system led to higher rates for procedures than makes sense based on objective measures involving time, training, or relative expertise. Preliminary evidence suggests, however, that the RBRVS system has led to less change in relative payment rates than originally anticipated.

Paying Hospitals

There are two major mechanisms for hospital reimbursement, retrospective and prospective, although there are numerous variations within these two categories.

Retrospective Payment

In the retrospective payment system, the amounts paid to hospitals by third-party payers and individuals are set after the services have been provided to patients over some time period, usually a year. Reimbursement was based, variously, upon "charges" and "costs." The former system has generally gone by the board. The more sophisticated retrospective payment model is based on costs. The determination of cost never involves individual patients; rather, it is a matter of negotiation between hospitals and third-party payers such as Blue Cross and Medicaid. Cost reimbursement is used when insured patients receive their benefits from the insurer as service rather than as dollar indemnities (reimbursement to individual patients for out-of-pocket payments they have already made). To determine reimbursable costs, third-party payers must sum total hospital costs, decide which costs are "allowable," then, using a formula, reimburse hospitals on a per-patient-day gross-costs basis.

Prospective Payment

The most significant change in hospital payment method in the past 20 years has been the expansion in the use of prospective payment. Of special importance were the changes in the method used by Medicare to pay hospitals. In the Tax Equity and Fiscal Responsibility Act (TEFRA) of 1982, Congress established a cost-per-case basis for hospital payment. TEFRA also placed a ceiling on the rate of increase in hospital revenues that would be supported by the Medicare program. The 1983 amendments to the Social Security Act further defined the case payment system. These amendments created a revolutionary method of paying hospitals for inpatient care to Medicare patients, based on "Diagnosis-Related Groups" or DRGs. Under this system, hospitals are paid a preestablished amount per case treated, with payment rates varying by type of case. The DRGs measured hospital output by first classifying patients into 23 major diagnostic categories (MDCs), based on major body systems. The MDCs were divided further into 47 diagnostic groups based on the patient's diagnosis or the surgical procedure used and on age, sex, and other clinical information. There is one additional group used for cases in which the admitting diagnosis and surgical procedure performed does not match (Grimaldi & Micheletti, 1982).

Two aspects of this payment system depart significantly from previous methods used to pay for Medicare patients. First, the DRG concept holds that the "best" measure of hospital output is the diagnosis treated rather than what individual services are provided (lab, X ray, operating room, and so forth) or length of hospital stay. That is, the basis of payment is the type of case treated (taking into account the usual and customary treatment pattern for that case), rather than totaling the costs of all the ancillary routine and inputs to hospital care.

Second, DRG payments are determined prospectively and are fixed. Although a portion of the initial rates for fiscal year 1984 were determined by historical costs, subsequent rates of increase in the payments have been controlled before payment is made. Hence, Medicare now has the ability to control the rate of cost increase for Medicare patients.

The use of DRGs has spread to other payers. At least 21 states, such as Pennsylvania, Utah, Ohio, Michigan, and Washington, have adopted case-based systems to pay for hospital care received by Medicaid patients. In 32 states, including Arizona, Oklahoma, and Kansas, a DRG system is employed to pay for Blue Cross patients. As of 1998, Maryland was the only state that uses a DRG system for all third-party payers.

The use of DRGs has been an important factor, although not the only one, in the decline in in-patient hospital utilization that has occurred since the mid-1980s. The reduction in hospital use has not been without side effects, however. In particular, evidence consistently indicates sharp increases in post-hospital use of services, including home health care and nursing home care, as well as increased readmissions (Guterman, Eggers, Riley, Greene, & Terrell, 1987). The tighter regulation of Medicare payment rates also may be responsible for part of the rapid growth in cost of private insurance as hospitals shift some of their costs from Medicare to private insurance. That is, higher rates may be charged for individuals with private insurance to compensate for any operating losses associated with care delivered to Medicare patients.

Whereas inpatient care under Medicare relies on prospective case payment, outpatient care reimbursement remains largely a cost-based system. A major problem in changing outpatient hospital spending to a per-visit or per-episode format is the ongoing problem of defining a clinically relevant case-mix system. However, as part of the 1997 Balanced Budget Act, Congress has directed the Department of Health and Human Services to accelerate the development of prospective payment systems for hospital outpatient care, as well as certain post-acute care benefits (i.e., skilled nursing facilities, home health care).

THE RISING PAYMENTS FOR HEALTH CARE

National spending for health care grew an average of 12.4% per year from 1970 to 1991. Between 1991 and 1995, however, the growth in national spending decreased to 6.7% per year, and in the last half of the decade spending rose at 5.9% per year on the average. The slower growth in health care spending of late is traced largely to the rise in managed health care, as well as federal legislation slowing the growth in Medicare and Medicaid. Despite this lower rate of growth, the rate of increase in health care costs has still consistently far exceeded the rate of inflation in the general economy. Thus, health care expenses each year account for an increasing share of the nation's GNP.

Furthermore, the most recent data, for the year 2000, show a reversion to sharp increases in health care spending, particularly in the private sector (Kaiser Family Foundation, 2000). Health insurance premium increases approaching double digits resumed during 1998 and were projected to continue through 2001. A key element in the resurgent growth in health care spending is the rising cost of prescription drugs, led largely by several expensive new drug therapies (see also chapter 10). The spike in drug costs placed the issue of prescription drug coverage center stage in the 2000 U.S. presidential campaign.

Several other factors have contributed to the rise in medical costs: general inflation in the economy, population growth, the development of new medical technology, and an increased "intensity" of services provided to all patients. Over the last 40 years, both the rapid development of medical technology and the increasing depth and breadth of medical care services provided to individual patients for any given medical diagnosis have been encouraged by growth in the extent of health insurance coverage and previous retrospective, cost-based payment systems that rewarded higher reported costs with higher payments (Feldstein, 1971). As insurance coverage increased, the out-of-pocket cost to the patient was reduced, leading to increases in demand for higher quality medical care, and hence to rising prices. The growth in the comprehensiveness of third-party insurance coverage was stimulated in part through the federal government's tax law (Phelps, 1984). Under current tax law, employer payments to employees for health insurance are not considered taxable income. Because these tax subsidies reduce the price of health insurance, they provide incentives to purchase more health insurance.

Although the spread of new technology undoubtedly offers unprecedented medical benefits, some innovations are of marginal value. Further, facilities and services unavailable in the late 1970s or found only in medical centers are now offered in a substantial number of community hospitals. The increase in diagnostic imaging by computerized axial tomography (CAT) was, for example, impressive, more than doubling since 1980 (Office of Technology Assessment, 1981). Similarly, rapid diffusion of the use of magnetic resonance imaging (MRI) occurred. The medical benefits of CAT scanning are well-known; for instance, it has reduced the need for exploratory surgery. Yet growth in new technology has expanded the potential pool of recipients as well as symptoms diagnosed. Thus, although it is true that new technology provides unprecedented medical benefits, the downside is that new technology increases expenditures.

Nevertheless, advances in medical technology continue at a rapid pace. Indeed, the recent spike in the growth in health care spending is driven largely by the growth in prescription drug spending. At the end of the 1990s, spending for pharmaceutical drugs was increasing at the rate of 15%–20% per year. That was well above the overall health care spending inflation rate and accounted for approximately one third of the overall rise in national health care spending. Advances in genomics, such as those achieved by the Human Genome project, will expand greatly our science base, as well as medical opportunities for treatments and cure. These include continued innovations in drug therapies, the treatment of autoimmune diseases, advances in molecular cell biology, and the study of genetics and its implications for the incidence of disease. Each of these promising innovations will yield substantial improvements in the quality and length of life. They are likely, however, to be accompanied by a high price tag. Thus, the debate will continue concerning the ability of public and private payers to "appropriately" balance their desires to control the growth in spending, while encouraging the diffusion of new and promising technologies.

CONCLUSIONS

Obviously, money funds the health care delivery system, but the routes dollars take from consumers to providers can be labyrinthine. Some dollars arrive directly, some via the government, and some through insurance companies. Most health care providers are paid by salary, but some, usually the higher-priced ones, are paid on a piecework basis. Hospitals are paid in numerous ways for services provided to patients. Some insurers base payments on what the hospital charges, whereas others pay on the basis of allowable average costs. Still others, notably Medicare and some Medicaid and Blue Cross plans, pay hospitals on a per-case basis, with the payment rate set in advance.

In the United States in the 1960s and 1970s a health insurance system that emphasized coverage for hospital care, with physician service in hospitals generally being more lucrative than in the office setting, tilted the system in the direction of utilization of the most expensive component of the system. Technological change, a significant factor in rising health care costs, was often poorly planned and evaluated, with decisions frequently made on the basis of universal access rather than cost-effectiveness.

In the 1980s and 1990s, however, the United States witnessed a virtual revolution in the financing and structure of medical care delivery. Fundamental changes in the methods used to pay health care providers, growing involvement by employers and employees in direct negotiation with providers, and a projected aggregate surplus of physicians have led to the changes in the structure of the delivery system. Notable has been the move from retrospective to prospective modes of payment. Although prospective per-case payment systems are generally restricted to inpatient hospital care, and considerable research and development efforts—aimed at designing prospective case payment systems for long-term care, home health care, and outpatient care—are currently under way. In some quarters, across-the-board capitation payments may prove feasible.

The 1980s also heralded the beginning of dramatic changes in the organization of medical practice. The growth in prepaid group practice, ambulatory surgery, and the "unbundling" of hospital services are indicative of the magnitude of recent changes in the delivery system. New alignments between providers, employers, and employees—in the form of HMOs, PPOs, and self-insurance ventures—also reflect the recent entrance of the consumer into direct financial negotiation with health care providers. Efforts by providers to unbundle services designed in part to increase revenues have been supplemented by the rise in capitation and integrated delivery systems. The impressive rise in efforts by purchasers to control costs, accompanied by the new dominance of managed care, truly represents a major change in the organization and delivery of services in the 1990s.

These changes accelerated during the 1990s. Managed care became the dominant force by which consumers receive their care (see chapter 11). Indeed, by the end of the decade, 91% of working Americans, 40% of Medicaid beneficiaries, and nearly 15% of the Medicare population received coverage through some form of managed care. The shift to managed care has been credited by many as the primary factor accounting for the substantial reduction in the growth of health care costs, though the precise role that managed care has played in these savings remains an issue. Impact of this major change in the delivery system on the quality of care and access to come will, however, have to be carefully monitored.

The rise in managed care has also produced tensions in our system, however. While managed care has slowed the growth in health spending, pleasing the purchasing community, the public has been less impressed. The tools used by managed care plans to control the growth in spending—restricted networks of physicians, prior authorization, and discounted fees—have raised concerns among the public over the quality of care, as well as access to care. This mounting tension over "patients' rights" within managed care plans has surfaced as a major legislative and political issue.

What remains unresolved, however, is the future for the 44 million Americans, as of the year 2000, who lack health insurance. Although Congress passed an important new insurance program designed to provide insurance to low-income children (as part of the 1997 Balanced Budget Act), it left unresolved how the remaining uninsured will access the system as the desire to control spending intensifies.

We currently finance health care services for the uninsured through direct funding of hospitals (for instance through the disproportionate share program in Medicare and Medicaid), state and local tax levy support, and profits generated from private health plans. This approach for financing the costs of treating indigent patients may make it difficult if not impossible to simultaneously pursue our cost-containment initiatives. Indeed, efforts by both the public sector and private health insurance to slow the growth in spending will continue to increase financial pressure on hospitals. As cost-containment efforts have increased, hospital operating margins have continued to fall (Medicare Payment Advisory Committee, 2000). A continued decline in hospital operating margins would make it increasingly difficult for hospitals to finance costs of treating the uninsured through "profits" generated on private health plans. Indeed, absent approaches that reduce substantially the number of uninsured, the move toward a more competitive marketplace will eventually eliminate cross-subsidies within hospitals, raising substantial concern over our future ability to care for the uninsured.

CASE STUDY

The private sector has dramatically increased its desire and ability to extract cost savings from providers largely through the use of managed care. These savings were generated, however, during a time when hospitals were making substantial profits from Medicare. The Balanced Budget Act of 1997 has reduced substantially the rate of growth in Medicare payments to providers.

What impact has this legislation had on

1. the ability of the private sector to sustain its cost-containment efforts?
2. pressures for even more productivity from the health care industry?
3. consolidations among health plans and providers?
4. access to care for the uninsured (i.e., the amount of charity care and bad debt provided by hospitals and other providers)?

DISCUSSION QUESTIONS

1. One of the more significant changes in the structure of insurance over the past 2 decades has been in the economic sectors that are at risk for higher health care spending. How has risk shifted throughout the system over the past 2 decades, and to what extent do these changes influence the yearly growth in health care spending?

2. What processes would be effective or desirable to balance society's desire to promote the introduction and diffusion of new lifesaving or quality-enhancing technologies, with an assurance that health care costs will not continue to rise even faster?

3. In addition to health care, several other sectors of the economy are rising at a faster rate than the overall rate of economic growth. For instance, like health care, the computer and information industry continues to account for a rising share of Gross Domestic Product (GDP). Despite the rising share of GDP assumed by the information and computer industry, however, there is not a substantial concern or body of literature examining options for "computer cost containment." Why the concern in the health care industry?

REFERENCES

Arnett, R. H., & Trapnell, G. (1984). Private health insurance: New measures of a complex and changing industry. *Health Care Financing Review, 6*(2), 31–42.

Armould, R., Debrock, L. W., & Pollard, J. W. (1984). Do HMO's produce services more efficiently? *Inquiry, 21,* 243–254.

Balanced Budget Act of 1997, Pub. L. No. 105-33. (1997).

Carroll, M. S., & Arnett, R. H., II. (1979). Private health insurance plans in 1977: Coverage, enrollment and financial experience. *Health Care Financing Review, 1*(2), 3–22.

Congressional Budget Office. (1995). *The effects of managed care and managed competition.* Washington, DC: U.S. Government Printing Office.

Congressional Research Service. (1976). *Workmen's compensation: Role of the federal government.* (IB75054). Washington, DC: Library of Congress.

Feldstein, M. S. (1971). *The rising cost of hospital care.* Washington, DC: Information Resources Press.

Gabel, J., DiCarlo, S., Fink, S., & de Lissovoy, G. (1989, January). Employer-sponsored health insurance in America: Preliminary results from the 1988 survey. *Research Bulletin.* Washington, DC: Health Insurance Association of America.

Gibson, R. M. (1979). National health expenditures, 1978. *Health Care Financing Review, 1*(1), 1–36.

Gibson, R. M., Levitt, K., Lazenby, H., & Waldo, D. (1984). National health expenditures, 1983. *Social Security Bulletin, 6*(2), 1–29.

Grimaldi, P., & Micheletti, J. (1982). *Diagnosis related groups: A practitioner's guide.* Chicago: Pluribus Press.

Group Health Association of America. (1986). *HMO industry profile: Trends, 1985–1986 (Vol. 4).* Washington, DC: Author.

Gruber, L. R., Shadle, M., & Polich, C. L. (1988). From movement to industry: The growth of HMO's. *Health Affairs, 7*(3), 197.

Guterman, S., Eggers, P. W., Riley, G., Greene, T. F., & Terrell, S. A. (1987). The first 3 years of Medicare prospective payment: An overview. *Health Care Financing Review, 9*(1), 67.

Hellinger, F. (1985). Recent evidence on case-based systems for setting hospital rates. *Inquiry, 22*(1).

Interstudy, Competitive Edge. (1997). *HMO directory 7.1.* Excelsior, MN: Author.

Interstudy, Competitive Edge. (1999). *HMO directory 10.1.* Minneapolis, MN: Author.

Kaiser Family Foundation and Health Research and Educational Trust. (2000, September). *Employee Health Benefits, 2000.* Menlo Park, CA: Author.

Knickman, J. (1988). Private long-term care insurance: Alleviating market problems with public-private partnership. *Health Economics and Health Service Research, 9,* 13S.

Krizay, J., & Wilson, A. (1974). *The patient as consumer.* Lexington, MA: D. C. Health.

Law, S. A. (1974). *Blue Cross. What went wrong?* New Haven, CT: Yale University Press, 1974.

Letsch, S., Levit, K., & Waldo, D. (1988). National health expenditures, 1987. *Health Care Financing Review, 10*(Winter), 109.

Levit, K., Lazenby, H., Braden, B., Cowan, C., McDonnell, P., Sivarajan, L., Stiller, J., Wan, D., Donham, C., Long, A., & Stewart, M. (1996). National health expenditures, 1995. *Health Care Financing Review, 18*(1), 175–214.

Luft, H. (1978). How do health maintenance organizations achieve their savings? *New England Journal of Medicine, 298,* 1366.

Luft, H. (1981). *Health maintenance organization: Dimensions of performance.* New York: Wiley.

Manning, W. (1984). A controlled trial of the effects of a prepaid group practice on use of services. *New England Journal of Medicine, 310*(23), 1505–1510.

McCarthy, C. M. (1975). Incentive reimbursement as an impetus to cost containment. *Inquiry, 12,* 320.

Medicare Advisory Payment Committee. (2000, June). *Report to Congress: Selected Medicare issues.* Washington, DC: MedPac.

Newhouse, J. P., Manning, W., Morris, C., Orr, L., Duan, N., Keeler, E., Leibowitz, A., Marquis, K., Marquis, S., Phelps, C., & Brooks, R. (1981). Some interim results from a controlled trial of cost sharing in health insurance. *New England Journal of Medicine, 305,* 1501.

Office of Technology Assessment. (1981). *Policy implications of the CT scanner: An update.* Washington, DC: Author.

Phelps, C. E. (1984). Taxing health insurance: How much is enough? *Contemporary Policy Issues, 3*(2).

Price, D. N. (1979a). Workers' compensation programs in the 1970s. *Social Security Bulletin, 42*(5), 3.

Price, D. N. (1979b). Workers' compensation coverage, payments and costs, 1977. *Social Security Bulletin, 42*(10).

Roemer, M., & Shonick, V. (1973). HMO performance: The recent evidence. *Health and Society, 51,* 271.

Russell, et al. (1974). *Federal loyalty spending, 1969–1974.* Washington, DC: National Planning Association.

Thorpe, K. E., & Phelps, C. (1992). The social role of not-for-profit organizations: Hospital provision of charity care. *Economic Inquiry, 29,* 472–484.

U.S. National Commission on State Workmen's Compensation Laws. (1973). *Report.* Washington, DC: U.S. Government Printing Office, 1973.

White House Domestic Policy Council. (1993). *Health Security Act.* Washington, DC: U.S. Government Printing Office.

Wolinsky, F. (1980). The performance of health maintenance organizations: An analytic review. *Milbank Memorial Fund Quarterly, 58*(4), 4.

4

The Health Care Workforce

Christine T. Kovner and Edward S. Salsberg

LEARNING OBJECTIVES

- ☐ Describe the types of health care workers in the United States.
- ☐ Identify some of the major issues facing clinicians, managers, and health policy makers about the health workforce.
- ☐ Describe the impact of the changing health care system on the health workforce.
- ☐ Recognize the difficulties in estimating the future demand and supply of health care workers.
- ☐ Discuss professional licensure as a mechanism for health care worker quality assurance.

TOPICAL OUTLINE

The workforce
Counting health workers: Problems and pitfalls
Nursing
Medicine
Other health workers
Current issues
Conclusion

KEY WORDS

health workforce, health professional, supply, demand, need, registered nurse (RN), advanced practice nurse, nurse-practitioner (NP), physician, graduate medical education, international medical school graduate, allied health, full-time equivalent (FTE), certification, licensure

The health care workforce is the backbone of the health care delivery system. Even with major technological advances, it is the health care worker who ultimately determines the availability, quality, and cost of health services. Any effort to improve health care services or control costs must consider the supply, distribution, use, and education of the health care workforce. Conversely, any change in financing, organization, or technology will also impact health care personnel.

The rapidly changing health care system is having a dramatic impact on the health care workforce, including the number and types of workers that will be needed, and where and how they will practice and work. The transformation of health care is disrupting historic roles for physicians, nurses, and other health care professionals. Competition, managed care, the development of integrated delivery systems, increasing corporatization of health care, and new medical advances and technologies are all impacting the workforce. Health care workers are reassessing their role and their relationship to the delivery system and other workers, and health professions education programs are reassessing their curricula and approaches. While the American health care system is still evolving, many of the implications for workforce have already became apparent.

Among the factors affecting the workforce are the following:

- As competition expands, health care facilities and organizations are far more concerned with costs, productivity, and outcomes than in the past, leading to a reassessment of how many workers of what type are needed and how they are used.
- Hospitals, the setting with the largest number of health workers, are under pressure to reduce costs. Many are reducing staff and redesigning their operations.
- There is increasing concern with outcomes and quality of care.
- Many services are shifting from inpatient to ambulatory care settings.
- HMOs, other managed care arrangements, and other purchasers of service are constraining the roles of physicians, advanced nurse practitioners, and other providers, reducing their autonomy.
- Many settings are substituting lower-cost workers.
- All settings are concerned with customer relations and patient satisfaction, and most organizations want workers who are flexible, computer literate, and customer oriented.

THE WORKFORCE

The health care workforce is large and diverse. It includes many of society's most educated and highest paid professionals, such as physicians and PhD researchers. It includes a wide range of caregivers, from nurses to therapists. It includes millions of skilled technicians who work in hospitals, laboratories, and other settings; and it includes millions of support staff, such as aides, clerks, and housekeepers. Large numbers of managers, administrators, lawyers, computer operators, security guards, maintenance personnel, and other nonhealth professionals also work in the health care industry.

Health services are labor intensive. This is true whether the services are provided in hospitals, in nursing homes, or in physicians' offices. In 1998, nearly 14 million people were employed in health care settings and/or as health professionals, approximately 10% of the nation's total workforce (U.S. Bureau of Labor Statistics, 2000).

Over the last 50 years, health care employment has consistently grown at a faster rate than the overall employment in the American economy. From 1988 through 1998, employment in health care settings grew by 36% (U.S. Bureau of Labor Statistics, 2000b). Even during national recessions, health care employment has risen.

The changes now under way in health care may slow the growth in jobs. However, the aging of the population, and efforts to address specific health problems, such as high rates of infant mortality, will contribute to the need for additional health personnel. While the federal Bureau of Labor Statistics projects that employment in health care settings will continue to rise over 25% between 1998 and 2008 (U.S. Bureau of Labor Statistics, 2000b), others believe that the changing health care system will slow the growth in jobs and may even lead to a loss of them (Berliner & Kovner, 1994; Pew Health Professions Commission, 1995).

Health care employment can be viewed in two ways: by work location or by occupation. Health care professionals and others workers are typically employed in settings such as hospitals, nursing homes, and ambulatory care facilities. Figure 4.1 shows the distribution of the total health workforce by practice setting, including those health professions working outside of the health industry. Although the vast majority of health personnel work in health settings, nearly 17% of the total health workforce are in settings that are not considered part of the health industry. For example, physicians teach at medical schools; nurses work in school health offices; and pharmacists work for pharmaceutical firms.

Table 4.1 presents the distribution of the health workforce in and out of the health industry. Between 1988 and 1998, the total U.S. workforce (non-farm) grew 19%; the total health industry workforce grew 36% (U.S. Bureau of Labor Statistics, 2000a), nearly twice as much. It is noteworthy that during this period the hospital workforce (public and private) grew by 21%, reflecting the impact of the changing health care system, including the shift in care from more costly institutional settings to ambulatory care settings. Figure 4.1 shows the distribution of the health workforce by practice setting.

COUNTING HEALTH WORKERS: PROBLEMS AND PITFALLS

Counting and tracking health workers can be very confusing. Often figures on health care employment just report health "sector" employment,

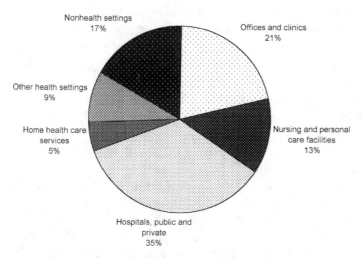

FIGURE 4.1   Distribution of the health workforce by practice setting, 1998.
Source: U.S. Bureau of Labor Statistics, 2000b.

excluding health professionals in other settings. As noted above, though, close to 17% of health professionals work outside of health settings.

Some data sources count the number of individuals in a setting or occupation regardless of how much they work. This is a body count—such as there are *x* nurses licensed in a state. Other data sets, in order to account for the fact that some people work only part-time, count full-time equivalents (FTEs). Two half-time workers represent two individuals but only one FTE. The American Hospital Association reports FTEs, allowing analysts and hospitals to compare staffing across hospitals. The Department of Labor uses a third method of counting: they count the number of paychecks. This is similar to a body count, except a person working at two

TABLE 4.1   The U.S. Workforce, 1999

Setting	Health professionals	Other workers	Total
Health service settings	8,485,358	4,064,745	12,550,104
Other work settings	2,103,557	124,713,945	126,817,502
Total	10,588,915	128,778,690	139,367,605
Health professionals working in health service settings	8,485,358	6.1%	
Health professionals working in other settings	2,103,557	1.5%	
Other workers in health service settings	4,064,745	2.9%	
U.S. health workforce	14,653,661	10.5%	
U.S. civilian labor force	139,367,605	100.0%	

Source: Current Population Survey (1999).

facilities would be counted twice. If hospitals substitute part-time workers for full-time workers, the Labor Department data might show an increase in employment while the AHA data might show a decrease in FTEs.

Another problem is defining the organization or reporting unit. As integrated delivery systems develop, the distinction between hospitals and other settings, such as ambulatory and long-term care is likely to blur, especially as some workers may move among sites. Also, if a facility contracts or outsources a work activity, for example food service, then these workers may no longer be reported as health workers, even if they still work in the same location.

State licensing boards count all individuals with a license in those occupations that require a license. However, not all of these individuals practice in their field. The number of licensed individuals sets the upper limit on the number that can practice that profession in a state. The percentage that are actually working or actively looking for work is generally referred to as the "labor force participation rate."

There is no single "right" way to count. This is not meant to discourage data analysis but to caution the reader to be aware of these differences and comparisons across data sources. For additional information on health workforce data issues, see the U.S. Department of Health and Human Services, Health Resources and Services Administrations, *State Health Workforce Data Resource Guide* (2000).

NURSING

This section presents an overview of the nursing profession. After a brief history of nursing, the section looks at how nursing is defined in law and by professional nurses. The various educational programs for nurses are described, as well as the levels of practice. Finally, current issues in nursing are analyzed within the context of the health care system. Nurse is a generic term that is applied to a variety of practitioners from nurses' aides and assistants to nurse researchers with PhDs. The focus of this section will be the professional registered nurse and the licensed practical nurse.

Definition of Nursing

A classic definition of nursing was given by Virginia Henderson (1966), who states:

> The unique function of the nurse is to assist the individual (sick or well), in the performance of those activities contributing to health or its recovery (or peaceful death) that he would perform unaided if he had the necessary strength, will, or knowledge. And to do this in such a way as to help him gain independence as rapidly as possible. (p. 15)

The American Nurses Association (1995) suggests that authority for nursing is based on a social contract between society and the profession. The regulation of health professionals is a state responsibility. As such, each state has its own legal definition of the practice of nursing. Each state board of nursing defines and interprets the authority and scope of practice of registered nurses, although nursing is usually defined as the diagnosis and treatment of human responses. By 1923 legislation was enacted in all states for voluntary registration (Bullough, 1975). The first mandatory licensing law went into effect in New York State in 1947. It required, with certain exceptions, that only licensed professional nurses could legally use the title Registered Nurse.

For example, in New York State a registered professional nurse is defined as

> . . . diagnosing and treating human responses to actual or potential health problems through services as case-finding, health teaching, health counseling, and provision of care supportive to or restorative of life and well-being, and executing medical regimes prescribed by a licensed or otherwise legally authorized physician or dentist. A nursing regimen shall be consistent with and shall not vary from any existing medical regimen. (New York Education Law, 1989)

All states require that prospective registered nurses attend an approved nursing program and take a national licensing exam, the National Council Licensure Examination for RN (NCLEX-RN), developed by the National Council of State Boards of Nursing. In 1999, of the 76,607 first-time candidates educated in the United States and its territories taking the exam, almost 84.47% passed, while only 47.7% of the 6,381 foreign-educated applicants passed the exam (Nursing Regulation Examination Pass Rates and Licensure Statistics, 2000).

In some states, nurses (or certain categories of nurses) may prescribe pharmacologic agents or deliver a baby. In other states they may not. In addition, some states require continuing education for license renewal.

Licensed Practical Nurse

Licensed Practical Nurses (LPNs)/Licensed Vocational Nurses (LVNs) work under the supervision of RNs or physicians and perform caregiving tasks such as medication administration and wound dressing change. LPN/LVNs must pass a national examination and are licensed in each state. In 1998, 40,195 people took the exam and 87.2% passed (Nursing Regulation Examination Pass Rates and Licensure Statistics, 2000).

Like other states, New York differentiates professional nursing from practical nursing, defining the latter as "performing tasks and responsibilities . . . under the direction of a registered, professional nurse or licensed or otherwise legally authorized physician or dentist" (New York Education Law, 1989).

Other Nursing Personnel

Other nursing personnel include a variety of unlicensed assistive personnel (UAP) such as nurse aides, assistants, orderlies, and technicians. These personnel also work under the supervision of registered nurses and perform such simple tasks as temperature taking and comfort measures such as bathing and linen change. These occupations are not licensed by the states, although federal regulations require that nurse aides who work in long-term care facilities that are reimbursed by Medicare and Medicaid must complete a specified educational program and pass a written and practical test. In addition, Medicare certified home health agencies have to hire certified home health aides. More than half of the states have regulations or guidelines for RNs who supervise UAPs. Some states have specific educational requirements for some of these workers (Thomas, Barter, & McLaughlin, 2000).

Education of Nurses

One of the most confusing aspects of nursing is the variety of programs for educating nurses. Unlike medicine, which has consistent educational requirements, nursing offers the student a number of options. Although the American Nurses Association recommends that states require a baccalaureate degree to practice nursing, students can attend a 2-year college program, a 3-year hospital-based (diploma) program, a 4-year college program, a 2-year master's degree program, or a nursing doctoral (ND) program. North Dakota requires a baccalaureate degree, while all other State Boards of Nursing accept any of these programs as appropriate preparation for the RN licensing exam. Practical nurse education occurs in high schools, hospitals, junior colleges, or vocational schools.

Registered Professional Nursing

There is no longer one reliable and valid current source of data about nurse education programs. Both the National League for Nursing (NLN) and the American Association of Colleges of Nursing (AACN) accredit nursing programs. The AACN accredits and obtains data on baccalaureate and graduate programs. The NLN accredits and obtains data on all nursing programs. Neither organization has complete data. In 2000, there were 1,666 basic educational programs to prepare RNs in the United States, at the following educational levels: associate degree (885); baccalaureate degree (695); diploma (86) (*Directory of Accredited Nursing* Programs, 2000). In addition, there were programs at the graduate level to prepare students for professional licensure. Total enrollments in baccalaureate nursing programs decreased from 1998 to 1999, the fifth year that enrollments decreased (American Association of Colleges of Nursing [AACN], 2000);

this trend was consistent across the United States. No U.S. data were available on the other types of programs, although regional reports indicated that enrollments were down over this same period. Accreditation standards do not specify individual course requirements. Consequently, curricula vary widely from school to school, and transfer of nursing course credits is extremely difficult.

The first associate degree program was opened in 1952 (Anastas, 1984). The typical associate degree program requires basic liberal arts courses such as English and sociology. In addition, science courses such as anatomy and physiology are required. Nursing courses usually include fundamentals of nursing (clinical skills), maternal and child health, and care of acutely ill hospitalized adult patients. Experience is gained by practicing skills in the campus laboratory and caring for patients in institutional settings such as hospitals. The nurses enrolled in associate degree programs are educated to be direct providers of care at the patient bedside. The programs are 2 academic years to 2 calendar years in length.

The typical diploma program is similar to the associate degree program, though it is usually under the auspices of a hospital. The practical experience sessions are usually longer than in the associate degree program, and the entire course takes about 3 years, with an emphasis on acute care (hospital-based) nursing. Often students are required to take liberal arts courses at a local college, and they receive college credit that can later be transferred to other colleges. However, diploma graduates who attend college often are not able to transfer the credits earned in the diploma program because until recently most of these programs were not degree-granting institutions.

The curriculum of the baccalaureate program is similar to that of liberal arts programs in other fields. Because the program is at least eight semesters long, the student takes more nonnursing courses than in either the associate or the diploma program. Students take liberal arts courses such as English, math, and psychology, and are required to take science courses such as microbiology, anatomy, and physiology. In addition, approximately half of the credits are usually in nursing courses. The organization of these courses varies from school to school. Some schools organize curricula developmentally and have courses devoted to care of infants, children, adults, and older people. Others base the curriculum on the relative health of populations and offer courses on prevention, episodic care, continuous care, and critical care. In addition, students learn to read and interpret research. Baccalaureate-prepared nurses are prepared to work in community settings and leadership positions as well as in acute care settings. They are generalists who can provide care to individuals, groups, families, and communities. Graduates are also prepared for advanced education in nursing.

Another opportunity for education in nursing is the external degree program, such as that offered by the Board of Regents of New York State. In 1971 an external associate degree program was begun, followed by a baccalaureate degree program in 1976. Students obtain either degree by completing equivalency testing in liberal arts, sciences, and nursing.

Students also must complete a practical exam. The program's philosophy centers on a person's knowledge and skills, rather than how the information and these skills were acquired. Graduates of these programs are eligible for state licensure.

Little recent data are available about nursing students. The vast majority of baccalaureate students continue to be female (90.5%), although this percentage is down slightly from 1998. In 1999, baccalaureate nursing students were primarily white (75.5%), followed by black (10.7%), Asian, and Hispanic (each 4.4%) and Native American (0.7). These percentages were about the same as they had been in 1998 (AACN, 2000).

Licensed Practical Nursing

Licensed Practical Nurses (LPN/LVN) are educated in one of approximately 1,100 state-approved programs in the United States (Directory of Accredited Nursing Programs, 2000). More than half of these programs are in trade, technical, or vocational schools, whereas the remainder are in colleges, community colleges, high schools, and hospitals. The programs typically are 1 year long and include classroom and clinical education. Many of those who take the LPN licensing examination were actually students in professional nursing programs. They take the examination to become LPNs prior to taking the RN examination. The typical LPN program takes about 1 year and includes basic courses in physical and social sciences, and simple nursing procedures.

Other Nursing Personnel

Educational requirements for other nursing personnel, such as nurses' aides, vary by employment setting. Some are educated in the setting in which they work, some in programs in high schools, and others in not-for-profit or for-profit vocational schools. Training takes from a few hours to six months or more.

Graduate Nursing Education

Nursing degree programs at the master's and doctoral level concentrate on nursing courses, with the assumption that the nurse baccalaureate graduate has had the basic liberal arts and science courses. Historically, specialists in nursing were educated in specialized hospitals or became specialists based on clinical practice with a particular type of patient. In the 1950s colleges and universities began offering academic programs for specialty education. By the 1960s, postgraduate education for clinical practice specialization was concentrated in universities.

Registered nurses with baccalaureate degrees can earn master's degrees in advanced clinical practice, teaching, and nursing administration/management.

Within these three broad areas students usually focus on a nursing content area such as adult health, maternal-child health, psychiatric-mental health, or community health. Specific programs include everything from nursing informatics (computers), home health care management, and geriatrics, to pediatric nurse practitioners. Most students choose to focus on advanced clinical practice. In a few programs people with a baccalaureate in another field can earn a master's degree to prepare them for professional practice.

Within the generic category of advanced practice nurses, those with a clinical practice focus include: Clinical Nurse Specialist (CNS), Nurse-Practitioner (NP), Nurse Midwife (NMW), and Certified Registered Nurse Anesthetist (CRNA). Clinical nurse specialists have advanced degrees with expert skills in a particular area, such as mental health, cancer, or women's health. Nurse-practitioners are educated to perform an expanded nursing role and diagnose and manage most common and many chronic health problems, often in primary care. In most states they can prescribe medicines. Their scope of practice, however, including whether or not they must have a collaborating relationship with a physician, varies from state to state. Nurse-midwives are educated to provide pre-, intra-, and postpartum care, provide family planning services, and routine gynecological care, as well as caring for newborns. Nurse anesthetists are educated to administer anesthetics.

By 2000 there were 358 programs offering a master's degree in nursing, an increase of 50 over 1995 (Directory of Accredited Nursing Programs, 2000). Because the AACN does not obtain data from all graduate programs, the exact number of enrollees and graduates of these programs is not available. Based on their sample and comparing the same programs from year to year, however, the AACN reported that enrollments decreased from 1996 to 1999. In addition to clinical practice, master's programs also prepare RNs in management and teaching. Graduate education in nursing continues to be populated primarily by women, with 91.4% of master's students being female. In terms of race, most master's graduates were white (83.4%), followed by black (6.7%), Asian (2.9%), Hispanic (2.7%), and Native American (0.6%). These percentages are far lower than these groups' percentage proportion of the U.S. population. The percentage of nonwhite enrollees in baccalaureate programs was 24.5% by 1999. This increase may add to the nonwhite percentage of master's students in the future. By 1999, NP programs had almost 65% of graduates from master's programs. Family NP is the most popular specialty both in terms of enrollments and graduations (AACN, 2000).

Doctoral Programs

Nurses can also earn doctoral degrees in nursing. There are three types of degrees offered. The ND (Doctor of Nursing) is similar to the MD, that is, it is the first professional degree, building on the earlier liberal arts or scientific education and preparing the student to take the state licensing exam to practice as a registered nurse. The DSN and DNSc are professional doctorates that prepare the nurse for advanced clinical practice. The PhD is a research degree, with requirements similar to the PhD in other fields; it requires extensive preparation in a narrow field and a dissertation. In 1999 there were 74 doctoral programs in nursing in the U.S., having grown from five programs in 1967 (AACN, 2000). In 1999, 94.6% of the almost 2,800 students enrolled in doctoral programs were female and most were white (77.6%) followed by black (6.2%), Asian (2.8%), Hispanic (1.5%), and Native American (0.4%). An additional 11% were nonresident alien or of unknown race (AACN, 2000).

Geographic Distribution and Educational Preparation

The National Council of State Boards of Nursing reported that in 2000 there were 3,054,215 licenses for RNs. An unknown number of RNs have licenses in more than one state. About 2.7 million people had licenses to practice as registered nurses in the United States in 2000 (Health Resources and Services Administration [HRSA], 2001). About 2.2 million (82%) were employed in nursing (an increase of about 86,000 over 1996); 59% were working full time. There is wide variation in the number of RNs in relation to the population. California, the state with the lowest ratio, had 554 RNs per 100,000 while Massachusetts, the state with the highest ratio, had 1,194 RNs per 100,000. Registered nurses are getting older with a mean age of 45.2 years in 2000. Only 18% of RNs were under 35 years of age. In part, this aging results from the average age at graduation of associate degree nurses. As shown in Figure 4.2, about 10% were minorities (defined as nonwhites), although the percentage of men employed in nursing was almost 6%, a slight increase from 1996. The percentage of minority RNs is inconsistent with their representation in the general population and has been a concern of nursing and government for many years.

The 2.2 million employed registered nurses were prepared in a variety of educational programs, with 55% having less than a baccalaureate degree. The number of graduates from associate degree programs exceeded those from baccalaureate programs. Although fewer nurses are now prepared at the diploma level, about 22% of employed RNs had a diploma as their highest level of education. Thirty-three percent had a baccalaureate degree.

Employment Settings

Although the percentage has decreased from 1996, most registered nurses continue to work in hospitals. As shown in Figure 4.3 about 1.3 million (59.1%) of RNs worked in hospitals, while only 151,900 (6.9%) worked in nursing homes in 1996. About 9.5% of RNs worked in ambulatory care settings. Staff nurses typically work in direct patient care, where they provide nursing care to individuals who may be acutely ill, as in a hospital; chronically ill or recovering from illness, as in a home setting; or well but

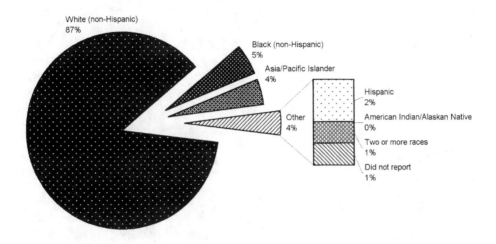

FIGURE 4.2   Distribution of RNs by racial/ethnic background, 2000.

Source: Health Resources and Services Administration (HRSA). (2000). *The Registered Nurse Population National Sample Survey of Registered Nurses.* Rockville, MD: Author.

requiring preventive care, as in a health department or health maintenance organization (HMO) (HRSA, 2000).

The average salary for full-time nurses was $46,782 per year in 2000 (HRSA, 2000). When adjusted for inflation, however, average salaries have been relatively flat since 1992. Salaries varied by geographic area, setting, and position. Nurses with more education had higher average salaries than those with less education.

Advanced Practice Nursing

There were about 196,275 (7.3%) advanced practice RNs in 2000 (HRSA, 2000). There were about 88,186 nurse practitioners, 29,844 nurse anesthetists, and 9,232 nurse midwives. The numbers of all but nurse anesthetists increased from 1996. As discussed earlier, advanced practice nurses practice in a variety of settings. About 89% of NPs were employed in nursing. Legal limitations on such practice vary considerably from state to state. Numerous studies support the position that nurse practitioners provide health care equal in quality to that provided by physicians (Brown & Grimes, 1995), and it costs substantially less to educate a NP than a physician.

Nurse midwives (NMW) provide health care to women. In particular, they provide care to women before, during, and after childbirth (Kovner & Burkhardt, 2001). In 1999, there were more than 5,700 NMWs. The typical NMW was 46 years old, female, Caucasian, and held a master's degree in nursing. Graduate education is not required to become a NMW. Almost

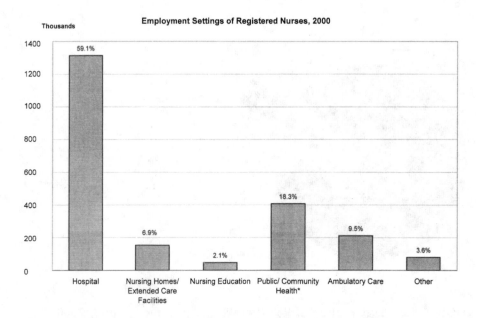

FIGURE 4.3   Employment settings of registered nurses, 2000.

Source: Health Resources and Services Administration. (2001). *The National Sample Survey of Registered Nurses March 2000: Preliminary Findings.* Rockville, MD: Author.

70% of the NMWs provided full-scope clinical midwifery practice including antepartum, intrapartum, and gynecologic care. More than 87% of NMWs attend births in hospitals. The remainder attend births in birthing centers (8.2%) and at home (4.6%) (Kovner & Burkhardt, 2001).

There were about 27,000 Certified Registered Nurse Anesthetists (CRNAs) in 2000. They are advanced practice nurses who provide anesthesia. CRNAs give about 65% of the 26 million anesthetics given to patients in the United States yearly and are the sole anesthesia providers in two thirds of rural hospitals. RNs attend 24–36-month graduate programs to become nurse anesthetists and then must pass a national certification examination (*Nurse Anesthetists at a Glance*, 2000).

State regulations on nurses prescribing pharmaceuticals are inconsistent. In Oregon, NPs can prescribe pharmaceuticals, with no conditions of physician oversight (Safriet, 1992). In some states advanced practice nurses (clinical nurse specialists and NPs) can prescribe without physician collaboration or authorizations, while in other states the NP must have a practice arrangement with a physician, and in some states clinical nurse specialists do not have prescriptive privileges. Some states limit prescriptive authority to central sites, to formularies, or to specific drugs.

Reimbursement continues to be a restriction on practice. Although RNs can bill patients for services, as they have been able to do since RNs performed private duty care in patients' homes in the early part of the 20th century, third-party reimbursement continues to be a problem. Many managed care organizations do not include NPs or NMWs on their primary care panels (Mason, Cohen, O'Donnell, Baxer, & Chase, 1997). This means that these nurses are not eligible for reimbursement for care provided. Medicare reimburses advanced practice nurses for care that is within their scope of practice. In terms of NMWs, Medicaid reimbursement is available in all states; however, services covered varied from state to state (Declercq, Paine, Simmes, & DeJoseph, 1998). HCFA issued a rule in 2001 that defers to state professional practice laws and hospital bylaws to determine which licensed professionals can administer anesthesia. This would allow for more autonomy and direct reimbursement for CRNAs. Physician groups, including the American Medical Association, are vehemently opposed to this regulatory change. As third-party reimbursement expands advanced practice nursing care will expand. As reimbursement decreases, it is likely that care will decrease. While RNs, including NPs, NMWs, and CRNAs, can bill clients directly for care, they cannot be reimbursed for all services by government, insurers, and other third-party payers.

The focus for the 21st century will likely be on the issues of scope of practice, prescriptive authority, and reimbursement. If the United States moves to a system which financial barriers to health care are removed, the use of advanced practice nurses, especially nurse practitioners and nurse-midwives, will likely expand. It remains to be seen what physician reaction will be.

Organized Nursing

The American Nurses Association (ANA) is the national professional organization for nurses. Founded in 1897, its members are not nurses but state or territorial nurses associations. The "tri-level" system is composed of individual nurses who may join local and/or district nurses associations. City or county associations are organized into state associations. Delegates from the state associations meet annually at a national convention to set policy for the ANA.

The ANA also offers voluntary certification exams in a variety of nursing specialty areas, such as community health nursing, mental health nursing, and nursing administration. It serves as a lobbying association for nursing: Its headquarters are in Washington, DC.

Sigma Theta Tau International is the honor society for nursing. An international organization located in St. Louis, its primary purpose is to foster scholarship in nursing. Membership is by election and restricted to those nurses who meet its academic and community service criteria. RNs and LPNs are also organized for collective bargaining by traditional labor unions. Among those with the largest number of nurses is the Services Employees International Union.

In addition to the general organizations described above, nurses belong to numerous specialty groups. The groups tend to have as a focus the specialty area or site of practice for nurses. The first such organization was the American Association of Nurse Anesthetists. Examples of other organizations include the American College of Nurse-Midwives, the National Nurses Society of Addictions, the National Black Nurses Association, and the Society for Nursing History.

MEDICINE

American medicine is undergoing a major transformation. Changes in the health care system are challenging physicians and transforming their traditional role in health care from the dominant, controlling force, to one of many players. The world of solo practice, fee-for-service medicine is rapidly being replaced with group practice, integrated delivery systems, managed care, and capitation. The increased use of nurse practitioners, physician assistants, and other health care professionals is forcing greater collaboration and cooperation. Physicians still play a central role in determining what type of care is provided, admitting patients to health facilities, ordering tests, prescribing medicine, and referrals to therapists, but they must now share the responsibility with other professionals and managed care organizations.

Undergraduate Medical Education

There are two types of medical education: allopathic (MD) and osteopathic (DO). Allopathic medicine is "a system of medicine based on the theory that successful therapy depends on creating a condition antagonistic to or incompatible with the condition to be treated" (Slee & Sell, 1986). Osteopathic medicine "emphasizes a theory that the body can make its own remedies, given normal structural relationships, environmental conditions, and nutrition. It differs from allopathic primarily in its greater attention to body mechanics and manipulative methods in diagnosis and therapy" (Slee's Health Care Teams, 2001). Once educated and trained, allopathic and osteopathic physicians are licensed by each state and have the same scope of practice.

There are 125 allopathic medical schools in the United States. The majority are part of academic medical centers that include tertiary hospitals and medical complexes. These medical schools graduated 15,824 physicians in 2000 (see Table 4.2; "Appendix IA," 2000). In addition, there are 19 osteopathic schools, which graduated 2,193 physicians in 1999 (American Association of Colleges of Osteopathic Medicine [ACOM], 1999). Of the 125 allopathic schools, 74 (59%) are publicly sponsored medical schools. The remainder are privately operated, not-for-profit schools. Medical school, the first formal step in the professional education of physicians, usually requires 4 years following baccalaureate education. The first 2 years are usually didactic (instruction taught in the classroom), and the second 2 years are primarily clinical. Questions have been raised regarding the adequacy and appropriateness of the traditional medical education model and curriculum. Medical schools have been criticized for not encouraging primary care, for overemphasizing high-tech tertiary care, for emphasizing organ systems rather than the whole patient, for not educating more underrepresented minorities, and for not preparing physicians to work in ambulatory settings or in managed care environments.

As a result of these criticisms, there has been a major reassessment of medical school curricula and many schools have modified or are considering modifying the traditional curriculum. For example, many schools have added instruction on alternative/complementary medicine and many have added coursework related to cultural competence (Barzansky, Jonas, & Etzel, 2000). In other cases, schools are beginning clinical training earlier in the education process.

Enrollment

Despite high tuition and a lengthy education, medicine is still a highly sought profession and applicants far exceed available slots. While the total number of applicants to allopathic medical schools has been declining over the past several years, from 46,968 in 1996–1997 to 38,529 in 1999–2000, only 17,445 were accepted in 1999–2000, a ratio of 1 acceptance for every 2.2 applicants (Barzansky et al., 2000).

Allopathic medical school graduations have been relatively stable since 1980, with graduations ranging between 15,300 and 16,300. (The difference from the number accepted reflects the fact that some accepted students do not attend and some students drop out.) As indicated in Table 4.2, however, female graduates have increased, rising from 23.1% of graduates in 1979–1980 to 42.4% in 1999–2000. In 1999–2000, 46% of new medical students were female (Barzansky et al., 2000). This has implications for the health care system, as female physicians have different specialty and practice patterns than male physicians (Forte & Salsberg, 1999).

The Association of American Medical Colleges (AAMC) defines underrepresented minorities as African Americans, Native Americans, Latino/Hispanics from Puerto Rico, and Mexican Americans. They exclude other Latino/Hispanics and Asians. The failure of American medical schools to enroll underrepresented minorities consistent with their representation in the general population has been of concern for many years. These concerns relate to issues of equity, access, and quality of care. It has been documented that underrepresented minority physicians are more likely to serve in underserved communities; serve underserved populations; as well as be more sensitive to cultural and social differences of their race and ethnicity, which can be critical in diagnosis and treatment and patient compliance (Komaromy et al., 1996).

In 1979–1980, 7.1% of allopathic medical school graduates were underrepresented minorities as defined by the AAMC. In 1989–1990, they represented

TABLE 4.2   Allopathic Medical School Enrollment and Demographics

Academic year	Number of applicants	Applicant acceptance ratio	Graduates	Percentage of women graduates	Percentage of underrepresented minority graduates
1979–1980	36,141	2.1	15,113	23.1	7.1
1989–1990	26,915	1.6	15,398	33.9	8.2
1999–2000	38,529	2.2	15,824	42.4	11.7*

Source: Barzansky, B., Jonas, H., & Etzel, S. (2000). Educational Programs in U.S. Medical Schools, 1999–2000. *Journal of the American Medical Association, 284,* Table 4, p. 1116.

8.2% of graduates, and in 1999–2000, 11.7% of medical graduates (in 1999–2000, another 3.1% of the graduates were other Latino/Hispanics not counted in the AAMC definition) (Association of American Medical Colleges, 1997, 1999; Barzansky et al., 2000). This slow progress has been discouraging to the medical education community as in 2000 an estimated 24% of all Americans were African American, Native American, and Latino/Hispanic (U.S. Census Bureau, 2000). This percentage has grown and is expected to continue to increase in future years.

Financing

Because medical schools are part of educational/service enterprises, it is extremely difficult to determine what it actually costs to educate a physician. In 1998–1999, allopathic medical schools reported revenues of $39.7 billion; the major sources of funding were faculty practice plans (34.5%), grants and contracts (30.1%), and hospital support (14.6%) (Krakower, Coble, Williams, & Jones, 2000). This includes patient care services, research, and other related health professions education. By this method of accounting, student tuition accounted for only 3.7% of medical school revenues.

Tuition in private allopathic medical schools went up nearly $10,000 per year in the past decade, rising from an average of $17,794 in 1989–1990 to $27,000 in 1999–2000. Over the same period, tuition in public medical schools nearly doubled, increasing from $5,810 for in-state students to $11,375 (Association of American Medical Colleges, 1999). Scholarship funding did not keep pace with this rise in tuition. The mean debt of graduating medical students increased from $35,621 in 1987 to $80,462 in 1997 (Association of American Medical Colleges, 1997).

Although physicians can anticipate higher than average incomes once they begin practice, the very lengthy period for education and training, with its relatively low salaries, combined with most loans coming due in the second year of post-graduate training, may discourage medical students from choosing primary care, a relatively low-paying group of specialties (Ginzberg, Ostow, & Dutka, 1993).

Graduate Medical Education

To be licensed as a physician and to be recognized by the profession as fully prepared, a physician must complete at least some formal supervised practical clinical experience through graduate medical education (GME), known as residency training. Until the early part of the 20th century, most physicians went directly from medical school to clinical practice. In response to the 1910 Flexner Report, a period of a year or two of internship was established to provide physicians with practical experience (Flexner, 1960, 1910). Following this internship, most physicians practiced as generalists, providing a full range of services to their patients. As medicine has become more complex and the number of physicians has grown, there has been greater specialization and more advanced training. After specialty training, a physician may choose to subspecialize. For example, after training for 3 years in internal medicine, a physician can choose 2 years additional training and subspecialize in cardiology or gastroenterology.

GME is a central determinant of the number and types of physicians available in a region. It is a major source of funding for teaching hospitals, and in many states, it has a major impact on Medicaid costs. The expansion of managed care, growing competition in health care and other developments have brought a series of GME issues to the foreground nationally, in-state capitals, and at teaching hospitals. The federal government and many states are considering legislation related to the financing of GME.

Historically, the vast majority of GME has taken place in large teaching hospitals. These hospitals offer residents an opportunity to see a wide range of patient conditions, and in many cases, these hospitals are where medical schools and their faculty are located. Although the primary purpose of graduate medical education is the education of the resident, residents are also extensively involved in patient care, research, and teaching medical students. The concentration of training in large teaching hospitals has been criticized as resulting in the overuse of high-cost technology and inpatient services (Physician Payment Review Commission, 1993). As services shift to ambulatory settings, there is a growing effort to provide more training outside of hospitals to better prepare physicians for future practice and encourage primary care.

The Growth of Residency Programs and Specialties

In 1999, there were 7,946 allopathic residency programs accredited by the Accreditation Council for Graduate Medical Education (ACGME) ("Appendix II," 2000). The ACGME is a private national body that oversees the accreditation of allopathic residency programs. In each specialty, a Residency Review Committee (RRC) establishes standards and assesses individual residency program performance against those standards. In 1999, there were 581 osteopathic internship and residency programs accredited by the American Osteopathic Association (AACOM, 1999).

In 1999, there were more than 97,989 physicians in training in ACGME accredited allopathic residency programs. This included 22,320 new first-year residents of whom 16,853 were graduates of U.S. and Canadian medical schools; the remaining 5,467 were graduates of foreign medical schools ("Appendix II," Brotherton, 2000). Thus, there were 32% more first-year residents than graduates from U.S. medical schools. There were 3,590 residents in osteopathic training programs (AACOM, 1999). All of these were graduates of U.S. schools.

Women are far more likely to go into those specialties generally considered to be in the realm of primary care. While women made up 38% of all residents in 1999, they constituted 47% of the residents in family practice, 65% in pediatrics, and 67% in obstetrics. On the other hand, they represented only 15% in cardiology and 8% in orthopedic surgery ("Appendix II," Brotherton, 2000).

International Medical Graduates

Graduates of medical schools outside of the U.S. and Canada, referred to as international medical school graduates (IMGs), are eligible to apply for residency training if they pass specific examinations testing medical knowledge and English proficiency, and meet other conditions. Because of the concern with shortages in the 1950s and 1960s, immigration requirements for physicians were reduced. Resident supply problems have existed since that time, however. As noted above, in 1995, the number of new, allopathic residents was nearly one third above the number of U.S. allopathic medical graduates. This gap was filled primarily by IMGs. Numerous groups have recommended that the total number of residency slots in the U.S. be sharply reduced (Consensus statement, 1997, Council on Graduate Medical Education, 1997, Physician Payment Review Commission [PPRC], 1993).

In 1999, 31% of IMGs in training in the United States were on exchange or temporary visas that allowed them to study American medicine but required that they return to their native country (Brotherton, 2000). Many of these physicians have obtained waivers, however, and have been permitted to stay in the United States.

Financing Graduate Medical Education

Historically, generous federal, state, and private insurance reimbursement rates for hospitals, a robust hospital sector, and federal investment in research supported the training of physicians as part of the basic function of academic medical centers and hundreds of other hospitals. Today, these hospitals are facing major challenges because the new competitive marketplace leaves little room for expenditures that are not directly related to patient care.

Embedded in complex hospital reimbursement formulas used by Medicare and most Medicaid programs is support for GME. In federal fiscal year

1998, Medicare provided an estimated $7 billion (Council on Graduate Medical Education, 2000), Medicaid an estimated $2.4 billion dollars (Henderson, 2000), and private payers an estimated $5 billion dollars (Mullan, Rivo, & Politzer, 1993). The total reimbursement in 1993 was estimated to be equal to $184,000 for each resident for each year of training (Mullan et al., 1993). Residents and teaching hospitals are involved in a number of activities, such as research and care for the poor. Despite numerous attempts, there is no consensus on what are the actual or the reasonable costs of training a physician (Salsberg, 1997).

The evolution of the health care system, particularly with increased competition, is leading to major pressures for fundamental changes in the financing of GME. In the long run, it may not be possible to pay for the higher costs of teaching hospitals through generous and hidden reimbursement policies. As pressures continue to mount to constrain costs, those such as from managed care, Medicaid, and Medicare, there is growing pressure to revise the financing of GME.

Physician Supply and Distribution

In 1998, there were approximately 620,000 allopathic physicians involved in patient care in the U.S. (American Medical Association, 2000). As seen in Table 4.3, the majority of these physicians are in office-based practice, which includes solo and group practice, as well as other ambulatory care settings, such as HMOs.

The number of allopathic patient care physicians nearly doubled between 1975 and 1998 (American Medical Association, 2000). As shown in Table 4.4, the physician-to-population ratio increased from 163 patient care physicians per 100,000 people in 1980, to 229 in 1998, or by about 40%.

Geographical Distribution

The supply of physicians is not evenly distributed across the U.S. The majority of physicians are concentrated in urban areas. In 1999, there were nearly 2,800 urban and rural areas that were classified by the federal government as Health Professional Shortage Areas (HPSAs) (http://www.bphc.hrsa.gov/databases/newhpsa/newhpsa.cfm). The lower physician-to-population ratio in most rural areas reflects, in part, the need for a minimum population base required to support a physician specialty practice and to maintain skill levels for certain specialties.

Doubling the total number of U.S. physicians over time has led to some dispersal of physicians to rural areas, but the vast majority of new physicians still locate in urban areas. From 1980 to 1998, the supply of allopathic physicians grew by 289,682 in metropolitan statistical areas, an increase of 75%. During the same period, the number of physicians in nonmetropolitan

TABLE 4.3   Distribution of Allopathic Physicians by Activity in 1998

Activity	Number	Percentage
Patient Care	621,736	79.9
Office-Based Practice	468,788	60.3
Hospital-Based Practice	152,948	19.7
Residents/Fellows	92,992	12.0
Full-Time Staff	59,956	7.7
Other Professional Activity	45,264	5.8
Medical Teaching	10,512	1.4
Administration	16,457	2.1
Research	14,479	1.9
Other	3,816	0.5
Not Classified		
Inactive	69,889	9.0
Address Unknown	938	0.1
Total	777,859	100.0

In 1998 there were approximately 620,000 allopathic physicians involved in patient care. The number of allopathic patient care physicians doubled between 1975 and 1998. The physician-to-patient population ratio increased from 159 patient care physicians per 1000,000 population in 1980 to 227 in 1998, or about 43%.

Source: American Medical Association. (2000). *Physician Characteristics and Distribution in the U.S., 2000–2001 Edition.* Chicago, IL: Department of Physician Data Services, Table 1.1, p. 16.

areas went up 23,745, an increase of 41% (American Medical Association, 2000). Despite the increase in total physician supply, serious access problems still exist in rural areas.

Gender, Ethnicity, and Nationality

One of the most striking recent changes in the physician supply in the U.S. has been the steady growth in the number of female physicians. The percentage of female patient care physicians grew from 7.8% in 1975 to 23.5% in 1998, as seen in Table 4.5. This trend will continue as the number of women entering medical school continues to increase. Because most physicians practice for 30 to 40 years, however, and only a small percentage leave or enter practice each year, it takes many years to significantly modify the composition of the physician workforce (Kindig & Libby, 1996). The growth in the number of IMGs has been steady, although far less dramatic than for women. This growth is likely to continue for several years, given the current number of IMGs in training.

Specialty Distribution

Table 4.5 presents the number of allopathic physicians in selected specialties from 1975 to 1998. Although in 1998 there were more than 267,000

TABLE 4.4   Allopathic Patient Care Physicians. Total, Total to Population Ration, Female, and IMGs

Year	Total patient care physicians	Physician to population ratio	Female physicians		IMGs	
			Number	Percentage	Number	Percentage
1975	311,937	142	224,345	7.8	61,416	19.7
1980	376,512	163	39,969	10.6	72,935	19.4
1985	448,820	185	64,424	14.4	95,362	21.2
1990	503,870	200	86,376	17.1	106,515	21.1
1995	582,131	222	126,583	21.7	136,812	23.5
1998	621,736	229	146,297	23.5	149,792	24.1

The percentage of female patient care physicians grew from 7.8% in 1975 to 23.2% in 1995.

Source: American Medical Association. (2000). *Physician Characteristics and Distribution in the U.S., 2000–2001 Edition.* Chicago IL: Department of Physician Data Services, Tables 5.9, 5.13, 5.16.

physicians in the four specialties generally considered to comprise primary care (internal medicine, family practice, pediatrics, and general practice), nonprimary care physicians comprised two thirds of all practicing physicians. This distribution is significantly different from most other countries, such as Canada, Great Britain, and Germany, where more than 50% of physicians are in primary care specialties (PPRC, 1993).

Through the 1980s and early 1990s, the number of physicians in nonprimary care specialties grew far more rapidly than those in primary care specialties. In recent years, there has been a resurgence of interest in primary care specialties and a higher percentage of new physicians have selected primary care. Some of this increase in interest may reflect the increase in managed care and its emphasis on primary care and prevention. It now appears, however, that interest by U.S. medical school graduates in primary care specialties may have peaked in 1999 (Association of American Medical Colleges, 2000). It is not clear whether the interest in primary care will level off at its current level or continue to decline again.

Physician Income

Figure 4.4 indicates the median net income after expenses but before taxes for some of the major specialties in 1997. Of particular interest is the much lower level of net income for primary care physicians. Physicians are among the highest paid professionals in the U.S., and their income through the 1980s grew faster than that of any other profession (Pope & Schneider, 1992). After that, market forces may have affected the income of physicians. In 1994, average physician income declined almost 4% from the prior year (Simon & Born, 1996). This was the first time since the AMA

TABLE 4.5   Allopathic Physicians by Specialty 1975, 1985, 1995, and 1998

Specialty	1975	1985	1995	1998	Percentage change (1985–1998)
Primary Care	131,080	191,939	242,000	267,897	39.6
Family Practice	12,183	40,021	59,345	66,900	67.2
General Practice	42,374	27,030	16,867	16,385	−39.4
Internal Medicine	54,331	88,862	115,168	127,574	43.6
Pediatrics	22,192	36,026	50,620	57,038	58.3
Obstetrics/Gynecology	21,731	30,867	37,652	39,512	28.0
Medicine Subspecialities	9,314	19,141	28,549	29,526	54.3
Cardiology	6,933	13,224	18,998	19,623	48.4
Gastroenterology	2,381	5,917	9,551	9,903	67.4
General Surgery	31,562	38,169	37,569	40,448	6.0
Surgery Subspecialties	34,920	48,150	58,473	60,636	25.9
Ophthalmology	11,129	14,881	17,464	18,035	21.2
Orthopedic Surgery	11,379	17,166	22,037	23,178	35.0
Otolaryngology	5,745	7,267	9,086	9,255	27.4
Urology	6,667	8,836	9,886	10,168	15.1
Facility-Based Specialties	26,791	48,383	64,782	68,042	40.6
Emergency Medicine	0	11,283	19,112	21,233	88.2
Pathology	11,720	15,456	17,824	18,046	16.8
Radiology	15,071	21,644	27,846	28,763	32.9
Psychiatry	23,922	32,355	38,098	39,494	22.4
Other Specialties	21,653	36,379	52,813	55,247	51.9
Anesthesiology	12,861	22,021	32,853	33,947	54.2
Dermatology	4,661	6,582	8,563	9,239	40.4
Neurology	4,131	7,776	11,397	12,061	55.1
Total physicians	393,742	552,716	720,325	777,859	40.7

Although in 1998 there were 267,897 physicians in primary care, nonprimary care physicians comprised nearly two thirds of all practicing physicians.

Source: American Medical Association. (2000). *Physician Characteristics and Distribution in the U.S. 2000–2001 Edition.* Chicago, IL: Department of Physician Data Services, Table 5.2.

collected this data that income had declined. Physician incomes again rose, however: nationally between 1995 and 1997, their average income rose 2% (American Medical Association, 1997; 1999b); and new physicians completing training in New York State in 1999 had starting incomes 1.3% above those who graduated just 1 year earlier (Center for Health Workforce Studies, 2000).

Physician Assistants

Physician Assistants (PAs) work under the direct supervision of physicians. While regulation of PAs varies from state to state, supervision does not mean on-site supervision. In most states the amount of delegation to a PA is a decision between the physician and the PA.

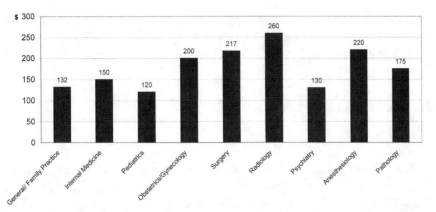

FIGURE 4.4   Median physician net income (in thousands of dollars) after expenses before taxes, by specialty, 1997.

Source: American Medical Association. (1999b). *Physician Socioeconomic Statistics, 1999–2000 Edition.* Chicago, IL: Center for Health Policy Research, p. 86.

Both demand and supply of PAs have been increasing rapidly. PAs can expand access to primary care and improve physician productivity, both of which are promoted by the expansion of managed care; PAs can substitute for physicians in hospitals; and in some areas, PAs may replace residents in training.

Physician Assistant Education

Physician Assistant is a relatively new profession. The first PA educational program was established by Duke University Medical Center in 1965, in part to allow an opportunity for medics who had gained clinical experience in the Vietnam War to practice in the health care system. In 1971, with the passage of the Comprehensive Health Manpower Act, federal financial support became available and contributed to the rapid expansion of programs. In 1998, 3,712 PAs graduated from 93 accredited PA programs (American Academy of Physician Assistants, 1999). PA programs are located in a number of academic settings and offer a variety of credentials. Most programs are 24 months in length.

Practicing Physician Assistants

In 1998, there were about 34,192 PAs practicing in the U.S. PAs work in a wide variety of specialties. The largest number of PAs (13,677) works in family practice (40%). The second largest concentration, with 5,470 PAs, is surgery (16%). As the effectiveness and efficacy of PAs is demonstrated in more and more specialty areas, PAs may be drawn away from primary care specialties. The PA to population ratio varies widely between states from 391 per 100,000 population in Alaska, to 15.9 per 100,000 population in Mississippi. PAs work in a wide array of practice settings, and in 1998, the average of total annual income for full-time clinically practicing PAs was $64,791 (American Academy of Physician Assistants, 1999).

OTHER HEALTH WORKERS

Other Doctors

In addition to physicians, there are a variety of other health professionals educated in graduate programs beyond the baccalaureate that use the title "doctor." These doctors tend to specialize in specific areas of the body. Each specialty has its own body of knowledge, professional association, and educational requirements.

Dentists

In 1998, there were approximately 155,500 practicing Doctors of Dental Science (DDSs). The number of dentists in the United States declined 5% between 1991 and 1998, while the population of the country grew by 7%, resulting in a 12% decline in dentists per capita (American Dental Association, 1998; U.S. Census Bureau, 2000). While 12% of dentists in practice in 1998 were female, 37% of dental school graduates in 1996–1997 were female (American Dental Association, 1998; U.S. Department of Education, November, 1999). Dentistry has far fewer graduate training opportunities than medicine and there are more dental school graduates who would like advanced training than there are opportunities (American Dental Association, 1997).

Podiatrists

Podiatrists diagnose, treat, and prevent abnormal foot conditions. Educated at one of the seven podiatric medicine schools in the U.S., they perform surgery, and prescribe and administer pharmaceuticals. Licensed by individual states, they deliver a wide range of medical and surgical services. There were about 13,000 practitioners in 1997 (American Podiatric Medical Association, 1997; U.S. Department of Health and Human Services, 1992).

Chiropractors

These doctors treat problems of the body's structural and neurological systems. Chiropractors are educated in 4-year programs, that follow at least 2 years of undergraduate education. There are 17 chiropractic schools; the Council on Chiropractic Education (CCE) has accredited 14 (U.S. Department of Health and Human Services, 1992). Their graduates are eligible for licensure in all 50 states. In 1996, there were approximately 58,000 licensed chiropractors (Federation of Chiropractic Licensing Boards, 1999).

Optometrists

Optometrists are licensed to diagnose and provide selective eye treatment. In some states, they are licensed to prescribe a limited range of pharmaceuticals. There were about 24,000 practicing optometrists in the U.S. in 1998 (U.S. Bureau of Labor Statistics, 2000a). Educated at one of the 16 schools of optometry, students have 4 years of professional training following undergraduate school. Optometrists, while having far less formal education than ophthalmologists (physicians with residency training in ophthalmology), provide many of the same services as these physicians, usually at a lower cost. As state government considers increasing the scope of practice of optometrists, and as managed care expands, there has been conflict about the overlapping roles of optometrists and ophthalmologists.

Allied Health Personnel

The Committee on Allied Health Education and Accreditation, of the American Medical Association, which oversees nearly 3,000 educational programs, defines allied health as ". . . a large cluster of health care related professions and personnel whose functions include assisting, facilitating, or complementing the work of physicians and other specialists in the health care system, and who choose to be identified as allied health personnel" (U.S. Department of Health and Human Services, 1992, p. 177). Although this is a general definition, it allows for occupations to be added and subtracted as the health care system evolves.

Allied health occupations are among the fastest growing in health care. The number of allied health professionals is difficult to estimate and depends on the definition of allied health. The U.S. Department of Health and Human Services and the Bureau of Health Professions estimate that there were approximately 1.8 million allied health personnel in the U.S. in 1990 (U.S. Department of Health and Human Services, 1992). Unlike medicine, women dominate most of the allied health professions, representing between 75% and 95% of most of the occupations.

For some allied health professions (physical therapists) all states require licensure, while for others (occupational therapy) only some states require licensure. Other occupations usually included under the allied health rubric are clinical laboratory personnel and speech-language pathology and audiology personnel. In addition to physicians, nurses, and allied health personnel, there are a variety of other health care practitioners. Space does not permit a thorough discussion of each of these workers, but several examples will be given.

Pharmacists

Pharmacists have traditionally prepared pharmaceutical prescriptions; however, their role has expanded to include providing information to patients about pharmaceuticals and drug interactions. All states require pharmacists to be licensed. Pharmacists are educated in 5-year Bachelor of Science programs or 6-year Pharm D. programs. In 1995, there were 75 colleges of pharmacy, with only 25 offering just the BS degree. Pharmacists can specialize by obtaining advanced degrees in pharmacy and through residency programs. Pharmacy technicians assist pharmacists with activities not requiring the judgement of a pharmacist (U.S. Bureau of Labor Statistics, 1997).

Public Health Personnel

Public health personnel include a variety of health workers. Whereas most health practitioners work with individual patients, public health workers are concerned with the health of entire communities and population groups. Many work in state and local health departments. There are approximately 448,254 public health workers (Gebbie, 2000). Of these, a substantial proportion were educated in a specific clinical discipline, such as nursing, medicine, or other professions discussed in this chapter. Some public health professionals are graduates of the nation's 24 accredited Schools of Public Health (U.S. Department of Health and Human Services, 1992). Their graduates are prepared in such areas as epidemiology, nutrition, health education, environmental health, health administration, and health policy. Other schools also prepare students in these areas.

Midwives

In addition to nurse-midwives, a few states have laws that allow direct entry into midwifery practice, without any nursing education, but with a multiyear academic program. People attend a midwifery program and then are eligible for certification by the American College of Nurse-Midwives and licensure in the state. In addition to these midwives are so called "lay midwives," who have no formal academic training and are not eligible for licensure, but practice midwifery.

Alternative Healers

Alternative healers include naturopaths and practitioners of acupuncture and oriental medicine. Several states now license these alternative healers.

ISSUES

The rapid changes in health care in the U.S. present both a crisis and an opportunity in terms of the health care workforce. There are many issues that remain to be resolved during the 21st century. Among the issues are the following: (a) accountability of the professions, (b) duplication and coordination among the professions, (c) assuring an adequate supply of physicians, and (d) assuring an adequate supply of nurses.

The Accountability of the Professions

Historically, the nation has relied heavily on licensure, accreditation, and certification of health professionals to assure that health care was of high quality. But as the health care system has become more internally competitive and consumers demand improved outcomes, the health care system's efforts to improve quality have expanded significantly. They are reviewed in depth in chapter 14. This section briefly reviews the role of professionalism and individual certification in assuring quality. As managed care expands, it is likely that there will be numerous skirmishes among professionals, government, and managed care organizations as to who should determine who is qualified to perform what activities and who should monitor the quality of care. Freidson (1973) stated that the autonomy of medicine is a characteristic of a profession:

> First, the claim is that there is such an unusual degree of skill and knowledge involved in professional work that nonprofessionals are not equipped to evaluate or regulate it. Second, it is claimed that professionals are responsible—that they may be trusted to work conscientiously without supervision. Third, the claim is that the profession itself may be trusted to undertake the proper regulatory action on those rare occasions when an individual does not perform his work competently or ethically. (p. 137)

Health professional licensure is the government's primary method of assuring qualified professionals. Most health professions are licensed by states. Licensure requires graduation from an approved school, passage of an examination, and, in certain cases, a minimum period of practical experience. In addition to formal licensure, government also exerts considerable control over the practice of health professionals through requirements for and monitoring of performance under Medicaid and Medicare. Government also impacts on practitioners through its regulation of health facilities, such as hospitals that provide care.

Another way to promote quality is through certification and accreditation. Beyond licensure, physicians can be certified for specialty practice in medicine and nurses can be certified for specialty practice in nursing. Each medical specialty establishes standards for physicians seeking to be board certified. This includes, at a minimum, satisfactory completion of an accredited residency program and passage of an exam. It may also include several years of practice and completion of a minimum number of specific procedures. In a few specialties, such as family practice, a physician must periodically pass an exam or demonstrate continuing competency. Board certification provides professional recognition within a specialty and sets minimum qualifications for practice as a board-certified physician. This is an important example of the self-regulation of the medical profession by physicians. Likewise, RNs can be certified for specialty practice.

Yet another approach to promoting high quality of care is through the regulation of health facilities, including requiring that they monitor the professionals who practice in their facility. For example, the Joint Commission on Accreditation of Health Care Organizations (JCAHO) requires that hospitals and other facilities monitor health professionals who practice in their facilities. The JCAHO requires hospitals to set criteria for staff privileges. For example, the hospital's medical bylaws may state that only "board eligible" or "board certified" surgeons may conduct surgery. They may further state that only physicians with certain training or experience, as evaluated by the hospital's medical board, may perform certain complex procedures. In this way, although all physicians in the same state may have the same license, physicians are restricted by health facilities in the types of care they can provide. Unlike licensure, which is usually for life, health facilities are expected to monitor performance on an ongoing basis. Nevertheless, as indicated in chapter 14, the public's concern with quality is likely to go well beyond relying on the profession to regulate itself.

Medical Errors

Medical errors and patient safety gained increasing attention in the early part of the 21st century. In part the interest was fueled by the Institute of Medicine's (IOM) report on medical errors (Kohn, Corrigan, & Donaldson Molla, 2000). In their report the IOM used Reason's definition of error, "An error is defined as the failure of a planned action to be completed as intended (i.e., error of execution) or the use of a wrong plan to achieve an aim (i.e., error of planning)" (Reason, 1990, p. 9).

The concern about medical errors results from the apparently large number of them that are thought to result in adverse patient events (Chassin, 1998; Declercq et al., 1998; Keepnews, 1998). Chassin (1998) suggests that the health care industry build on work in other industries, such as aviation and manufacturing, to achieve a six sigma level of quality, which is fewer than 3.4 defects or errors per million events (e.g., surgical procedures).

The health care industry historically has used the "name, blame, and shame" approach to identify the cause of errors. In that approach one or more individual providers are named as responsible for the error. Those providers are then blamed, often in court, in terms of a malpractice lawsuit, and then shamed, sometimes by losing their job. At other times the perpetrator is publicly shamed, perhaps by a reprimand by a supervisor or suspension of a license to practice a profession. In those industries that have successfully decreased errors the approach has been to analyze systems rather than blame individuals. Anesthesia is one area of medicine that has had enormous success in decreasing errors, reducing its error rate dramatically.

As more research becomes available about approaches to decreasing errors, many health professionals are devoting time and effort to reducing mistakes. Approaches include the use of engineering or technology. For example, having physicians enter medication orders directly into a computer can decrease transcription errors.

Duplication and Coordination Among the Professions

There is a growing recognition throughout the health care field that optimal care requires extensive collaboration among health care personnel, including doctors, nurses, physical therapists, pharmacists, aides, and even nontraditional caregivers, like acupuncturists and massage therapists. In their training and education programs, an increasing number of health professions are trying to incorporate "interdisciplinary" or "multidisciplinary" aspects into the curriculum in recognition that professionals will need to work with other personnel in the caregiving world. This development also recognizes the complexity and many facets of healing, and that a team can be more effective than any profession working alone.

Despite this move towards collaboration, there is also likely to be greater competition between and among professions. Attractive professional careers, good incomes, professional autonomy, and/or an opportunity to help others have helped to fuel an increasing supply of health professionals. When combined with pressures from purchasers and insurers to constrain costs, this growing supply is likely to lead to conflicts, which are likely to be greatest where different professions or subgroups provide similar or overlapping services. For example, this would include the following:

1. Advanced practice nurses, including nurse practitioners, are likely to increasingly compete with physicians. The conflict is expected to be especially strong between those physicians and nurses who provide primary care because of the overlap in the nature of the care they provide.

2. Many primary care physicians argue that specialists do not have the skills or orientation to provide primary care. At the same time, some specialists, having gone through a generalist education before subspecializing, believe they are qualified to provide primary care. For example, a gastroenterologist completes an internal medicine residency program before subspecializing.

3. Some primary care physicians may also provide services that the specialist believes only the specialist should provide. For example, primary care physicians can treat many patients with allergies, especially with the development of new medications, but a physician trained in the specialty of allergy and immunology is best qualified to treat complex cases; however, there may be differences in how each would define which cases should be referred to the specialist.

4. Psychiatrists, psychologists, and social workers have scopes of practice that overlap and each may believe they are the best qualified to treat certain types of patients.

In addition to competition among professionals, there will be increased competition between professionals and assistive personnel because of the overlap in the care they provide. Examples include physical therapy assistants and physical therapists, and unlicensed assistive personnel and registered nurses. Although most people would agree that it is clear that for some activities, such as making a patient bed, an unlicensed person can provide the same quality of care as registered nurses, for other activities, such as starting an intravenous line, the quality comparison is less clear and research evidence sparse. The competition between different professions and occupations can spill over to the legislative and/or regulatory arena where different groups may argue for or against an expansion of the scope of practice for a particular occupation or profession. Reimbursement policies for Medicaid and/or private insurance companies can be another battleground since it can have a major impact on the economic health of an occupation or profession. Regrettably, there are few studies of the impact on outcomes of permitting different occupations to perform specific activities. Thus, the debates between professions are often publicity campaigns rather than substantive policy discussions.

Assuring an Adequate Supply of Physicians

One of the more hotly debated recent health workforce policy issues has been physician workforce planning. At the core of the debate is how to encourage the production of a physician workforce that can best meet the health needs of the nation. The debate has been fueled by a lack of agreement as to whether the current and projected supply is adequate to meet the nation's needs, as well as whether the marketplace, without specific government interventions, will produce the appropriate role, number, mix and distribution of physicians. The National Council on Graduate Medical Education (COGME) has been in the forefront of efforts to encourage a physician supply and distribution better able to meet the medical needs of the nation. The Council, by statute, advises the Department of Health and Human Services and the Congress on physician workforce issues.

Since about 1980, the national policy goal has been to limit the growth in the supply of physicians, in part, in response to an expected surplus of physicians. The supply of physicians has been growing steadily since the 1950s. In the 1990s, simultaneous with the growth in supply, managed care was expanding rapidly. A number of studies found that HMOs, which were the model for managed care, used less physician resources than the fee-for-service system. For example, several studies have found HMO staffing to range from 120 to 138 per 100,000 (Politzer, Gamliel, Cultice, Bazell, Rivo, & Mullan, 1996). The COGME estimated that there is generally a need for between 145 and 185 physicians per 100,000 population (Council on Graduate Medical Education, 1996). This compares to the national average in 1998 of nearly 200 physicians per 100,000 population. (Dill, Salsberg, Wing, Rizzo, Krohl, Fields, et al., 2000). There were signs, such as the drop in physician incomes (Simon & Born, 1996), that the surplus was beginning to be felt by practicing physicians.

There are some benefits of a surplus: it may drive prices down; it may make it easier to get physicians to underserved areas; and it may make physicians more sensitive to patients. On the other hand, physicians could generate their own demand by ordering tests and revisits. In a surplus, physicians may not have sufficient volume to maintain their skills; society and individual physicians will have wasted a large investment; and there is little public benefit for the investment (Wennberg, Goodman, Nease, & Keller, 1993).

Another reason for concern has been the high level of public financing for GME. Medicare and Medicaid provided an estimated $10 billion in 2000 (Council on Graduate Medical Education, 2000). If there is a physician surplus, it is hard to justify massive public support. In 1997, the Balanced Budget Act did reduce the amount of Medicare funding for GME; however, other efforts to decrease GME financing have been blocked by concerns with the impact on teaching hospitals and care for the poor in inner cities that are served by residents (Iglehart, 1996).

Although the nation's physician supply is still growing, there is some concern now emerging that the nation may face a shortage in the next decade. This reflects several factors, including the aging of the baby boom generation, the growing supply of female physicians (who work fewer hours over the course of their professional life than males), the evolution of managed care to a less restrictive form than expected, the general growth in the nation's population, and the aging of the nation's physician workforce (Council on Graduate Medical Education, 1999; Cooper, 2000; Cooper, McKee, Lard, & Getzer, 2001). There have even been calls to increase the number of medical school slots in America (Mullen, 1999).

Assuring an Adequate Supply of Nurses

Cyclical shortages and surpluses of registered nurses have occurred during the 20th century. This reflects a number of factors, including a lag in response of prospective students and the educational system to changes in demand. In response to severe shortages in the late 1980s, salaries for registered nurses rose significantly; these higher salaries led to an increase in the numbers of RNs being educated in the early 1990s. In addition, in response to higher RN salaries and shortages, as well as pressures to reduce costs from managed care, health facilities increasingly sought ways to substitute lower-cost personnel for RNs. Throughout the late 1990s, enrollment in nursing programs fell.

By the beginning of the 21st century, there were again RN shortages (Brewer & Kovner, 2001). In previous shortage periods some health care organizations have reorganized to decrease the demand for nurses. Approaches included case management, work redesign, and the use of technology. Case management had as its goal the prudent use of health resources. Redesign interventions varied from increased use of assistive personnel and health care teams, to rethinking the components of care required by patients during an episode of illness. An example of a technology intervention was the use of computerized information systems to improve communication and decrease paperwork.

Responses to the shortage of the early 21st century included similar approaches to those used in the past; however, there is some concern that as this latest shortage may be different than previous ones. There is concern that as the RN workforce ages (the average age of RNs is mid-40s), shortage periods will become more common and more severe. With a full economy and the growing business aspects of health care, there have been growing opportunities for nurses not involving direct patient care. In addition, the physical demands of the job may lead some of the most experienced nurses to leave health facilities.

KEEPING CURRENT ABOUT THE HEALTH WORKFORCE

Although we used the latest available data at the time of publication of this book, it is clear that some of the data may appear outdated. In some cases, the data are not outdated; it is the most recent information available. In other cases, more recent data have appeared since publication. We therefore include a list of sources that provide recent data about the health workforce:

U.S. Department of Health and Human Services:
   Health Resources Services Administration (www.hrsa.gov)
   Health Care Financing Administration (www.hcfa.gov) (http://bhpr. hrsa.gov/healthworkforce/)
American Academy of Physician Assistants (www.aapa.org)
American Dental Association (www.ada.org)
American Medical Association (www.ama-assn.org)
American Nurses Association (www.ana.org)
American Osteopathic Association (www.am-osteo-assn.org)
American Physical Therapy Association (www.apta.org)
National Center for Health Statistics (www.cdc.gov/nchs/)
National Council of State Boards of Nursing (http://www.ncsbn.org)
New York State (http://chws.albany.edu/)
U.S. Department of Commerce:
   U.S. Census Bureau (www.census.gov)
U.S. Department of Labor:
   Bureau of Labor Statistics (www.bls.gov)

CONCLUSIONS

The rapid changes in the health care delivery system will undoubtedly lead to changes in the roles and relationships of health professionals. Managed care and managed competition will require greater collaboration among health professionals. It will also mean greater supervision and management of health professionals by nonhealth professionals. Some health professionals may resist this inevitable oversight as an intrusion on their professionalism. New relationships and even a new definition of professionalism may need to be developed.

The provision of health care in the early 21st century will require the cooperation and coordination of the many health workers currently providing health care, and those who will be educated in these health careers in the future, and will likely include health care workers educated in new careers. There are large areas of overlap in the care provided by health professionals. Physicians, nurses, and physical therapists all work with patients in performing range of motion exercises. Physicians, nurses, and pharmacists all teach patients about medications and their side effects. Nurses and respiratory therapists teach and supervise patients to deep breathe following surgery. It is not surprising that patients in hospitals complain because they cannot tell who is who—everyone is wearing a white uniform or lab coat; or more recently, many health care workers are wearing street clothes.

Most health care professionals today are educated in their own professional schools, in health facilities, and divisions of colleges and universities. Most health professionals currently do not take any courses together, nor do many even share the same faculty. In many cases, students in a variety of professions receive their clinical training in the same institutions; however, there is rarely any shared clinical teaching or learning. To provide effective care in the future, health care professionals should share much of their initial academic health experiences. If most health professionals take pathophysiology, why shouldn't they take it together? Others suggest that there should be a core curriculum for health professionals, with specialization into physical therapy, respiratory therapy, or imaging occurring at the upper division in the undergraduate curriculum.

It seems clear that as health care moves from the hospital to the community, even more coordination of patient care and cooperation among health providers will be required. It is also likely that any one of a variety of health professionals may be the primary caregiver or coordinator and this will vary depending on the health problems of the clients.

CASE STUDY

The State Hospital Review and Planning Council (SHRPC) in New York has responsibility for codes for hospitals and nursing homes in New York. Committees make many decisions with recommendations to the full council. The federal government requires a 75-hour training course for all nurses' aides who work in nursing homes that receive Medicaid and Medicare funding. The nursing home advocacy group in the state has provided you with the following information: Massage therapists must have 1,000 hours of training, barbers 1,500 hours, and manicurists 400 hours to obtain a license. A recent government report demonstrates that those nursing homes with lower staffing levels have higher rates of citations for poor care. Another report states that nursing homes with higher staffing levels have fewer adverse patient events. The advocacy group urges the committee to set the state standards for required hours of training for nurses' aides at 150 hours rather than the 75 hours that the federal government requires.

Nursing home owners say that the federal government knows what it's doing and that nursing homes in the state should just have to meet federal standards. Nursing home owners say that they are already strapped for money because of the state's low reimbursement rates for Medicaid patients in nursing homes. Raising the hours of training would cost them money because they would have to pay for the training and give staff time off from work to attend training. Secondly they say that it is already very difficult to find nurses' aides to work in nursing homes. The average vacancy rate in nursing homes in the state is 15%. They say that requiring more hours of training would make it more difficult to hire staff.

You are a member of the Code Committee of the SHRPC. The governor of New York has said that his goal is to decrease state regulation and not increase the state budget. The governor appoints members of the SHRPC and your term is up in 1 year and you can be appointed to a second term. Staff from the Health Department have proposed that required training be increased to 100 hours, and have provided a very detailed curriculum. What would you do?

DISCUSSION QUESTIONS

1. What role should the federal government have in assuring an adequate supply of health professionals? State government?
2. Some people have proposed that institutions and/or organizations should be able to decide what health professionals should be able to do rather than state boards of licensure. Discuss pros and cons.
3. How should health professional education be funded?
4. What role should professional associations have in assuring that their professional members and nonmembers provide safe care?
5. Discuss the pros and cons of interstate licensure compacts.
6. What responsibility do individual practitioners have for medical errors?

7. Should the federal government set mandatory staffing levels for health workers in the organizations for which the government (e.g., HCFA) pays for care? Why?

REFERENCES

American Academy of Physician Assistants (1999). *Physician assistants: Statistics and trends, 1991–1998.* Alexandria, VA: Author. Division of Research and Data Services.

American Association of Colleges of Osteopathic Medicine (AACOM). (1999, August). *AACOM/AOHA Graduate Medical Education Survey, 1998–1999 academic year.* Chevy Chase: MD: Author.

American Association of Colleges of Nursing. (2000). *1999–2000 Enrollment and graduations in baccalaureate and graduate programs in nursing.* Washington, DC.

American Dental Association. (1997). *A dental education and career information fact sheet* [on-line]. Available: http://www.ada.org/prac/careers/fs-dent.html>.

American Dental Association. (1998). 1998 Distribution of dentists in the United States by region and state. *The survey of dental practitioners.* Chicago: ADA survey center.

American Medical Association. (1997). *Socioeconomic characteristics of medical practice, 1997.* Chicago, IL: Center for Health Policy Research.

American Medical Association. (1999). *Physician socioeconomic statistics, 1999–2000 edition.* Chicago, IL: Center for Health Policy Research.

American Medical Association. (2000). *Physician characteristics and distribution in the U.S., 2000–2001 Edition.* Chicago, IL: Department of Physician Data Services.

American Nurses Association. (1995). *Nursing social policy statement.* Washington, DC: Author.

American Podiatric Medical Association. (1997). *Podiatric medicine: The physician, the profession, the practice,* [on-line]. Available: http://www.apma.org/podit.html.

Anastas, L. (1984). *Your career in nursing.* New York: National League for Nursing.

Appendix IA, (2000, September 6). *Journal of the American Medical Association 284,* 1154–1157.

Appendix II, Tables 1, 3, 4, and 6, (2000, September 6). *Journal of the American Medical Association, 284,* 1159–1166. Graduate Medical.

Association of American Medical Colleges. (1997, January). *AAMC data book statistical information related to medical education.* Washington DC: Association of American Medical Colleges.

Association of American Medical Colleges. (2000, March 16). *Report of the National Resident Matching Program* [on-line]. Available: http.aamc.org/nrmp.

Association of American Medical Colleges. (1999). *Tuition and student fees, first-year medical school students, 1999–2000.* Table 1 [on-line] http://www.aamc.org/findinfo/infores/ datarsc/tuitfees/992000/tab1.htm.

Barzansky, B., Jonas, H., & Etzel, S. (1996). Educational programs in U.S. medical schools, 1999–2000. *Journal of the American Medical Association, 284,* 1114–1120.

Berliner, H. S., & Kovner, C. T. *The supply and demand for health workers in New York City: 1995–1997.* New York: New York State Department of Health.

Brotherton, S. E., Simon, F. A., & Tomany, S. C. (2000). U.S. graduate medical education, 1999–2000. *Journal of the American Medical Association, 284,* 1121–1126.

Brewer, C., & Kovner, C. (2001). Is there another nursing shortage? What the data
tell us. *Nursing Outlook, 49*(1), 20–26.

Brown, S. L., & Grimes, D. (1995). A meta-analysis of nurse practitioners and
nurse midwives in primary care. *Nursing Research, 44*(6), 332–339.

Bullough, N. (1975). Barriers to the nurse practitioner movement: Problem of
women in a women's field. *International Journal of Health Sciences, 5,* 225.

Center for Health Workforce Studies and New Century Concepts. (2000, March).
Residency training outcomes by specialty in 1999 for New York state. New
York: Author.

Chassin, M. R. (1998). Is health care ready for six sigma quality? *A Journal of
Public Health and Health Care Policy, 76*(4), 1–16.

Cooper, R. A. (2000, September). *Evaluation of specialty physician workforce
methodologies.* Rockville, MD: U.S. Department of Health and Human
Services, Health Resources and Services Administration.

Cooper, R. A., McKee, H. J., Lard, P., & Geten, T. E. (2001). *Economic and demographic trends affecting physician supply and utilization signal on impending
physician shortage.* (Manuscript submitted for publication.)

Consensus Statement on Physician Workforce (1997, February 28). Association of
American Medical Colleges, American Association of Colleges of Osteopathic
Medicine, American Medical Association, American Osteopathic Association,
Association of Academic Health Centers, National Medical Associations.

Council on Graduate Medical Education. (1996). *Patient care physician supply and
requirements: Testing COGME recommendations. Eight report,* DHHD Pub.
NO. HRSAP-P-DM95-3). Rockville, MD: Bureau of Health Professions,
Health Resources and Services Administration.

Council on Graduate Medical Education. (1997). *1997 recommendations to the
congress and the Secretary of Health and Human Services on graduate medical education payment reform.* Rockville, MD: U.S. Department of Health
and Human Services.

Council on Graduate Medical Education. (2000). *Fifteenth report—COGME
physician workforce policies: Recent developments and remaining challenges
in meeting national goals.* Rockville, MD: U.S. Department of Health and
Human Services, Health Resources Services and Administration.

Council of Graduate Medical Education. (2000). *Fifteenth report: Financing med-
ical education in a changing health care environment.* Rockville, MD: U.S.
Department of Health and Human Services, Health Resources and Services
Administration.

Declercq, E. R., Paine, L. L., Simmes, D. R., & DeJoseph, J. F. (1998). State regulation, payment policies, and nurse-midwife services. *Health Affairs, 17*(2),
190–200.

Dill, M., Salsberg, E., Wing, P., Rizzo, A., Krohl, D., Fields, A., Moore, J., Tsao,
H., Marzan, G., Myers, V., Acoma, C., Beaulieu, M., Szczepkowski, C., Forte,
G., Dionne, M., Ayers, M., & Otto, L. (2000). *HRSA state health workforce
profiles.* Rockville, MD: U.S. Department of Health and Human Services,
Health Resources and Services Administration, Bureau of Health Professions,
National Center for Health Workforce Information and Analysis.
Directory of Accredited Nursing Programs. (2000). Available: http://www.
NLNAC.org/Directorymainpl.htm.

Fawcett, L. (1989). *Analysis and evaluation of conceptual models of nursing* (2nd ed.). Philadelphia: F. A. Davis.

Federation of Chiropractic Licensing Boards. (1999). *Official directory, chiropractic licensure and practice statistics 1994–1998.* Greeley, CO: Author.

Flexner, A. (1960). *Medical education in the United States and Canada.* Washington, DC: Science and Health Publications. (Original work published 1910).

Forte, G., & Salsberg, E. (September, 1999). Women in medicine in New York state: Preliminary findings from the 1997–2000 New York state physician re-registration survey. *News of New York* (Newsletter of the Medical Society of the State of New York), *54*(9), 7, 14.

Freidson, E. (1973). *Profession of medicine.* New York: Dodd, Mead & Company.

Gebbie, K. M. (2000). Preparing currently employed public health nurses for changes in the health system. *American Journal of Public Health, 90,* 722–727.

Ginzberg E., Ostow, M., & Dutka, A. (1993, March). *The economics of medical education.* New York: Josiah Macy Jr. Foundation.

Health Professional Shortage Areas. (Accessed October 29, 2001). [On-line]. Available: http://www.bphc.hrsa.gov/databases/newhpsa/newhpsa.cfm.

Health Resources and Services Administration (HRSA). (2000). *The Registered Nurse Population National Sample Survey of Registered Nurses.*

Henderson, V. (1966). *The nature of nursing.* New York: Macmillan.

Henderson, T. M. (2000). Medicaid's role in financing graduate medical education. *Health Affairs, 19*(1), 221–229.

Iglehart, J. K. (1996). A health policy report, the struggle to reform Medicare. *The New England Journal of Medicine, 334*(16), 1071–1075.

Keepnews, D. (1998). New opportunities and challenges for APRNs. *The American Journal of Nursing, 98*(1), 62–64.

Kindig, D. A., & Libby, D. L. (1996). A domestic production vs. international immigration. Options for the U.S. physician workforce. *Journal of the American Medical Association, 276*(12), 978–982.

Kohn, L. T., Corrigan, J. M., & Donaldson Molla, S. (Eds.). *To err is human: Building a safer health system.* Washington, DC: National Academy Press.

Komaromy, M., Grumbach, K., Drake, M., Vranizan, K., Lurie, N., Keane, D., & Bindman, A. B. (1996). The role of black and Hispanic physicians in providing health care for underserved populations. *New England Journal of Medicine, 334,* 1305–1310.

Kovner, C., & Burkhardt, P. (2001). Findings from the American College of Nurse-Midwives annual membership survey, 1995–1999. *Journal of Midwifery and Women's Health, 46,* 24–29

Krakower, J. Coble, T., Williams, D., & Jones, R. (2000). Review of U.S. medical school finances, 1998–1999. *Journal of the American Medical Association, 284*(9), 1127–1129.

Mason, D., Cohen, S., O'Donnell, J., Baxter, K., & Chase, A. (1997). Managed care organizations' arrangements with nurse practitioners. *Nursing Economics, 15,* 306–314.

Mullan, F., Rivo, M., & Politzer, R. (1993). Doctors, dollars and determination: Work-force policy. *Health Affairs,* (Suppl.), 138–151.

Mullan, F. (2000). The case for more U.S. medical students. *New England Journal of Medicine, 343,* 213–217.

New York Education Law, Article 139, § 6902, (1989).

Nurse Anesthetists at a Glance. (2000). Available: http://www.AANA.com/CRNA/ataglance.asp.

Nursing Regulation: Examination Pass, Rates and Licensure Statistics. (2000). Available: http://www.ncsbn.org/public/regulation/licensure_stats.htm.

Pew Health Professions Commission. (1995, December). *Critical challenges: Revitalizing the health professions for the twenty-first century.* San Francisco: UCSF Center for the Health Professions.

Physician Payment Review Commission (PPRC). (1993). *Annual report to Congress 1993.* Washington, DC: Author.

Politzer, R., Gamliel, S., Cultice, J., Bazell, C., Rivo, M., & Mullan, F. (1996). A matching physician supply and requirements: Testing policy recommendations. *Inquiry, 33,* 181–194.

Pope, G., & Schneider, J. (1992). Trends in physician income. *Health Affairs,* 181–193.

Reason, J. T. (1990). *Human error.* Cambridge, MA: Cambridge University Press.

Safriet, B. (1992). Health care dollars and regulatory sense: Role of advanced practice nursing. *Yale Journal on Regulation, 9*(2), 149–220.

Salsberg, E. (1997). *State strategies for financing graduate medical education.* New York: United Hospital Fund.

Simon, C. J., & Born, P. H. (1996). TRENDS: Physician earnings in a changing managed care environment. *Health Affairs, 15,* 124–133.

Slee, V. M., & Slee, D. A. (2001). *Slee's health care terms—e-edition* [on-line]. Available: http://Tringa.swdata.com/

Thomas, S. A., Barter, M. & McLaughlin, F. E. (2000). State and territorial boards of nursing approaches to the use of unlicensed assistive personnel. *JONA's Healthcare Law, Ethics, and Regulation, 2*(1), 13–21.

U.S. Bureau of Labor Statistics. (1997, June 16). *A occupational outlook handbook* [on-line]. Available: http://www.bls.gov/oco/ocos079.htm

U.S. Bureau of Labor Statistics. (2000a, January 1). *Current employment statistics* [on-line]. Generated by M. Dill, using Selective Access System. Available: http://stats.bls.gov/ceshome.htm

U.S. Bureau of Labor Statistics. (2000b, January 31). *Office of Employment Projections* [on-line]. ftp://ftp.bls.gov/pub/special.requests/ep/IND-OCC.MATRIX

U.S. Census Bureau. (2000, March 31). *Detailed state projections by single year of age sex race and Hispanic origin: 1995 to 2025* [on-line]. Available: http//www.census.gov/population/www/projections/st_yr95to00.html

U.S. Department of Education, National Center for Education Statistics (1999). *Integrated Postsecondary Education Data System, Completions Data— 1989–1990 through 1996–1997* [on-line]. Available: http://nces.ed.gov/IPEDS/complations.htm//data.

U.S. Department of Health and Human Services. (1992). *Health personnel in the United States eighth report to Congress: 1991* (DHHS Pub. No. HRSPOD 92-1). Washington, DC: U.S. Government Printing Office.

U.S. Department of Health and Human Services, Health Resources and Services Administration. (2000). *State health workforce data resource guide.* Washington, DC, U.S. Government Printing Office.

U.S. Department of Health and Human Services, Health Resources and Services Administration, Bureau of Primary Health Care. (2001). *Health professional shortage area database* [on-line]. Available: http://bpnc.hrsa.gov/databases/newhpsg/newhpsa.fcfn.

Wennberg, J. E., Goodman, D. C., Nease, R. F., & Keller, R. B. (1993). Finding equilibrium in U.S. physician supply. *Health Affairs, 12,* 89–103.

5

Comparative Health Systems

Victor G. Rodwin

LEARNING OBJECTIVES

- ☐ Analyze conceptual and methodological issues in the study of health systems.
- ☐ Identify common problems of health policy in diverse health systems.
- ☐ Highlight key features of health systems in France, Canada, and Britain.
- ☐ Describe the U.S. health system in comparative perspective.
- ☐ Examine the uses of comparative analysis in learning from abroad.

TOPICAL OUTLINE

Issues in the study of comparative health systems
Common problems of health policy in three countries
The U.S. health system: A comparative perspective

KEY WORDS

health systems, inputs and outputs, outcomes, inefficiency in the allocation of resources, determinants of health policies, national health insurance (NHI), national health service (NHS), socialized health service, direct vs. indirect third-party payment, policy learning

Comparative analysis of health systems in industrially advanced nations has produced a large and growing literature that provides profiles and improves our understanding of health care systems abroad. This chapter begins with an overview of general issues in the comparative study of health systems. Next it assesses some common problems of health policy in three countries: France, Canada, and Britain. Finally, it analyzes the U.S. health system from a comparative perspective and examines the uses of comparative analysis for Americans, in learning from abroad.

ISSUES IN THE STUDY OF COMPARATIVE HEALTH SYSTEMS

Three stages may be distinguished in the evolution of comparative health systems research (Dumbaugh & Neuhauser, 1979), all of which are apparent in contemporary studies of health systems abroad. The first stage dominated until the mid-1960s, and continues today in the form of "travelogues" written by physicians returning from overseas tours. During the second stage, researchers described health systems from a variety of perspectives—often with hopes of promoting health care reform. During the third stage there has been an attempt to make the comparative study of health systems into a kind of social science. The research has focused largely on explaining variation across health systems on the basis of received theories within such disciplines as anthropology, sociology, political science, and economics.

The social science approach to comparative analysis of health systems has the inherent defect of its virtues. To achieve a rigorous study design, it has classified descriptive data on health systems, formulated hypotheses, and tested them against available evidence. Among economists, for example, the focus has been largely on cross-sectional comparisons of health services utilization and expenditures, thus narrowing the scope of research questions and eroding the ideals shared by stage 2 scholars, who were more motivated by the pragmatic concerns of improving the delivery of medical care in their countries.

Social scientists tend to display more interest in the theoretical concerns of their disciplines than in social change. Nevertheless, some excellent studies have been produced and this has raised some conceptual and methodological issues that remain at the center of health services research.

Conceptual Issues

The concept of a "health system" is clearly central to efforts to compare health services across nations. And yet there is no fully satisfactory definition of this concept, for it is difficult to agree both on the boundaries of the system and on a definition of health. Blum (1981) has provided a visual model of health, suggesting that health care services are merely one input into health among three others—heredity, behavior, and environment (see Figure 5.1). Weinerman (1971) defined the health system as "all of the activities of a society which are designed to protect or restore health, whether directed to the individual, the community, or the environment" (p. 273). Anderson (1972) outlined more concretely the "boundaries of a

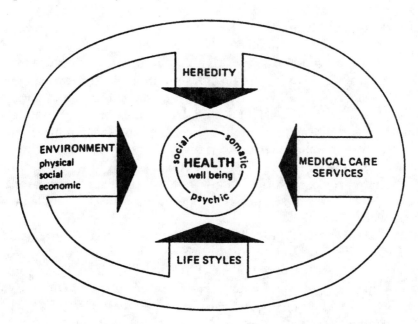

FIGURE 5.1   Inputs to health.

Adapted from: Blum, H. (1981). *Planning for Health* (2nd ed.). New York: Human Sciences Press, p. 3.

relatively easily defined system with entry and exit points, hierarchies of personnel, types of patients"—in short what he calls "the officially and professionally recognized 'helping' services regarding disease, disability and death" (p. 22).

Viewing the concept of health system at a macrosociological level, Field (1973) proposed the following formal definition: "that societal mechanism that transforms generalized resources . . . into specialized outputs in the form of health services" (p. 768). He added that "the 'health system' of any society is that social mechanism that has arisen or been devised to deal with the incapacitating aspects of illness, trauma, and (to some degree) premature mortality . . . the five D's: death, disease, disability, discomfort, and dissatisfaction" (p. 772).

Another approach to the concept of health system is to define it implicitly by postulating a causal model of it. Thus, drawing on Weinerman's definition and on Elling and Kerr's (1975) proposed framework for studying health systems, De Miguel (1975) outlines four subsystem levels that influence health status: individual, institutional, societal, and environmental. Such an approach allows one to analyze a health system by investigating the effects of a hierarchy of independent variables on the dependent variable, health status. It also raises questions about the most effective levels at which to effect system change.

Methodological Issues

The fundamental methodological issue in comparative health systems research involves devising a study design and selecting two or more national systems that allow the analyst to hold some variables constant, while manipulating experimental ones. In the area of health policy, for example, how does one evaluate the success of cost-containment efforts in health systems characterized by diverse patterns of financing and provider reimbursement? Quasi-experimental research designs would suggest matching two health systems on all but a few policy-related factors. But "matching," let alone a real experiment, is rarely feasible in policy research.

One response to this difficulty has been to match health systems on at least some criteria (e.g., levels of health resources) and then to call for "in-depth studies of contrasting cases" (Elling & Kerr, 1975). Another response has been to use the language of natural experiment and view "most similar systems" as laboratories in which to assess the effects of alternative policy options at home (Marmor, Bridges, & Hoffman, 1978). A more recent response has been to adopt a "modular approach" that examines systematically and sequentially diverse components of health systems, for example, needs, inputs, the delivery process, and health system outcomes (Ellencweig, 1992).

Another methodological concern in the social science approach to comparative health systems research is whether the descriptive studies and data collected during stages 1 and 2 (see above) are actually comparable. If they are not, this casts great doubt on the utility of making international comparisons. If they are, qualifications must usually be made.

The most difficult methodological issues arise in evaluating health systems, for this involves specifying the relationship between the elements of a health system (inputs and outputs) and their impact on health status (outcomes). But how does one distinguish the effect of health services on health from the effects of improvements in social services, income security, education, and transportation, not to mention the social and physical environments? This question raises the problem of devising indicators of health status. It also explains why, in his comparative study of the United States, Sweden, and England, Odin Anderson (1972) found it impossible to attribute differences in the usual health indices of morbidity and mortality to patterns of medical care organization in these countries. There has been little progress on this score over the past 28 years. To evaluate health systems, it is necessary to agree on consistent definitions of health system inputs and outputs and to devise health status indicators to measure outcomes. The World Health Organization (WHO) recently published a study of health system performance in which member health systems were ranked on the basis of eight measures (WHO, 2000). The results, however, are controversial and this study is likely to be followed by many more.

Learning from Abroad

Comparative studies of health policy are sparse. Most often, they describe an experience in a range of policy areas; only rarely have they interpreted, let alone evaluated, this experience. Exceptions to this general rule are of interest because they have contributed at least three ideas with implications for learning from abroad.

First is the idea of evolutionary progress in health systems. Medical sociologists such as Field (1973) and Mechanic (1976) argued that health systems in Western industrialized nations evolve in similar directions. Drawing on Field's five system typology—the private health system, the pluralistic one, the national health insurance (NHI) system, the national health service (NHS), and the socialized health service—such views suggest that the direction of change in modern societies is from the system of Type 1 to that of Type 5 (see Table 5.1). Unlike Field and Mechanic, who were not convinced that such change necessarily implies "progress," Milton Roemer (1977) described the evolution of health systems as a march toward a health ideal.

The second idea, the notion of public policy learning, is methodological in nature. It is highlighted in Glaser's studies of health policy in Western Europe and Canada. *Paying the Doctor* (1970) analyzed systems of physician remuneration. *Health Insurance Bargaining* (1978) explained how alternative administrative arrangements affect the process of bargaining between the medical profession and the state. *Paying the Hospital* (1987) describes systems of hospital reimbursement and assesses the implications for the United States. *Health Insurance in Practice* (1991) reviews a wide range of issues related to the financing and organization of national health insurance in cross-national perspective. Each of these studies starts with the presumption that the United States has many problems and that the policies and experience of Western Europe and Canada can shed light on and provide a useful range of solutions for the United States.

The third idea focuses on understanding either determinants of health policies or at least their effects. Leichter (1979), for example, analyzed the determinants of health policies in Britain, Germany, Japan, and the former Soviet Union. Similarly, Altenstetter (1974) and Stone (1981) showed how different structures and processes explain the differences in policy between the United States and West Germany; and Hollingsworth (1986) attempts to relate differences in structure and performance by comparing the United States and Britain. This approach views "most similar systems" as laboratories in which to assess the effects of alternative policy options at home (Teune, 1978). It is exemplified by Evans (1984) and Marmor and his colleagues (1978), who used this approach in their studies of Canada.

The idea of evolutionary progress in the development of health systems suggests that the United States can learn about future policy issues by studying nations whose systems are more advanced. Similarly, the idea that policy learning brings foreign solutions to bear on American problems is a

TABLE 5.1   The Evolution of Health Systems

Health system	Type 1: Private	Type 2: Pluralistic	Type 3: National health insurance	Type 4: National health service	Type 5: Socialized health service
General definition	Health care as item of personal consumption	Health care as predominantly a consumer good or service	Health care as an insured, guaranteed consumer good or service	Health care as a state-supported consumer good or service	Health care as a state-provided public service
Position of the physician	Solo entrepreneur	Solo entrepreneur and member of variety of groups, organizations	Solo entrepreneur and member of medical organizations	Solo entrepreneur and member of medical organizations	State employee and member of medical organizations
Role of professional associations	Powerful	Very strong	Strong	Fairly strong	Weak or nonexistent
Ownership of facilities	Private	Private and public	Private and public	Mostly public	Entirely public
Economic transfers	Direct	Direct and indirect	Mostly indirect	Indirect	Entirely indirect
Prototypes	U.S., Western Europe, Russia in the 19th century	U.S. in 20th century	Sweden, France, Canada, Japan in 20th century	Great Britain in 20th century	Soviet Union in 20th century

Sources: Rodwin, V. G. (1984). *The Health Planning Predicament: France, Quebec, England, and the United States.* Berkeley: University of California Press, p. 245, Field, M. G. (1978). *Comparative Health Systems: Differentiation and Convergence,* Final Report under Grant No. HS-00272. Rockville, MD: National Center for Health Services Research.

variation on this theme. Finally, the idea of using comparative analysis to understand the determinants and effects of policies abroad can assist us in evaluating alternative policy options at home.

There is, however, an important caveat to these views. The ideas summarized above, indeed most of the literature in comparative health policy, often minimize or overlook the substantial problems of health systems abroad. An alternative, problem-oriented approach might be to reverse this emphasis. For example, another way to think about learning from abroad is to begin with the recognition that most countries, irrespective of their particular health system, face serious common problems with regard to the efficient and equitable allocation of scarce health care resources. The Organization for Economic Cooperation and Development (OECD) and the World Bank have published important comparative studies that reflect this approach (see Suggested Readings). Within this problem-oriented approach there are at least three ways of viewing the problems.

Economists, for example, emphasize the problem of inefficiency in the allocation of health care resources. They point out that cost containment should not be confused with allocative efficiency in the use of health care resources, and they study the possibilities of obtaining more value for the money spent on health care. This applies not only with regard to improving health status but also with respect to altering input mixes in the provision of health services taking advantage of cost-effective treatment settings (e.g., ambulatory surgery) and personnel (e.g., nurse practitioners).

Public health and medical care analysts criticize the lack of integration among primary, secondary, and tertiary levels levels of care. Although health planners have called for redistributing resources away from hospitals to community-based ambulatory care services and public health programs, the allocation of resources within health regions has been notoriously biased in favor of more costly technology-based medical care at the apex of the regional hierarchy (Fox, 1986; Rodwin, 1984). The consequence of this allocational pattern has been to weaken institutional capability for delivering primary care services, and has exacerbated the separation between primary, secondary, and tertiary levels of care, thus making it difficult for providers to assure that the right patient receives the right kind of care, in the right place, and for the right reason.

Consumers have noted the inflexibility of bureaucratic decision-making procedures and the absence of opportunities for exercising what Hirschman (1970) calls "voice" in most health care organizations. Indeed, the problem of control and how it should be shared among consumers, providers, managers, and payers is at the center of most criticisms leveled against the current structure of health systems in Western industrialized nations. In all of these systems, decisions about what medical services to provide, how and where they should be provided, by whom, and how often are separated from the responsibility for financing medical care.

COMMON PROBLEMS OF HEALTH POLICY
IN THREE COUNTRIES

Drawing on the problem-oriented approach presented above, this section provides an example of how to assess common problems with regard to the efficient and equitable allocation of scarce health care resources in four nations: France, Canada, Britain, and the United States (see Table 5.2). The three other countries are far smaller than the United States in terms of population size. They have slightly lower gross domestic product (GDP) per capita and spend less on health care as a percentage of GDP. But all three countries represent important models of health care financing and organization. France is a prototype model of a traditional European national health insurance (NHI) system; Canada is an example of a newer NHI system operating in a federal institutional structure that resembles more closely that of the United States; Britain is the model par excellence of a national health service (NHS).

Other than the system of health care financing in the United States (see chapter 3), there are two principal methods of health care financing: compulsory payroll taxes and general revenue taxation. France is an example of an employment-based NHI system financed by payroll taxes on employers and employees. Canada and Britain both rely on general revenue taxation. Whereas Canada uses national and provincial general tax revenues to finance a federal decentralized NHI system, Britain relies overwhelmingly on central government funds to finance an NHS. Despite these differences in health care financing and the differences in health care spending noted above, there are also some notable points of convergence between the United States and at least two of the selected countries with regard to certain health system characteristics, as well as health outcome characteristics (see Table 5.2).

France

The French health system combines NHI with solo office-based fee-for-service private practice in the ambulatory care sector and a mixed hospital care sector, of which two thirds of all acute beds are in the public sector and one third are in the private sector (Rodwin & Sandier, 1993). Physicians in the ambulatory sector and in private hospitals (known as *cliniques*) are reimbursed on the basis of a negotiated fee schedule. Roughly 30% of all physicians selected the option to extra-bill beyond the negotiated fees that represent payment in full for the remaining 70% of physicians (Rodwin & Sandier, 1993). They may do so as long as their charges are presented with "tact and measure," a standard that has never been legally defined but which has been found, empirically, to represent a 50%–100% increase to the negotiated fees. Physicians based in public hospitals are reimbursed on a part-time or full-time salaried basis. *Cliniques* used to be reimbursed on

TABLE 5.2 Country, Health System, and Health Outcome Characteristics: France, Canada, United Kingdom, and United States

Country characteristics	Year	France	Canada	UK	U.S.
Total population in thousands	1999	59,099	30,491	59,333	272,878
Percent of population age 65 and over	1997	15.7%	12.3%	15.8%	12.5%
GDP $ per capita[a]	1999	$22,465	$25,428	$22,459	$31,935
Health system characteristics					
Health expenditure as a percent of GDP	1998	9.6%	9.5%	6.7%	13.6%
Per capita health expenditures[a]	1998	$2,077	$2,312	$1,461	$4,178
Doctors' consultations per capita	1995	6.4	6.6	6.1	5.8
Acute care bed days per 1,000 population	1996	1,200	1,300	800	800
Health outcome characteristics					
Health system perceived as "bad"[b]	1994	10.0%	12.0%	17.0%	28.0%
Infant mortality per 1,000 live births	1997	4.7	5.5	5.9	7.2
Life expectancy (females) at age 65	1997	20.8	20.1	18.5	19.2
Life expectancy at birth (males)	1997	74.6	75.8	74.6	73.6
Self-evaluation as "very good" or "good," pop. 15 and over[c]	1996	NA	90.10%	88.10%	89.00%
Adverse effects from medicine, per million population[d]	1993	17.6	0.6	1.1	0.6

Source: OECD. (2000). *HealthData.* Paris: Author.

[a] In purchasing power parities.
[b] Percentage of population that perceives health systems as "bad" based on surveys reported by Blendon, Leitman, Morrison, & Donelan (1990).
[c] Percentage of population that evaluates their own health status as "very good" or "good" based on national surveys.
[d] Number of deaths caused by adverse effects from medicines as reported by WHO *World Statistics Manual* and complemented by national sources, and cited by OCED HealthData.

the basis of a negotiated per diem fee; in the late 1990s they gradually moved to a case-mix reimbursement system. Before 1984, public hospitals were reimbursed on the basis of a retrospective, cost-based, per diem fee; since then they receive prospectively set "global" budgets adjusted for patient case mix.

Although the French NHI was rated No. 1 on the basis of its overall efficiency and fairness, by the recent WHO study of health system performance (WHO, 2000), there are still several problems with the system. From a public health point of view, there is inadequate communication between full-time salaried physicians in public hospitals and solo-based private practice physicians working in the community. Although general practitioners in the fee-for-service sector (roughly one half of French physicians) have informal referral networks to specialists and public hospitals, there are no formal institutional relationships that assure continuity of medical care, disease prevention and health promotion services, posthospital follow-up care, and more generally systematic linkages and referral patterns between primary-, secondary-, and tertiary-level services.

From an economic perspective, there still remain problems of economic efficiency. On the demand side, two factors encourage consumers to increase their use of medical care services: the uncertainty about the results of treatment, and the availability of universal and comprehensive insurance coverage. To reduce the risk of misdiagnosis or improper therapy, physicians are always tempted to order more diagnostic tests. Since NHI covers most of the cost, there is no incentive—neither for the physician nor for the patient—to balance marginal changes in risk with marginal increases in costs. This results in excessive (and often inappropriate) use of services.

On the supply side, fee-for-service reimbursement of physicians provides incentives for them to increase their volume of services so as to raise their income. Likewise, case-based reimbursement of *cliniques* provided incentives to increase patient admissions so long as revenues exceed costs. The imposition of global budgets, in 1984, eliminated this problem for the pubic hospitals. The move toward using indicators of case mix for setting public hospital budgets and negotiating per diem fees for *cliniques* has also weakened the incentives to increase hospital services. The budgets for public hospitals represent a blunt policy tool, however—one that tends to support the existing allocation of resources within the hospital sector and possibly to jeopardize the quality of public hospital services. It is relatively easy for a hospital to receive an annual budget to maintain its ongoing activities but extremely difficult to receive additional compensation for higher service levels, institutional innovation, or improvements in the quality of care. Since 1996, even with prospectively set budgets for hospitals, as well as *cliniques,* all hospital institutions naturally seek to maximize the level of their annual allocations and to resist budget cutbacks.

In summary, under French NHI, providers have no financial incentives to achieve savings while holding quality constant or even improving it. Nor are there incentives—in public hospitals, for example—to increase service activity in exchange for more revenues. Consumers have few incentives, other than minimal co-payments, to be economical in their use of medical care. And there are no incentives to move the French system away from hospital-centered services toward new organizational forms that encourage teamwork between general practitioners, specialists, and hospitals, and greater responsiveness to emerging market demands (Rodwin, 1997).

In 1996, as part of a broader reform of the social security system, Prime Minister Juppé attempted the most far-reaching reform of the French health sector since 1958. The central state's supervisory role over the national health insurance system was reinforced. In addition, the French Parliament was made accountable for health expenditures. It was required to set a global expenditure target for total health care expenditures reimbursed by French NHI and to set targets for each of France's 21 regions. To advise Parliament in this new responsibility and assist the Ministry of Health in overseeing the health system, a slew of new institutions were created: the National Committee on Public Health, a National Agency for Hospital Accreditation and Quality, and Regional Agencies for hospital planning and control.

Although President Chirac dissolved Parliament shortly after the national strikes in protest to the social security reforms, almost all of the health care reforms have been maintained by the new socialist government of Prime Minister Jospin. Perhaps most noteworthy has been the increased role of' the National Agency on Health Accreditation and Evaluation in setting standards for the quality of hospital care and developing national medical guidelines for physicians in private practice, which the NHI Administration is trying to enforce. The problems identified earlier are hardly resolved; but the central government is increasingly intervening to modernize and rationalize the French health care system (Le Pen & Rodwin, 1996).

Canada

Under Canadian NHI, although coverage for prescription drugs is far less generous than in France (only two provinces have a program to cover prescription drugs), there are no co-payments for any covered hospital and medical services. This means that patients are not required to pay a proportion of their medical bills; there is "first-dollar" coverage for a comprehensive "package" of hospital and medical services. Physicians in ambulatory care are paid predominantly on a fee-for-service basis, according to fee schedules negotiated between physicians' associations and provincial governments. All physicians must accept these fees as payment in full. In contrast to France, where physicians in public hospitals are largely paid on a salary basis, most physicians in Canadian hospitals are paid on a fee-for-service basis, as in the United States.

There are few private, for-profit hospitals in Canada, like the French *cliniques* and American proprietary or "investor-owned" institutions.

Most acute care hospitals in Canada are private, nonprofit institutions. But their operating expenditures are financed through the NHI system, and most of their capital expenditures are financed by the provincial governments. In the United States, among advocates of NHI, Canada's health system has often been depicted as a model for NHI (Himmelstein & Woolhandler, 1989). Its financing—through a complex shared federal and provincial tax revenue formula—is more progressive than the European NHI systems financed on the basis of payroll taxes. Canada's levels of health status are high by international standards. In comparison with the United States, it has achieved notable success in controlling the growth of health care costs. What, then, are the problems in this system?

From the point of view of health care providers, Canada's successful cost-containment program is perceived as a crisis of "underfinancing." Physicians complain about low fee levels. Hospital administrators complain about draconian control of their budgets. And other health care professionals note that the combination of a physician "surplus" and excessive reliance on physicians prevents an expansion of their roles.

Although Evans (1992) contends that Canadian cost-control policies cannot be shown to have jeopardized the quality of care, providers and administrators alike claim that there has been deterioration since the imposition of restrictive prospective budgets. Leaving aside the issue of quality, the same issues discussed in the context of France are present in Canada with respect to economic efficiency. Neither the hospital, the physician, nor the patient has an incentive to be economical in the use of health care resources. On the demand side, because patients benefit from what is perceived as "free" tax-financed first-dollar coverage, they have no incentive to choose cost-effective forms of care. For example, in the case of a demand for urgent care, there is no incentive for a patient to use community health centers rather than rush directly to the emergency room.

On the supply side, physicians lack incentives to make efficient use of hospitals, which are essentially a free good at their disposal. There are no incentives for altering input mixes to affect practice style. Nor are there incentives for providers to evaluate service levels and the kinds of therapy performed in relation to improving health status. It could be argued that these problems are common to all health systems, but they are especially acute in a system characterized by concentrated political interests—health care providers, on the one hand, and a "single payer," on the other—that tend to support the status quo. On the one hand, providers organized in strong associations have strong monopoly power, which they use to defend their legitimate interests; on the other, the monopoly power of sole-source financing (NHI) keeps provider interests in check at the cost of not intervening in the organizational practice of medicine.

Stoddard (1984) characterized the problems of the Canadian health system as "financing without organization" and this is still a fundamental problem in the Canadian system. In his view, Canadian provinces "adopted a 'pay the bills' philosophy, in which decisions about service provision—

which services, in what amounts, produced how, by whom and where—were viewed as the legitimate domain of physicians and hospital administrators" (p. 3). The reason for this policy is that provincial governments were concerned about maintaining a good relationship with providers. This concern has not avoided tough negotiations and periodic confrontations. But there have been only limited efforts to devise new forms of medical care practice, for example, health maintenance organizations (HMOs) or new institutions to handle long-term care for the elderly. The side effect of Canadian NHI has been to support the separation of hospital and ambulatory care and to reinforce traditional organizational structures.

As in France there are, in essence, two strategies for managing the Canadian health system and making adjustments. The first involves greater regulation on the supply side: even stronger controls on hospital spending, more rationing of medical technology, and more hospital mergers and eventually closures. The second involves increased reliance on market forces on the demand side: various forms of user charges such as co-payments and deductibles now advocated as a form of privatization. Neither strategy is likely to succeed on its own. The former will control health care expenditures in the short run, but it fails to affect practice styles. Its effectiveness runs the risk of exacerbating confrontations between providers and the state and jeopardizing health care needs. The latter deals with only part of the problem—the demand side—and neglects the issue of supply-side inefficiency. It provides no mechanism by which consumer decisions can generate signals to providers to adopt efficient practice styles. Moreover, to the extent that it has been used, it has raised the level of private expenditures.

Between these two strategies, there is increasing recognition among Canadian policy makers that the health sector requires significant reorganization. In Ontario, in 1996, the Health Services Restructuring Commission (HSRC) was formed; in Quebec, the federation of GPs formed a task force on the reorganization of primary care. Both of these efforts reinforced a trend toward "integrated health systems" and the use of gatekeepers in primary care. In Ontario, the main accomplishment of HSRC was to devise a seven-point plan to restructure the balance of resources among hospitals and community health services. In Quebec, the main accomplishment of the task force was also limited to planning for needed reforms. The Canadian system has been remarkably resistant to organizational reform, in practice.

Throughout the 1990s, the major health policy battles, in Canada, were fought over the problem of funding health services. Hospital budget cuts held per capita public spending on health care roughly constant from 1992–1997 but total health care spending, as a percent of GDP, fell by a full percentage point (Naylor, 1999). The combination of escalating drug costs and hospital cuts has eroded public confidence in the system (Evans, 2000). But in the spring of 2000, contentious meetings between provincial health ministers and federal officials resulted in a deal to restore federal cash payments for health care and other social welfare services.

Over the period of 2000–2004, the federal government has agreed to provide 1 billion Canadian dollars to purchase medical equipment in hospitals and 800 million Canadian dollars to support projects that reform the delivery of primary care services (Kondro, 2000). The strings attached to this deal commit the provinces to develop a formulary service for prescription drugs and to produce annual "report cards" on the performance of their respective systems. Thus, the pressure is still on to produce some organizational reform and hold the supply side more accountable to those paying the bill.

Britain

There are many models of an NHS in Europe, ranging from decentralized systems in Sweden, Norway, Finland, and Denmark, to more centralized systems in Spain, Greece, Portugal, and Italy. Because the British NHS is one of the oldest and most thoroughly studied models, it stands as an exemplar. It is financed almost entirely through general revenue taxation and is accountable directly to the central government's Department of Health and Social Security (DHSS) and Parliament. Access to health services is free of charge to all British subjects and to all legal residents. But despite the universal entitlement, health expenditures in the UK represent only 6.7% of the gross domestic product (GDP)—less than one half that in the United States (see Table 5.3).

Although the NHS is cherished by most Britons, there are, nevertheless, some serious problems concerning both the equity and efficiency of resource allocation in the health sector. With regard to equity (defined as "equal care for those at equal risk") in 1976, the Resource Allocation Working Party (RAWP) developed a formula for narrowing inequalities in the allocation of NHS funds among regions (Townsend & Davidson, 1982). The formula (DHSS, 1976) represented one of the most far-reaching attempts to allocate health care funds because it incorporated regional differences in health status based on standardized mortality ratios. Some progress was made in redistributing the aggregate NHS budget along the lines of the RAWP formula in the 1980s and it was eventually eliminated in the 1990s. But substantial inequities still remain, from the points of view of both spatial distribution and social class.

With regard to efficiency, the problems are even more severe because NHS resources are extremely scarce by OECD standards. Perhaps because there are fewer health care resources in Britain than in the rest of Western Europe or the United States, the British have been more aggressive in weeding out inefficiency than in these wealthier countries. And because the NHS faces the same demands as other systems to make available technology and to care for an increasingly aged population, British policy makers recognize that they must pursue innovations that improve efficiency. Numerous obstacles have been encountered, however: opposition by professional

TABLE 5.3   Total Expenditures on Health Care as a Percentage of GDP: 1997

Country	Total expenditure on health in GDP (%)
Australia	8.3
Austria	8.2
Belgium	8.6
Canada	9.3
Czech Rep.	7.1
Denmark	8.2
Finland	7.3
France	9.6
Germany	10.5
Greece	8.5
Hungary	6.9
Iceland	7.9
Ireland	7.0
Italy	8.4
Japan	7.4
Korea	5.0
Luxembourg	6.0
Mexico	4.7
Netherlands	8.6
New Zealand	7.6
Norway	8.1
Poland	6.2
Portugal	7.6
Spain	7.0
Sweden	8.5
Switzerland	10.3
Turkey	4.0
United Kingdom	6.7
United States	13.6

Source: OECD. (2000). *HealthData.* Paris: Author.

bodies, difficulties in firing and redeploying health care personnel, and the institutional separation between hospitals, general practitioners, and community health programs.

The tripartite structure of the NHS has, since its establishment in 1948, been a source of inefficiency:

1. Regional Health Authorities (RHAs) had been responsible (until the mid-1990s) for allocating budgets to districts and hospitals. Hospital-based physicians, known as "consultants," are paid on a salaried basis from these budgets, with distinguished clinicians receiving "merit awards." All consultants have the right to see a limited number of private, fee-paying patients in what are called "pay beds" within their service units.

2. Outside the RHA budget (until the mid-1990s) were the Family Practitioner Committees (FPCs) responsible for paying general practitioners

(GPs), ophthalmologists, dentists, and pharmacists. The GPs are reimbursed on a capitation basis, with additional remuneration coming from special "practice allowances" and fee-for-service payment for specific services (e.g., night visits and immunizations).

3. Separate from both the RHAs and the FPCs have been the local authorities (LAs), who are responsible for the provision of social services, public health services, and certain community nursing services.

This institutional framework has created perverse incentives—for example, to shift borderline patients from GPs to hospital consultants, to the community, and back to the hospital. Until the reforms introduced by the Thatcher government in 1991, GPs had no incentive to minimize costs and could even impose costs on RHAs by referring patients to hospital consultants or for diagnostic services. NHS managers could shift costs from the NHS to social security by sending elderly hospitalized patients to private nursing homes. And consultants could shift costs back onto the patient by keeping long waiting lists, thereby increasing demand for their private services. As in France and Canada, neither the patient nor the physician in Britain bears the cost of the decisions they make; it is the taxpayer who foots the bill.

Four strategies—all of them inadequate—attempted to deal with this problem. The first came promptly with the arrival of the first Thatcher government in 1981. After cautious attempts to denationalize the NHS by promoting a shift toward NHI and privatization, the conservative government backed off when they realized that such an approach would not merely provoke strong political opposition but also would increase public expenditure and therefore conflict with their budgetary objectives. Instead, the strategy was narrowed in favor of encouraging competition and market incentives in limited areas. To begin with, the government allowed a slight increase in private pay beds within NHS hospitals. In addition, it introduced tax incentives to encourage the purchase of private health insurance and the growth of charitable contributions. Also, the government encouraged local authorities to raise money through the sale of surplus property and to contract out to the private sector such services as laundry, cleaning, and catering.

The second response was the NHS Management Inquiry (Griffiths, 1983), which resulted in yet another reorganization in the long history of administrative reform within the NHS. Roy Griffiths, the former director of a large English department store chain, introduced the concept of a general manager at the department (DHSS), regional, district, and unit levels. This manager was presumably responsible for the efficient use of the budget at each level of the NHS. In summary, the report observed, in a sentence that has since become well known, "if Florence Nightingale were carrying her lamp through the corridors of the NHS today, she would almost certainty be searching for the people in charge" (Griffiths, 1983, p. 12). The problem, however, is that, following the Griffiths Report, the tripartite structure of the system remained largely unchanged; and the general managers had very little information about least-cost strategies (across the tripartite structure) for generating improvements in health status.

The third response to the problem of improving efficiency was to reduce the drug bill (Maynard, 1986). In April 1985, the government limited the list of reimbursable drugs and reduced the pharmaceutical industry's rate of return. These measures helped contain the costs of the formerly open-ended drug budget within the NHS, but there is no evidence that they had any impact on the efficiency of health care expenditures.

Finally, the fourth and most significant reform for improving efficiency was announced in a government White Paper, *Working for Patients* (1989), passed in 1990 (The National Health Service and Community Care Act) and implemented on April 1, 1991. The White Paper proposed a range of significant changes, all of which attempt to create "internal markets" within the public sector, by giving providers incentives to treat more patients and by having "money follow patients." On the demand side, the government proposed that, instead of operating as monopoly suppliers of services, district health authorities be required to purchase services for the patients they serve. On the supply side, the government proposed that NHS hospitals be given the option to convert from purely "public" status to that of independent, self-governing "trusts." Also, the government proposed that GPs be given the option to serve as "fundholders" for their enrolled patients and thereby serve as purchasers on their behalf for basic specialty and hospital services.

In July 1990, RHAs were streamlined and FPCs were transformed into newly named Family Health Service Authorities (FHSAs) with stronger management over primary care. In 1996 the districts were merged with the FHSAs into roughly 80 Health Authorities (HAs) and placed under a new National Health Service Executive (NHSE) with eight regional offices. The HAs were supposed to function as integrated purchasing coalitions, thereby strengthening the role of internal markets in the allocation of health resources. There have been some preliminary evaluations of these reforms, but they are still too recent to permit one to conclude very much about the effects of internal markets on efficiency of resource allocation, continuity of care, and responsiveness to patient demands. There is, however, general agreement that the reforms shifted the balance of power between GPs and hospital specialists, encouraged innovation in primary care, encouraged greater cost consciousness, and raised administrative costs (Smee, 2000).

Following Tony Blair's election as Prime Minister, the New Labour party's "third way" reforms focused more on collaboration and less on competition but the government's White Paper retained the major elements of the Thatcher reforms ("The New NHS," 1997). The purchaser/provider split was retained albeit with more emphasis on cooperation. All GPs have been brought into primary care groups (PCGs) thus bringing important elements of managed care to the NHS. Fundholders have now been largely absorbed by PCGs, and the HAs are losing their former purchasing role as they become increasingly responsible for providing a framework for PCG accountability (Dobson, 1999). Finally, as in France and Canada, there have been efforts to improve quality and standards. The National Institute for Clinical Effectiveness (NICE) is setting standards and the Council for Health Improvement (CHIMP) will enforce them (Legrand, 1999).

In retrospect, it is no exaggeration to suggest that the history of the British NHS is largely a story of successive organizational reforms to improve the efficiency and equity of resource allocation within the health care sector. An additional and more recent goal has been to increase the responsiveness of health care providers to consumers. Most astute observers of the NHS concur that even the most radical reforms under Prime Ministers Thatcher and Blair have had limited effects on the basic structure and problems of the system (Klein, 1998; Legrand, 1999). The fundamental tension between the push to introduce market mechanisms and the need for central control to preserve political accountability has remained intact. Moreover, the institutional power of central control appears to have the upper edge.

THE U.S. HEALTH SYSTEM: A COMPARATIVE PERSPECTIVE

How does the U.S. health care system measure up in comparison to the health systems in France, Canada, and Great Britain? To answer this question, we will review the ways in which the U.S. health system differs from and resembles that of other Western industrialized nations. Let us examine this issue from the perspectives of three characteristics that typically distinguish the United States from Western Europe and Canada: (a) values and popular opinion, (b) the structure of health care financing and organization, and (c) policy responses to health sector problems.

American Values and Popular Opinion

The prevailing image of American values and popular opinion is that of 19th-century liberalism, which has colored American perceptions of equity, the proper role of government, and citizenship. These perceptions represent a range of American values and popular opinions that distinguish the United States from Western Europe and Canada.

American attitudes about equity with regard to health care were formed in the 19th century as the country became populated in urban centers by immigrant populations. During this period the concept of "truly needy" emerged (Rosner, 1982). Many Americans developed a sense of responsibility to come to their aid, but there were also harsher attitudes inspired by social Darwinist notions that distinguished between the "truly needy" and the "undeserving" or "unworthy" poor. Whereas in Western Europe broadly based socialist parties viewed poverty as an outcome of the economic system, in the United States there was an inclination to regard poverty as an individual problem. Hence, the greater attention to *equality of opportunity* in the United States as compared with *equality of results* in the more left-leaning European social democracies.

As far as the proper role of government is concerned, in contrast to Western Europe and Canada, the United States has a history of antigovernment attitudes. The suspicion about excessive governmental authority and the attachment to individual liberties is a pervasive American value.

American perceptions of citizenship also present a striking contrast to western European perceptions. In the United States individualistic values, on the one hand, and social and ethnic heterogeneity, on the other, have resulted in more "fractionalized understandings of citizenship" (Klass, 1985). In western Europe and Canada, the understandings of citizenship are grounded in notions of solidarity and universal entitlements. The difference is that western Europe and Canada have largely succeeded in covering all of their citizens under some form of national health insurance (NHI); the United States has not.

There is a general aversion among Americans to universal entitlements. As Reinhardt (1985) observed, when Americans face a trade-off between establishing tax-financed entitlements and leaving the uninsured on their own, they prefer to do the latter. It would be misleading, however, to draw any conclusions about how generous Americans are or how much social welfare they provide based only on the image of liberalism outlined above. In contrast to western Europe and Canada, Americans prefer to promote redistribution policies through local assistance and indirect subsidies to the voluntary sector via tax exemptions.

Clearly, in comparison with western Europe and Canada, there are important differences in the United States with regard to values and popular opinion. But how much of a difference do these differences make?

The Structure of Health Care Financing and Organization

The prevailing image of the American health care system is one of a privately financed, privately organized system with multiple payers. These characteristics derive, in large part, from the absence of a publicly mandated NHI program. In comparison with western European nations, Japan, and Canada, the United States is last with respect to the public share of total health care expenditures (see Table 5.4). Although the United States has the highest per capita health care expenditures—public and private combined (Table 5.5)—and spends the highest percentage of its GDP on health care (see Table 5.3), it retains the lowest share of public expenditure as a percentage of total health expenditures (see Table 5.4).

The organization of health care in the United States is noted for being on the private end of the public-private spectrum. In comparison with western Europe, the United States has one of the smallest public hospital

TABLE 5.4   Sources of Finance and Health Care Expenditures: The Mix Between Public and Private in 1997 as a Percentage of Total Expenditure on Health

Country	Public	Private
Australia	68.2	31.8
Austria	70.9	29.1
Belgium	89.3	10.7
Canada	69.4	30.6
Czech Rep.	91.7	8.3
Denmark	82.4	17.6
Finland	76.1	23.9
France	76.4	23.6
Germany	76.9	23.1
Greece	57.7	42.3
Hungary	75.3	24.7
Iceland	83.9	16.1
Ireland	75.0	25.0
Italy	68.0	32.0
Japan	79.5	20.5
Korea	40.6	59.4
Luxembourg	92.5	7.5
Mexico	60.0	40.0
Netherlands	69.6	30.4
New Zealand	77.3	22.7
Norway	82.7	17.3
Poland	74.1	25.9
Portugal	67.1	32.9
Spain	76.5	23.5
Sweden	84.3	15.7
Switzerland	73.2	26.8
Turkey	72.8	27.2
United Kingdom	83.7	16.3
United States	45.4	54.6

Source: OECD. (2000). *HealthData.* Paris: Author.

sectors. In the organization of ambulatory care, American private fee-for-service practice corresponds to the norm, at least in comparison with NHI systems. The absence of an NHI program in the United States has resulted, however, in a system of multiple payers and has encouraged a more pluralistic pattern of medical care organization and more innovative forms of medical practice—for example, multi-specialty group practices, HMOs, ambulatory surgery centers, and preferred provider organizations (PPOs) (see chapter 11).

The United States is also different, in comparison to Canada and western Europe, with regard to the ways in which health resources are used. For example, the United States (along with Spain and the United Kingdom) is among those OECD countries with the lowest number of acute care

TABLE 5.5   Per Capita Health Care Expenditures, 1997 in $US Purchasing Power Parities (PPP)

Country	$US (PPP)
Australia	1,923
Austria	1,886
Belgium	1,973
Canada	2,185
Czech Rep.	930
Denmark	2,032
Finland	1,491
France	2,003
Germany	2,325
Greece	1,157
Hungary	672
Iceland	1,919
Ireland	1,432
Italy	1,754
Japan	1,809
Korea	766
Luxembourg	2,147
Mexico	356
Netherlands	2,004
New Zealand	1,347
Norway	2,154
Poland	448
Portugal	1,151
Spain	1,154
Sweden	1,712
Switzerland	2,697
Turkey	255
United Kingdom	1,406
United States	3,998

Source: OECD. (2000). *HealthData.* Paris: Author.

hospital beds per thousand population (see Table 5.6). These data should not necessarily lead one to the conclusion that the United States is less prone to institutionalize patients than Western Europe and Canada. They probably reflect the size of the American private nursing home industry, which has no equivalent in western Europe or Canada, where a portion of long-term care for the elderly is still provided in hospitals.

These are ways in which the American health care system is different from that of western Europe and Canada. But there are also some noteworthy points of similarity. For example, most health systems in industrially advanced nations are centered around the hospital. They allocate roughly one half of total health care expenditures to the hospital sector. The United States is only slightly below the norm in this regard (see Table 5.7).

There is also a high degree of similarity among the United States, Canada, and Western Europe in the broad structure of health care financing

TABLE 5.6   Acute Care Hospital Beds and Use of Inpatient Care, 1997

Country	No. of beds per 1,000 population	Bed days per 1,000 population
Australia	4.0	1,000
Austria	6.4	1,700
Belgium[a]	5.3	1,300
Canada[b]	3.6	1,400
Czech Rep.	6.8	1,800
Denmark	3.5	1,000
Finland	2.7	1,000
France	4.3	1,200
Germany	7.1	2,100
Greece[c]	3.9	N/A
Hungary	5.8	1,600
Iceland[a]	3.8	1,100
Ireland	3.3	1,000
Italy	5.2	1,400
Luxembourg[d]	5.6	1,800
Netherlands	3.7	1,000
Norway	3.3	900
Portugal	3.4	900
Spain[d]	3.2	800
Sweden[d]	2.8	800
Switzerland	5.8	1,800
Turkey	2.1	400
United Kingdom	2.4	1,000
United States	3.2	700

[a] 1995
[b] 1993
[c] 1992
[d] 1996

Source: OECD. (2000). HealthData. Paris: Author.

and provider reimbursement (see Figure 5.2). From the point of view of both consumers and providers, the essential feature of modern health care systems is the central role of third-party payment, by either government or health insurers. On the financing end, all health systems are supported primarily either by general revenue taxes or by payroll deductions in the form of compulsory taxes or voluntary health insurance premiums. On the payment end, the magnitude of third-party payment dwarfs the out-of-pocket payment by consumers.

For the consumer, what matters with regard to health care financing is not the relative public and private mix but rather the relative portion of *direct versus indirect* third-party payment. To emphasize that the largest portion of health care financing in the United States is private is misleading, for the more critical factor is that public and private health insurance are both forms of third-party payment.

TABLE 5.7   Components of Health Care Expenditure, 1997 (% of Total)

Country	Inpatient	Ambulatory	Pharmaceutical	Other
Australia	43.0	22.7	11.3	23.0
Austria[a]	22.7	23.6	10.6	43.1
Belgium	34.5	33.9	16.1	15.5
Canada	42.5	26.7	14.5	16.3
Denmark	68.9	18.2	8.5	4.4
France	44.6	24.2	20.9	10.3
Germany	33.7	29.5	12.2	24.6
Iceland	55.1	22.9	16.3	5.7
Italy	44.5	27.7	17.5	10.3
Japan	29.8	39.6	20.0	10.6
Luxembourg	35.9	50.1	12.6	1.4
Netherlands	52.5	20.5	10.3	16.7
Switzerland	50.8	39.7	7.7	1.8
United States	42.5	30.9	10.1	16.5

[a] 1996

Source: OECD. (2000). *HealthData.* Paris: Author.

This amount was equal to 78.3% of national health expenditures in 1999, leaving consumers with direct out-of-pocket contributions equal to 17% of total health expenditures (Smith, Heffler, & Freeland, 1999). The OECD does not routinely compare consumers' out-of-pocket payments to total expenditures. Available data on this important indicator suggest, once again, however, that the United States is different (see Figure 5.3). It has the highest share of direct out-of-pocket payments by consumers. Even under French NHI, consumers contribute roughly 14% of total health expenditures in the form of out-of-pocket payments. The difference is not as large as the image of a private financing system would suggest.

The image of a private organizational structure in American health care is well founded. But that view, too, is misleading and incomplete. In spite of a notable but small investor-owned hospital sector, a dominant investor-owned managed care sector, and the *relatively* small size of the public sector in the United States, in comparison to OECD nations, there is nevertheless an important role for the public sector in the United States health care system—both in ambulatory services for the noninstitutionalized patient and in the provision of hospital services.

With regard to ambulatory care, there is a maze of special federal programs and a network of local government services, largely for the poor. The services are provided either in county or municipal hospital emergency rooms, in local health departments, or in nonprofit community health centers receiving significant public financing from the federal, state, and/or local governments. As for hospitals, almost 30% of all registered hospitals (private, nonprofit, local, state, and federal institutions) are owned and operated by governments (American Hospital Administration, 2000). This includes the federal Veterans Health Administration hospitals, marine and

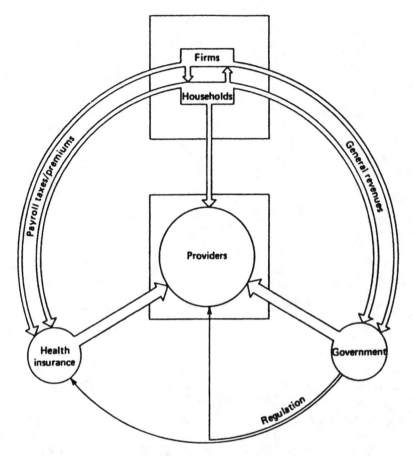

FIGURE 5.2   Health care financing and provider reimbursement.

military hospitals, as well as state, county, and municipal hospitals. Although Medicare and Medicaid were intended to bring the poor into "mainstream medicine" (i.e., into the private sector), local county governments continue to finance care for the "medically indigent" uninsured, either through private vendors or directly in public hospitals. These hospitals are a major source of care not only for Medicaid beneficiaries but also for more than half of the poverty population who do not meet Medicaid eligibility levels and consequently often do not have access to private physicians or voluntary hospitals.

To sum up, there are distinctive characteristics of health care financing and organization in the United States, but there are also striking points of similarity when compared with western Europe and Canada. The distinctive characteristics include the absence of an NHI program, preferences for institutional flexibility, and innovative forms of medical care organization. The points of similarity—the coexistence of both public and private provision and third-party payment—are structural features of the American health system as well as those of most other OECD health systems.

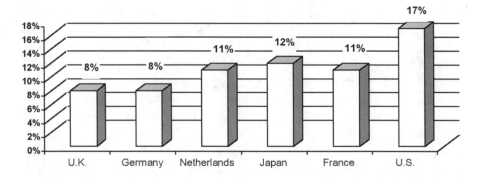

FIGURE 5.3   Share of patient out-of-pocket payments as a percentage of personal health care expenditures (1988–1999).

Sources: UK: Year 1989. OECD. (1992). *The Reform of Health Care: A Comparative Analysis of Seven OECD Countries.* Paris: Author, p. 116.

Germany: Year 1995. Busse, R., & Howorth, C. (1999). *Cost-containment in Germany, 1977–1997.* Unpublished paper, Department of Epidemiology and Social Medicine, Medizinishce Hochschule Hannover, Hannover, Germany.

Netherlands: Year 1988. OECD. (1992). *The Reform of Health Care: A Comparative Analysis of Seven OECD Countries.* Paris: Author, p. 89.

Japan: Year 1990. Kousei Tokeo Kyokai. *Kousei no Sninyou, 38*(9), 1991, p. 237, cited by Ikegami, The Economics of Health Care in Japan. *Science, 258,* 1992.

France: Year 1996. *Comptes nationaux de la santé,* 1996. Ministry of Health.

U.S.: Year 1999. Smith, S., Heffler, S., & Freeland, M. (1999). The next decade of health spending. *Health Affairs, 18*(4), 86–95.

Policy Responses to Health Sector Problems

In the mid-1980s, a keen foreign observer of the United States health care system, Brian Abel-Smith (1985) referred to the United States as the "odd man out" when he noted the divergence between Western European and American policy responses to the problem of containing health care costs. He suggested that Western Europe relies on regulation, whereas the United States seeks to promote competition and greater reliance on market forces. These differences remain strong. Abel-Smith pointed to three examples of American policy responses to health sector problems: (a) the growth of deductibles, co-payments, and other cost-sharing mechanisms; (b) the trend toward making those who benefit from insurance actually pay the whole cost. This implies, for example, reducing cross-subsidies in health care financing (see chapter 3), and making arguments for reducing the deductibility of health insurance premiums from employer and employee taxes on grounds that this will encourage employers and employees to shop more prudently for insurance coverage; and (c) the growth of competitive bidding as a mechanism of forcing competition among alternative providers.

There remain important insights in this interpretation of the American policy response to health sector problems. But there have also been some convergent trends since the 1980s. To begin with, the growth of cost-sharing was not limited to the United States. Many European countries have followed similar revenue-enhancing strategies. In fact, although the share of out-of-pocket payments by consumers, as a percentage of total health expenditures, is higher in the United States than in western Europe (Figure 5.3), the share in the United States has declined over the past 2 decades (Smith et al., 1999). Second, the U.S. arguments for reducing the deductibility of insurance premiums were largely rhetorical because employer health insurance premiums remain tax deductible and employee spending accounts—also tax deductible—have expanded greatly throughout the 1990s.

Third, despite the rhetoric and actual force of competition in the U.S. health system, there is probably more regulation in the highly regulated eastern states (e.g., New York, New Jersey, and Maryland) than in all of western Europe. Even in well-known "pockets of competition" (e.g., California, Arizona, and Minnesota) regulation is essential, if only to enforce the rules of the competitive game. The prospective payment system (PPS) for Medicare payment provides a good illustration. Although one of its effects was to intensify competition between hospitals, the use of diagnosis-related groups (DRGs) for hospital reimbursement was actually a highly regulatory strategy of centralized price controls, one that falls well within Western European policy traditions.

Despite the rhetoric of competition, with respect to physician payment, American policy remains highly regulatory. Since the creation of physician review organizations (PROs) under PPS, the regulation of physician behavior in the United States is surely stronger than any emerging European equivalent, including the French and Canadian systems of medical profiles, which are among the most developed outside the United States (Rodwin, 1989b).

In summary, three characteristics distinguish American policy responses from those of western Europe and Canada:

1. The United States has long been concerned about the dangers of monopoly power and has pursued (until the wave of industry consolidation in the health sector in the 1990s) a strong antitrust policy. A notable case in point is provided by the Federal Trade Commission's measures to curb the monopoly powers of physicians and hospitals and to eliminate restraints on trade in health care by allowing advertising (*Bates v. State Bar of Arizona*, 1977). Indeed, this remains a distinguishing characteristic of the U.S. health care system.

2. Following directly from the first characteristic of the American policy response is the absence in the United States of institutional structures for negotiating between major groups of health care providers and the government or an NHI board of directors, or both. In the United States, structural interests are not formally sanctioned and accepted as institutionalized

counterparts for purposes of negotiating with the government. Instead, the more typical response of American health policy is to advocate proposals to fragment powerful groups that are presumed, as a consequence, to compete with one another. This strategy of "divide and conquer" presents a striking contrast to the Western European and Canadian response that consolidates the organization of provider groups and confronts them with countervailing organizations. It serves as a severe constraint, in the United States, on the possibilities of negotiating a national fee schedule for physicians or a uniform hospital payment system for all payers and hospitals (Rodwin, 1989b). The constraint, however, has made it possible for individual payers (e.g., Medicare, Medicaid, and private health plans) to strike harder bargains with smaller groups and to foster competition and new organizational arrangements for medical care.

3. In contrast to Western European and Canadian strategies of comprehensive health care reform and strong centralized regulation, American strategies (with the exception of PPS for Medicare) are characterized by far greater decentralization and by more persistent social experimentation. Although major policy initiatives have usually come from the federal level and a range of government programs at the county and municipal levels, when compared to unitary European states (e.g., France and Britain), American federalism provides a striking contrast. But even in comparison to other federal states, such as Canada and Germany, the United States is still characterized by more decentralization and experimentation in the policy-making process.

These three characteristics of American policy responses to health sector problems highlight the ways in which the United States is different from Western Europe and Canada. But if one compares the evolution of American health policy over the past half century with that of Western Europe and Canada, there are also points of similarity.

For example, Brown (1988) identified four American policy responses to health sector problems: (a) the subsidy strategy—government grants on the supply side; (b) the financing strategy—third-party financing on the demand side; (c) the reorganization strategy—government inducements to promote new organizations for delivering medical care; and (d) the regulatory strategy—government attempts to influence the "use, price and quality of services, and the size, location, and equipment of facilities." Three of the four categories—subsidy, financing, and regulatory—are equally good descriptors of the western European and Canadian policy responses to their health sector problems.

In the 1950s and 1960s, during the expansion phase of health care systems, there was extraordinary convergence among Western industrialized nations around both the subsidy and financing strategies (De Kervasdoue, Kimberly, & Rodwin, 1984). In the mid-1970s and 1980s, during the containment phase, there was also convergence around the regulatory and reorganization strategies. Although one can point to examples of the reorganization strategy in all countries, Canada (particularly Quebec) and western Europe have focused more on administrative reorganizations in the public sector, whereas the United States has encouraged massive reorganization in the private sector at the level of the delivery system. The growth of large profit-making health corporations, particularly among managed care organizations (MCOs), is no doubt the most notable aspect of recent American health policy responses to health sector problems.

The Uses of Comparative Analysis in Learning from Abroad

Given the ways in which the health sector in the United States resembles that of western Europe and Canada and the ways in which it is exceptional, what inferences can one draw about the uses of comparative analysis for purposes of learning from abroad? If the United States is truly exceptional in the health sector, then one can argue that there is little to learn from western Europe and Canada. Countries often rely on this "assumption of uniqueness" to reject ideas from abroad (Stone, 1981). To the extent that the United States is unexceptional, however, a case can be made for drawing lessons from comparative experience.

For example, there is a widely shared belief among American policy makers that a national program providing for universal entitlement to health care in the United States would result in runaway costs. In response to this presumption, nations that entitle all of their residents to a high level of medical care while spending less on administration and on medical care than the United States, are often held up as models. The Canadian health system is the most celebrated example. French NHI, a prototype of western European continental health systems, is another case in point. Britain's NHS, although typically considered a "painful prescription" for the United States (Aaron & Schwartz, 1984), nevertheless assures first-dollar coverage for basic health services to its entire population and, as we have seen, spends less than half as much money, per capita, as the United States (see Table 5.5).

All of these countries have produced some of the leading physicians and hospitals in the world. Judging by various measures of health status, they are in the same league as, or better than, the United States (see Table 5.8). But in 2001, over 18% of the population in the United States remains uninsured for health care services, while spending, as a percentage GDP, surpasses that of all industrially advanced nations (see Table 5.3).

Should we adopt the western European or Canadian models of health care financing and organization? Or should we maintain our present system and recognize that it is a manifestation of American exceptionalism, that is, of the ways in which the United States is fundamentally different from western Europe and Canada? Both of these responses are probably inappropriate. The second response—that comparative analysis is not useful—insulates us from the experience of other nations. It smacks of ethnocentrism, makes

TABLE 5.8   Health Care Expenditures and Health Status: 1997

Country	Total expenditure on health as a % of GDP	Life expectancy At birth Females	Life expectancy At birth Males	Life expectancy At age 65 Females	Life expectancy At age 65 Males	Infant mortality per 1,000 live births
Canada	9.3	81.4	75.8	20.1	16.3	5.5
France	9.6	82.3	74.6	20.8	16.3	4.7
Germany	10.5	80.3	74.1	18.9	15.2	4.8
Italy[a]	8.4	81.3	75.0	19.7	15.7	6.2
Japan	7.4	83.8	77.2	21.8	17.0	3.7
Spain	7.0	82.0	74.6	20.2	16.2	5.0
United Kingdom	6.7	79.7	74.6	18.5	15.0	5.9
United States	13.6	79.4	73.6	19.2	15.9	7.2

[a] 1996

Source: OECD. (2000). HealthData. Paris: Author.

us conservative, and thereby supports the status quo in the United States. The first response—that we should adopt the western European or Canadian model—relies too heavily on the experience of those nations. It is misleading because, as we have seen, there are serious limitations in the western European and Canadian health systems. Moreover, many of the present institutional arrangements of health care delivery in the United States are superior to those abroad.

The proliferation of medical technology, combined with an aging demographic structure are trends common to all modern health care systems and have contributed to rising health care costs. Policy makers have responded largely by implementing systems with increasing control over expenditures on doctors' services as well as hospital budgets. Virtually no one in Canada or western Europe views the American system as a model to emulate. Even under the government of Prime Minister Thatcher there was no significant challenge to the principle of an NHS in Britain (*Working for Patients,* 1989). Nor is there any question about eliminating NHI in such countries as France, Canada, Germany, Belgium, or the Netherlands.

Despite these attitudes, one striking aspect about how some common problems are currently being dealt with abroad is the extent to which a number of fashionable American themes have drifted north to Canada and across the Atlantic to western Europe. In the context of the problems we identified earlier—inefficiency in the allocation of health care resources, lack of continuity between levels of care, and the absence of consumer "voice" in most health care organizations—the concept of a managed care organization (MCO), in combination with elements of market competition, has a certain appeal. Since an MCO is, by definition, both an insurer and a provider of health services, it establishes a link between the financing and provision of health services. Because its managers have a budget to care for an enrolled population, they have powerful incentives to provide needed services in a cost-effective manner while simultaneously maintaining quality to minimize the risk of disenrollment.

The idea of introducing MCOs or similar kinds of health care organizations into national systems that provide universal entitlement to health care resembles, in many ways, the American experience of encouraging Medicare beneficiaries to enroll in Medicare Choice (often called Part C). This idea involves two reforms. It spurs policy makers to combine regulatory controls with competition on the supply side; and it encourages them to design market incentives for both providers and consumers of health care.

To the extent that the insertion of MCOs into NHI or NHS systems represents an American "solution" to *foreign* problems, it may provide a way in which Canada and western Europe could learn from the United States (Rodwin, 1989a). It may also, paradoxically, have more practical implications for the United States than simply transposing a European NHI system into the American context. For example, the insertion of MCOs into NHI or NHS systems might provide insights on how managed care and universal coverage could be combined in the United States.

Alternatively, experience abroad with managed care and health care reform might highlight some of the obstacles faced in attempting to assure universal access in a system so reliant on decentralized control.

Just how policy learning occurs as a result of studying health care systems abroad is not thoroughly understood (Rodwin & Brecher, 1992). But there is no doubt that more policy research in the field of comparative health systems could potentially be helpful in learning from abroad.

CASE STUDY

You have just been hired by Health Care Associates (HCA), a large U.S. consulting firm specializing in health care management and policy analysis. HCA's clients range from government agencies to large health care providers, insurers, and purveyors of information-based administrative technologies. The firm has grown rapidly over the past decade and thrives on its stellar reputation for quality work and advice that has helped many clients achieve their goals.

Because many of HCA's private clients are entering the global marketplace, the CEO calls you one day and asks you to prepare a memorandum on the market opportunities for techniques of managed care in health care systems abroad. What would you advise her to do? Include in your answer a discussion of the possibilities in national health insurance systems (e.g., France and Canada), as well as national health services systems (e.g., Britain). Also, based on your understanding of the financing and organization of their respective health care systems, provide some advice on potential clients for introducing elements of managed care within each system. Finally, as an optional exercise, write a memorandum to HCA's CEO in which you explain what U.S. policy makers could learn from the cases in this chapter.

DISCUSSION QUESTIONS

1. What are the strengths and weaknesses of the social science approach to comparative health systems?
2. How can the analysis of health systems abroad be used to promote policy learning?
3. What are three common problems in health policy development found in different countries?
4. How does the French NHI system differ from the Canadian NHI system in its financing?
5. Compare the organization and financing of the British and U.S. health systems.
6. Is there evidence of policy convergence in the evolution of the French, Canadian, and British health systems?
7. Are policy responses to health sector problems different in the United States than in France, Canada, and Britain? If so, how? If not, why not?

ACKNOWLEDGMENT

I wish to thank Amy Chepaitis for general research assistance, including updating the OECD data and preparing the tables for this chapter.

REFERENCES

Aaron, H., & Schwartz, W. (1984). *The painful prescription: Rationing hospital care*. Washington, DC: Brookings Institution.

Abel-Smith, B. (1985). Who is the odd man out? The experiences of western Europe in containing the costs of health care. *Milbank Memorial Fund Quarterly: Health and Society, 63*(1), 1–17.

Altenstetter, C. (1974). *Health policy-making and administration in West Germany and the United States*. Beverly Hills, CA: Sage.

American Hospital Administration. (2000). *Hospital statistics*. Chicago, IL: Author.

Anderson, O. (1972). *Health care: Can there be equity? The United States, Sweden, and England*. New York: John Wiley.

Bates v. State Bar of Arizona, 433 U.S. 350 (1977).

Blendon, R. J., Leitman, R., Morrison, I., & Donelan, K. (1990). Satisfaction with health systems in ten nations. *Health Affairs, 2*(9), 185–192.

Blum, H. (1981). *Planning for health* (2nd ed.). New York: Human Sciences Press.

Brown, L. (1988). *Health policy in the United States: Issues and options*. New York: Ford Foundation.

De Kervasdoue, J., Kimberly, J., & Rodwin, V. (Eds.). (1984). *The end of an illusion: The future of health policy in western industrialized nations*. Berkeley, CA: University of California Press.

De Miguel, S. (1975). A framework for the study of national health systems. *Inquiry, 12,* 10.

Department of Health and Social Security (DHHS). (1976). *Sharing resources for health in England: Report of the resource allocation working party*. London: Her Majesty's Stationery Office.

Department of Health and Social Security (1989). *Working for patients*. London: Her Majesty's Stationery Office.

Dobson, F. (1999). Modernizing Britain's national health service. *Health Affairs, 18*(3), 40–41.

Dumbaugh, K., & Neuhauser, D. (1979). International comparisons of health services: Where are we? *Social Science and Medicine, 221,* 13B.

Ellencweig, A. (1992). *Analyzing health systems: A modular approach*. New York: Oxford University Press.

Elling, R., & Kerr, H. (1975). Selection of contrasting national health systems for in-depth study. *Inquiry,* (Suppl. 12), 2.

Evans, R. G. (1984). *Strained mercy: The economics of Canadian health care*. Toronto: Butterworths.

Evans, R. G. (1992). Canada: The real issues. *Journal of Health Policy, Politics and Law, 17,* 739–762.

Evans, R. G. (2000). Canada. *Journal of Health Politics, Policy and Law, 25*(5), 890–897.

Field, M. (1973). The concept of "health system" at the macrosociological level. *Social Science and Medicine, 7*, 763–785.

Field, M. G. (1978). *Comparative health systems: Differentiation and convergence.* Final report under Grant no. HS-00272. Rockville, MD: National Center for Health Services Research.

Fox, D. (1986). *Health policies, health politics.* Princeton, NJ: Princeton University Press.

Glaser, W. (1970). *Paying the doctor: Systems of remuneration and their effects.* Baltimore: Johns Hopkins University Press.

Glaser, W. (1978). *Health insurance bargaining: Foreign lessons for Americans.* New York: Gardner Press.

Glaser, W. (1987). *Paying the hospital.* San Francisco: Jossey-Bass.

Glaser, W. (1991). *Health insurance in practice: International variations in financing, benefits, and problems.* San Francisco: Jossey-Bass.

Griffiths, R. (1983). *NHS management inquiry.* London: Department of Health and Social Security.

Himmelstein, D., & Woolhandler, S. (1989). A national health program for the United States: A physician's proposal. *New England Journal of Medicine, 320,* 102–108.

Hirschman, A. (1970). *Exit, voice and loyalty.* Cambridge, MA: Harvard University Press.

Holliday, I. (1992). *The NHS transformed.* Manchester, UK: Baseline Books.

Hollingsworth, J. (1986). *A political economy of medicine: Great Britain and the United States.* Baltimore: Johns Hopkins University Press.

Klass, O. (1985). Explaining America and the welfare state: An alternative theory. *British Journal of Political Science, 15,* 427–450.

Klein, R. (1995). *The new politics of the NHS* (3rd ed.). London: Longman.

Klein, R. (1998). Why Britian is reorganizing its national health service—yet again? *Health Affairs, 17*(4), 111–125.

Kondro, W. (2000). Canada's ministers agree on health package. *The Lancet, 356*(9234), 1011.

Leichter, H. (1979). *A comparative approach to policy analysis: Health care policy in four nations.* Cambridge: Cambridge University Press.

Le Pen, C., & Rodwin, V. (1996). Le plan Juppe: Vers un nouveau mode de regulation des soins. *Droit Social, 9*(10).

Le Grand, J. (1999). Competition, cooperation, or control? Tales from the British National Health Service. *Health Affairs, 18*(3), 27–39.

Marmor, T. R., Bridges, A., & Hoffman, W. (1978). Comparative politics and health policies: Notes on benefits, costs, limits. In D. Ashford (Ed.), *Comparing public policies* (pp. 59–80). Beverly Hills, CA: Sage.

Maynard, A. (1986). *Annual report on the National Health Service.* New York: Center for Health Economics.

Mechanic, D. (1976). The comparative study of health care delivery systems. In D. Mechanic (Ed.), *The growth of bureaucratic medicine: An inquiry into the dynamics of patient behavior* (pp. 23–43). New York: John Wiley.

Ministry of Health. (1996). *Comptes nationaux de la santé.* Paris: Author.

Naylor, C. (1999). Health care in Canada: Incrementalism under fiscal duress. *Health Affairs, 18*(3), 9–26.

Organization for Economic Cooperation and Development (OECD). (2000). *HealthData.* Paris: Author.

Organization for Economic Cooperation and Development. (1992). *The reform of health care: A comparative analysis of seven OECD countries* (p. 116). Paris: Author.

Reinhardt, U., Marmor, T. R., Durham, A., Davis, K., & Blumenthal, D. (1985). Hard choices in health care: A matter of ethics. In L. Etheredge et al. (Eds.), *Health care: How to improve it and pay for it* (pp. 19–31). Washington, DC: Center for National Policy.

Rodwin, V. (1984). *The health planning predicament: France, Quebec, England and the United States.* Berkeley, CA: University of California Press.

Rodwin, V. (1989a). New ideas for health policy in France, Canada, and Britain. In M. Field (Ed.), *Success and crisis in national health systems: A comparative approach* (pp. 265–285). New York: Routledge.

Rodwin, V. (1989b). Physician payment reform: Lessons from abroad. *Health Affairs, 9*(1), 76–83.

Rodwin, V. (1997). The rise of managed care in the United States: Lessons for French health policy. In C. Altenstetter & J. Bjorkman (Eds.), *Health policy reform, national variations and globalization* (pp. 39–58). New York: St. Martin's Press.

Rodwin, V., & Brecher, C. (1992). Comparative analysis and mutual learning. In V. Rodwin et al. (Eds.), *Public hospital systems in New York and Paris* (pp. 3–8). New York: New York University Press.

Rodwin, V., & Sandier, S. (1993). Health care under French national health insurance: A public-private mix, low prices and high volumes. *Health Affairs, 12*(3), 110–131.

Roemer, M. (1977). *Comparative national policies health care.* New York: Marcel Dekker.

Rosner, D. (1982). Health care for the "truly needy": Nineteenth-century origins of the concept. *Milbank Memorial Fund Quarterly: Health and Society, 60*(Summer), 355.

Smee, C. (2000). United Kingdom. *Journal of Health Politics, Policy and Law, 25*(5), 945–951.

Smith, S., Heffler, S., & Freeland, M. (1999). The next decade of health spending. *Health Affairs, 18*(4), 86–95.

Stoddard, D. (1984, May). *Rationalizing the health care system.* Paper presented at the Ontario Council Conference, Toronto, Ontario, Canada.

Stone, D. (1981). Drawing lessons from comparative health research. In R. A. Straetz, M. Lieberman, & A. Sardell (Eds.), *Critical issues in health policy* (pp. 135–148). Lexington, MA: D.C. Heath and Co.

Teune, H. (1978). The logic of comparative policy analysis. In D. Ashford (Ed.), *Comparing public policies.* Beverly Hills, CA: Sage Publications.

Townsend, P., & Davidson, N. (Eds.). (1982). *Inequalities in health: The Black report.* London: Penguin.

Weinerman, R. (1971). Research on comparative health systems. *Medical Care, 11*(9), 3.

World Health Organization (WHO) (2000). *The world health report 2000. Health systems: Improving performance.* Geneva: Author. (Available: whr@who.int).

SUGGESTED READINGS ON COMPARATIVE HEALTH SYSTEMS AND POLICY

Altenstetter, C., & Bjorkman, J. (Eds.). (1997). *Health policy reform, national variations and globalization.* New York: St. Martin's Press.

Anderson, O. (1989). *The health services continuum in democratic states.* Ann Arbor, MI: Health Administration Press.

Bennett, A., & Adams, O. (1993). *Looking north: What can we learn from Canada's health care system?* San Francisco: Jossey-Bass.

Comparative health policy [Special issue]. (1992). *Journal of Health Policy, Politics and Law, 17*(Winter).

Ellencweig, A. (1992). *Analyzing health systems: A modular approach.* New York: Oxford University Press.

Field, M. (Ed.). (1989). *Success and crisis in national health systems.* New York: Routledge.

Graig, L. (1993). *Health of nations: An international perspective on U.S. health care reform.* Washington, DC: Congressional Quarterly Press.

Hurst, J. (1992). *The reform of health care: A comparative analysis of seven OECD countries.* Paris: Organization for Economic Cooperation and Development (OECD).

Investing in health: World bank development report. (1993). Washington, DC: World Bank.

Jerôme-Forget, M., White, J., & Weiner, J. (Eds.). (1995). *Health care reform through internal markets: Experience and proposals.* Washington, DC: Brookings Institute for Research on Public Policy.

Lassey, M., Lassey, W., & Jinks, M. (1997). *Health care systems around the world.* Upper Saddle River, NJ: Prentice Hall.

Merrill, J. (1994). *The road to health care reform.* New York: Plenum.

Organization for Economic Cooperation and Development (OECD). (1990). *Health care systems in transition: The search for efficiency.* Paris: Author.

OECD. (1992). *The reform of health care: A comparative analysis of seven OECD countries.* Paris: Author.

OECD. (1993). *Health systems: The socioeconomic environment (statistical references).* Paris: Author.

OECD. (1994). *Health: Quality and choice.* Paris: Author.

OECD. (1995a). *New directions in health policy.* Paris: Author.

OECD. (1995b). *Internal markets in the making: Health systems in Canada, Iceland and the United Kingdom.* Paris: Author.

OECD. (1996). *Health care reform: The will to change.* Paris: Author.

Payer, L. (1996). *Medicine and culture: Varieties of treatment in the United States, England, West Germany and France.* New York: Henry Holt, Owl Book Edition.

Pursuit of health systems reform (Special issue). (1991). *Health Affairs, 10*(Fall).

Raffel, M. (Ed.). (1997). *Health care reform in industrial countries.* University Park, PA: Pennsylvania State University Press.

Roemer, M. (1991). *National health systems of the world* (Vols. 1 and 2). New York: Oxford University Press.

Saltman, R. (Ed.). (1988). *The international handbook of health systems.* New York: Greenwood Press.

Saltman, R., & Von Otter, C. (1995). *Implementing planned markets in health care.* Bristol, PA: Open University Press.

Wall, A. (Ed.) (1996). *Health care systems in liberal democracies.* London: Routledge.

White, J. (1995). *Competing solutions: American health care proposals and international experience.* Washington, DC: Brookings Institution.

II

Settings

Part II, "Settings," is divided into six chapters, detailing hospitals and health systems, ambulatory care, long-term care, mental health services, drugs, and managed care. Settings are places where health care is provided. (Obviously, drugs are provided in various settings.) Integrated health care systems provide or arrange for care that includes all these settings, but more commonly care and payment for care is fragmented across settings such as hospitals, clinics, nursing homes, mental health centers, drugstores, and HMOs.

In chapter 6, Kovner explains how hospitals have developed in the United States and have increasingly become part of health systems. He differentiates among some important types of hospitals. Next he reviews hospital organizational structure and public and payer concerns with hospital cost and quality. Finally, he focuses upon new developments in hospital operations to include multiunit structures, clinical quality improvement, patient-focused care, restructuring, and hospital community benefit programs.

In chapter 7, Mezey reviews what is meant by ambulatory care and presents ambulatory care statistics. He describes how and where primary care is delivered, and how the delivery of primary care is changing in the face of managed care. In chapter 8, Feldman, Nadash, and Gurson define the key components of long-term care and discuss the factors that contribute to need and demand for service. They distinguish among the principal paid providers of long-term care and the populations they serve. Finally, the authors identify the major cost, quality, and access issues in long-term care, and discuss the strengths and weaknesses of alternative policy options.

In chapter 9, Sharfstein, Stoline, and Koran present definitions and an overview of mental disorders. They identify highlights in the development of the American mental health care system, and describe the key mental health professionals and their roles in the system. They analyze trends of the various settings for mental health care in use over time, and identify financing differences between general medical and mental health care.

In chapter 10, Strongin identifies the characteristics of the American pharmaceutical industry. She describes the approval process for a new drug. Next she analyzes pharmaceutical marketplace dynamics and the growth of prescription drug expenditures. In chapter 11, Smits identifies the causes of the growth of managed care in the United States. She describes the current impact of managed care on the health insurance marketplace, and distinguishes the major organizational types of managed care plans. Smits describes the use of "at-risk" subcontractors such as pharmacy benefits managers and managed mental health companies. She describes what large purchasers want and expect from managed care plans, analyzes current efforts to monitor plan quality, and discusses the issues of public policy and of health care markets that will drive the evolution of HMOs and managed care in the future.

6

Hospitals

Anthony R. Kovner

LEARNING OBJECTIVES

- ☐ Identify how hospitals have developed in the U.S.
- ☐ Differentiate among some important different types of hospitals.
- ☐ Understand public and payer concerns with the cost and quality of hospital care.
- ☐ Describe the organizational structure of hospitals and how physicians relate to them.
- ☐ Analyze the challenges facing hospitals and hospital responses to these challenges.

TOPICAL OUTLINE

Historical development
Hospital statistics and characteristics
Payer and public concerns with costs and quality
Hospital organizational structure
New developments in hospital organization
Organizational challenges and response
Conclusions

KEY WORDS

acute care, alliances, average daily census, clinical quality improvement, community benefit programs, continuous quality improvement (CQI), full-time equivalents (FTEs), hospitals, investor-owned hospitals, Joint

Commission on the Accreditation of Healthcare Organizations (JCAHO), medical staff organization, multiunit organizations, networks, organizational structure, ownership, patient-focused care, public hospitals, quality, rural hospitals, scope of services, systems, teaching hospitals, utilization

Smith and Kaluzny (1986) have characterized the health care system as a white labyrinth "so large, complex and subtle that it defies description." To many Americans, hospitals are just such white labyrinths. People often know little about how their local hospital or hospital system functions, and even those who work in hospitals often know little about the departments, occupations, or facilities in the system, other than their own. And hospitals, like other local organizations, open, grow, merge, and close.

In the 23 years that have spanned the seven editions of this book, the editors have struggled with ways to organize the materials by chapter. An example of a problem encountered would be whether mental hospitals be discussed in the "Mental Health" chapter or in this one. Hospitals provide "Ambulatory Care" (the title of another chapter). Also, many hospitals own a variety of long-term care facilities (the title of yet another chapter) ranging from nursing homes and subacute facilities to home care agencies and day care programs. Inpatient medical care doesn't warrant a chapter by itself. But the hospital and its culture remains a dominant one in health care delivery. Hospitals consume a smaller percentage of the health care dollar than they did in 1976, and inpatient utilization has decreased, but hospitals remain central to health care delivery and have grown into systems of many hospitals; and some systems are vertically integrated, to include facilities other than hospitals. These systems remained, for the most part, as of 2000, dominated by hospital culture, ownership, and control.

This chapter surveys the following topics concerning hospitals and hospital systems: (a) historical development; (b) statistics and characteristics; (c) concerns about hospital cost and quality; (d) organizational structure; and (e) challenges and responses. The primary focus remains on acute, short-term, general hospitals and hospital systems.

HISTORICAL DEVELOPMENT[1]

The development of American hospitals and hospital systems can be divided into five periods:

1. The beginning, before 1870.
2. The first period of rapid growth, 1870–1910.

---

[1] The Historical Development section of this chapter, through 1980, remains in large part the same as in the first and second editions and was authored by M. Enright and S. Jonas.

3. The first period of consolidation, 1910–1945.
4. The second period of rapid growth, 1945–1980.
5. The second period of consolidation, 1980–2000+.

The first hospitals were primarily of a religious and charitable nature, tending to provide care for the sick rather than providing for medical cure (Freymann, 1974; Rosenberg, 1987; Starr, 1982). In the American colonies, the earliest hospitals were actually infirmaries in poorhouses. Private voluntary hospitals (those provided or supported by community leaders) in the United States date back to the 18th century (Freymann, 1974). These institutions cared for the poor: Since hospitals could provide little effective medical treatment, there was no reason for doctors to use them for paying patients. By 1873, there were an estimated 178 such hospitals in the United States (Stevens, 1971).

From 1870 to 1910, as biomedical science and technology developed effective means of intervention, hospitals evolved into local physicians' workshops for all types and classes of patients. More effective hospital care was achieved primarily through advances in hygiene, including the development of trained nurses and techniques for asepsis and surgical anesthesia. Between 1870 and 1910 there was a period of spectacular growth, with the number of hospitals increasing from 178 in 1873, to more than 4,300 in 1909 (Stevens, 1971). Medical care became too complex for physicians to carry their entire armamentarium in their little black bags; special equipment and consultation with other medical specialists became essential.

According to Starr (1982), voluntary and public hospitals were established during the period of 1750 to 1850. From 1850 to 1890, many new hospitals were formed to meet the needs of specific religious or ethnic groups, or to specialize in the treatment of certain diseases or categories of patients, such as children and women. For-profit hospitals owned by physicians grew rapidly during the period of 1890 to 1920. Fewer new hospitals were built during 1910 through 1945 than during the periods before and after.

The types of patients in hospitals changed with medical discoveries. In 1923, the discovery of insulin drastically changed the character of diabetes treatment. Liver extract reduced the incidence of pernicious anemia in 1929. Sulfonamides began to affect treatment of pneumonia and some other infectious diseases in 1935, a trend that accelerated with the widespread use of antibiotics beginning in 1943, as well as the continuing development of immunization techniques. The development of rehabilitation services began to bring more disabled patients to the hospital. In the 1950s, hospitals increasingly treated chronic illness. As infectious diseases generally have been conquered (with the exception of HIV/AIDS), hospitals have increasingly focused on the pathology of trauma and degenerative and neoplastic disease.

The fourth period, 1945 to 1980, was a second major growth era for hospitals. It was marked by a tremendous increase in hospital services, costs, and technology and by a more modest expansion in the number of hospitals. Many small rural hospitals were built during this period, financed by federal monies under the Hill-Burton Act. A major factor influencing the increased breadth and intensity of inpatient hospital services was the rapid growth of hospital insurance. The Blue Cross system was originally developed during the Great Depression in order to assure payment to hospitals. Hospital insurance developed rapidly during World War II as a result of collective bargaining agreement. During this period, the federal government limited wage increases to workers but not fringe benefits. Finally, in 1965, Medicare and Medicaid programs were created, the former providing health insurance for the elderly and the latter providing health care benefits for the poor.

Since 1980, hospital occupancy rates have decreased for a smaller number of hospitals with less total beds. There has been an emergence in the industry of hospital systems, networks, and alliances, some of which are quite large, most particularly in local markets. In some cities, 40 or more independent hospitals have been collapsed into three or four competing health systems. At the same time, hospital services other than inpatient care have expanded rapidly. Such services include chronic care and ambulatory care, often with satellite sites dispersed over a wide geographic area.

HOSPITAL STATISTICS AND CHARACTERISTICS

Hospitals can be differentiated by capacity, utilization and ownership, and by scope of services and types of patients served.

Capacity, Utilization, and Ownership

Table 6.1 provides summary statistics on general acute care hospitals, and some key facts on size, utilization, employment, and expenditures. Hospitals other than general acute care include governmental mental health and long-term hospitals, of which there were 1,218 in 1998 (American Hospital Association [AHA], 2000). Acute care[2] hospitals admitted more than 31.8 million patients in 1998, with an average length of stay of 6 days. On any day, there was an average of almost 525,000 patients hospitalized. These represent substantial decreases from 1983, as shown in Table 6.1 (AHA, 2000).

The number of acute care hospitals (see Table 6.1) decreased from 5,783 in 1983 to 5,015 in 1998 (AHA, 2000). Hospitals vary in size. In 1998, there

---

[2] Same as "community" hospitals; all nonfederal, short-term, general, and special hospitals whose facilities and services are available to the public. A short-term hospital is one in which the majority of its patients are admitted to units where the average length of stay is less than 30 days (AHA, 2000).

TABLE 6.1   Acute Care Hospital Facts

Parameters	1983	1998
Total number of hospitals	5,783	5,015
Beds (thousands)	1,018	840
Patient Admissions (thousands)	36,152	31,812
Births (thousands)	3,490	3,726
Outpatients (thousands)	210,044	474,193
Average Length of Stay (days)	7.6	6.0
Average Daily Census (thousands)	749	525
FTEs (per 100 adjusted census)	358	468
Expenses (adjusted per inpatient day)	$369.49	$1,066.96

Adapted from: American Hospital Association. (2000). *Hospital Statistics.* Chicago, IL: Author.

were 1,193 hospitals of less than 50 beds and 254 acute care hospitals of 500 beds or more (AHA, 2000). Acute care hospitals employed 3.8 million full-time equivalent (FTE) staff in 1998. Acute care hospital expenditures in 1998 totaled $318.8 billion. Most acute hospitals are under nonprofit ownership, as shown in Table 6.2. (See also chapter 13 regarding governance and management.) Ownership patterns have not changed significantly during the last 15 years.

Scope of Services and Some Types of Acute Care Hospitals

Hospitals differ from one another with respect to size, mission, ownership, scope and complexity of services, competitive environment, population served, financial condition, participation in systems, networks and alliances, efficiency, and quality. For example, with regard to scope of services, according to the *AHA Guide* (AHA, 1999), Nor-Lea Hospital in Lovington, New Mexico had 28 beds and provided the following services: CT scanner, emergency department, health fair, home health services, hospice, outpatient care, nutrition programs, occupational health services, outpatient surgery, social work services, and ultrasound (AHA, 1999). Montefiore Medical Center in New York City had 1,032 beds and was listed as providing all the services that Nor-Lea provided. In addition, Montefiore provided alcoholism services, angioplasty, birthing room, breast cancer screening, cardiac catheterization, cardiac intensive care, case management, children wellness program, community health status assessment and service planning, community outreach, dental services, diagnostic radioisotope, drug abuse and outpatient services, lithotripter, freestanding outpatient center, geriatric, health information, health screenings, HIV/AIDS services, magnetic resonance imaging, medical surgical intensive care, neonatal intensive care, obstetrics, oncology, open heart surgery, patient education center, patient representative services, physical rehabilitation (inpatient and outpatient), positron emission tomography scanner, primary care department,

TABLE 6.2   Acute Care Hospital Ownership

Ownership	1983	1998
Nonprofit	3,347	3,026
State and Local Government	1,679	1,218
Investor-Owned	757	771

Adapted from: AHA. (2000). *Hospital Statistics.* Chicago, IL: Author.

psychiatric services (inpatient, child adolescent, consultation liaison, education, emergency, geriatric, outpatient, partial hospitalization), radiation therapy, reproductive health services, single photon emission computerized tomography, skilled nursing, sports medicine, support groups, teen outreach services, volunteer services, and women's health center/services (AHA, 1999).

Hospitals are similar to one another in that they provide inpatient care by nurses and physicians, the latter having a great deal of autonomy in deciding whom to admit and what services patients should receive. Over the long run, hospitals have to be financially solvent. Nearly all hospitals endeavor to survive and grow. Hospitals provide services every day and at every hour of the day. Some hospital services are difficult to quantify and measure; for example, how can one measure the amount of health education services a patient receives? But all hospitals must be organized so that standby capacity is available to meet medical emergencies and to deal with critical and life-threatening situations. Hospitals are characterized by hierarchy and rules. There is increasing standardization of patient care. And there is overall agreement about the principal objectives of hospitals: curing and caring.

Some Important Types of Hospitals

Teaching Hospitals

In 1997, there were 277 nonfederal, short-term, general hospitals belonging to the Council of Teaching Hospitals and Health Systems (COTH) of the Association of American Medical Colleges. These COTH hospitals (such as Montefiore Medical Center referred to previously) represent 6% of all hospitals. Relative to other hospitals, COTH hospitals are larger and are located in large, urban areas. They offer more specialized services and provide more uncompensated care than nonCOTH hospitals. Although COTH hospitals represent only 6% of the nation's hospitals, in 1997, 22% of the nation's total outpatient visits were to COTH hospitals, as well as 20% of the total surgical operations. COTH hospitals employed 25% of the total FTEs for all hospitals in 1997 (American Association of Medical Colleges [AAMC], personal communication, 1999).

Because of their commitment to the triad of teaching hospital missions—education, research, and patient care—COTH members also offer a large percentage of tertiary or highly complex services. For example, in

1997, 94% of COTH members reported having a cardiac catheterization lab (vs. 33% for nonCOTH members); 85% reported a megavoltage radiation facility (only 47% for nonCOTH hospitals); and 65% of COTH institutions reported the capability to perform kidney transplants (only 5% of nonCOTH hospitals reported the capability to perform kidney transplants).

In 1997, COTH members comprised 6% of the nation's short-term nonfederal hospitals, but claimed 44% of the total deductions for charity care (approximately $6.7 billion) and 26% of the deductions for bad debt (approximately $4.5 billion) (AAMC, personal communication, 1999). For more information about COTH, see http://www.aamc.org.

Networks, Systems, and Alliances

The AHA defines networks, systems, and alliances as follows. A network is defined as a group of hospitals, physicians, other providers, insurers, and/or community agencies that work together to deliver health services. A system includes both multihospitals (two or more hospitals owned, leased, sponsored, or contract managed by a central organization) and diversified single hospitals. The latter are defined as bringing into membership three or more nonhospital organizations, and at least 25%, of their owned and leased nonhospital pre-acute and post-acute health care organizations. An alliance is defined as a formal organization, usually owned by shareholders/members, that works on behalf of its individual members in the provision of services and products and in the promotion of activities and ventures (AHA, 1999). As of 1998, the AHA registered 2,176 acute care hospitals as being in health systems, 1,380 in networks, and 2,778 in group purchasing organizations (the dominant kind of alliance). The same hospitals can be registered in more than one category (AHA, 2000).

An example of a large nonprofit hospital that is part of a network, a system, and an alliance, is the Henry Ford Health System (HFHS) of Detroit, Michigan. By 1999, HFHS was a $1.9 billion corporation, with 17,550 employees serving almost 20% of the Detroit metropolitan area population. It included 6 hospitals and 34 outpatient care sites. HFHS had affiliations with six medical schools and had 1,500 research projects with $40 million in grant funding. HFHS was the sixth largest employer in Michigan (http://www.henryfordhealth.org).

Premier is an example of a hospital alliance formed for group purchasing and other activities, and represents, as of 1999, 215 owners and 950 other affiliated hospitals, and the 1,830 hospitals and health care facilities they operate. Premier's total purchasing volume reached $8.5 billion in 1998 (http://www.premierinc.com).

Public Hospitals

Public hospitals are owned by agencies of federal, state, and local government. Federal hospitals historically have been designed for special beneficiaries:

American Indians, merchant seamen, military personnel, and veterans. State hospitals typically have provided long-term psychiatric and chronic care, especially for patients with tuberculosis in the past. There are also state university or teaching hospitals that provide short-term general acute care. An example of a public hospital system is the Veteran's Administration (VA), one of the nation's largest health care systems. As of 1999, the VA had 172 hospitals, 551 outpatient clinics, 131 nursing homes, 40 domiciliaries, 206 counseling centers, and 215,468 employees. These facilities serve more than 10% of the total veteran population each year (http://www.va.gov).

There are two main types of acute care public hospitals. The first type has similar characteristics to smaller nonprofit hospitals, is located in small towns or cities of moderate size, is used by private attending physicians, and serves paying and indigent patients.

The second type is located in major urban areas. Physician staff are mostly salaried resident physicians in training. Hospital deficits are paid by taxes. As of 1998, there were 1,218 state and local government general and other special hospitals with a total of 139,355 beds (AHA, 2000). These 1,218 hospitals (24% of all acute care hospitals) provided 16.6% of the acute care hospital beds, 14.3% of the inpatient admissions, and 16.9% of the outpatient visits (AHA, 2000).

Rural Hospitals

Rural areas are areas falling outside a metropolitan statistical area, which is defined as containing a city with a population of at least 50,000 or an urban area with a population of at least 50,000 and a total metropolitan population of 100,000 (AHA, 1992). In 1998, 2,199 (43.8%) of the nation's hospitals were rural; 72.7% of these hospitals had fewer than 100 beds (AHA, 2000).

Between 1982 and 1997, admissions to rural hospitals dropped from 8.3 million to 5.1 million, a 39% decline. Between 1980 and 1990, 280 rural community hospitals stopped providing inpatient acute health services (AHA, 1992). Key problems of rural hospitals include threat of closure, thereby depriving local residents of access to care; the questionable financial viability of hospitals with fewer than 50 beds; difficulties in assuring quality of care in such hospitals when operated as independent units; and difficulties in attracting skilled professionals to work in isolated rural localities. Rural American counties face different kinds of problems depending on economic structure. Although they are often thought to consist of farm areas, rural counties can be classified as economically dependent on farming; manufacturing; mining, oil, and energy; large, governmental installations; federal lands; and retirement settlement communities, or characterized by persistent poverty (AHA, 1988).

To survive in more competitive hospital markets, rural hospitals have undertaken a variety of innovative measures. According to the AHA rural hospital assessment (1988), rural hospitals have tried to increase patient volume by introducing or expanding ambulatory or long-term services;

and many have sought to expand technological capabilities, increase referrals, or reduce costs through shared service or networking arrangements and consolidation activities.

PAYER AND PUBLIC CONCERNS WITH COSTS AND QUALITY

Hospital care is big business. In 1998 hospital acute and long-term expenditures amounted to $382.8 billion, representing 33% of the nation's health expenditures and 4.5% of the nation's gross national product, or $1,362 per American (Levit et al., 2000). Hospital expenditures have been growing slowly during the past few years and the hospital share of national health spending has been growing only modestly. Costs for a day of hospital care are very expensive and increasingly so, typically over $1,000 per day, and over 40 million Americans lack insurance or other coverage to pay these bills. Health plans, government, and commercial payers want to contain these costs.

What Does a Hospital Stay Cost Payers?

In a response to what are typical hospital charges for a long-stay inpatient, a financial manager of a large urban hospital abstracted four "typical bills," ranging from $42,612 to $76,574. A breakdown of hospital charges for the least expensive of these four, "Mrs. L" is shown in Table 6.3. This is a bill for a female inpatient, age 58, treated for simple pneumonia/pleurisy, who expired in the hospital after a stay of 25 days.

This case is at a large hospital, where charges are not among the highest in the city. Questions can be raised as to whether all of the services the patient received were necessary, and whether they could have been provided more cheaply, and whether Mrs. L's admission was necessary, although there is no reason to think other than that the services received were necessary and provided at reasonable cost, and that the admission and length of stay were justified. Private and governmental payers have responded to these charges by establishing fixed payments based on the type of case or the length of the patient's stay in the hospital.

Hospitals As Employers

The impact of hospitals on local economies can be very important. In small communities, hospital closure can remove a vital source of local employment and revenues to local hospital suppliers. Construction of a hospital means numerous jobs for construction workers and future hospital employees. Unions have a vital interest in continuing employment for their members, so it is no wonder that they, together with hospital associations and others, lobby vigorously not only against hospital closings, but also at

TABLE 6.3   Breakdown of Charges Rendered to "Mrs. L" During 25-day Hospitalization

	Charges for 1999
Room and Board	$26,050
Laboratory	1,631
Therapy	425
Drugs	9,222
X-Ray	4,575
Blood Service	262
EKG, EEG, etc.	67
Miscellaneous	380
Total	$42,612

Source: Valentine, R., personal communication (1999). Lutheran Medical Center.

the state level for governmental payment for the costs of charity care, bad debts, and graduate medical education, and push for increasing eligibility for Medicaid and Child Health coverage.

Concerns about the quality of hospital care have also become a national issue (see Kohn, Corrigan, and Donaldson, 1999). Quality is discussed at length in chapter 14. Because of the seriousness of the consequences of poor quality care in the hospital, this is of great concern to all Americans who may be admitted in any year or whose family or friends may be admitted. Hospital spokesmen may maintain that it is perhaps hard to believe that quality is as high as it is, given that hospitals are open 7 days a week, 365 days a year, while individual caregivers only work 40 hours a week, 48 weeks a year. Care is often very complex and requires teams of caregivers, including many physicians who are not salaried and spend most of their time away from the unit in which their patient is being treated. Chassin (1998) suggests that there are three main reasons for quality problems:

1. Overuse, providing a health service when its risk of harm exceeds its potential benefit.
2. Underuse, failing to provide an effective service when it would have produced favorable outcomes.
3. Misuse, avoidable complications of appropriate health care.

An example of overuse is unnecessary surgery. Underuse, for instance, is lack of access to needed care because of lack of health insurance. An example of misuse would be mistakes in medication distribution and use.

Leape (1994) argues there is much that physicians and nurses could learn from aviation, where designing for safety has led to an industry—which although highly complicated and risky—seems far safer. Leape suggests building in multiple safety checks, standardizing procedures, and institutionalizing safety. He suggests that hospital risk management activities should include all potentially injurious errors and seek out underlying system failures. Leape, like Berwick (1989), suggests focusing on system improvements rather than blaming individual providers.

Quality can be subdivided into two categories: technical medical quality and service quality. Technical quality would include proper diagnosis and treatment. Service quality would include patient convenience and control of medical treatment. Service quality considerations include patient understanding of treatment options and compliance regimens, patient choice of caregiver, relief from pain, and a quiet and clean hospital environment. (See Kenagy, Berwick, & Shore, 1999.)

HOSPITAL ORGANIZATIONAL STRUCTURE

The principal departments of the acute care hospital are medical and dental, nursing, other diagnostic and therapeutic support, financial, personnel, and hotel services. Most hospitals provide services to inpatients who are admitted and assigned a bed, and to outpatients who come to an emergency department, an outpatient clinic, or satellite center, for a diagnostic or therapeutic service for a procedure not requiring admission.

Medical and Dental Department Organization

Physicians and dentists relate to hospitals in different ways. Attending physicians on the hospital staff who are not salaried often conduct much of their business in private offices that they own or rent. These physicians may admit patients to more than one hospital and may compete with the hospital for patients or customers. Other physicians may be salaried or paid by the hospital, according to the amount of hospital work they do. These physicians often see patients or provide diagnostic services in offices that are provided for them by the hospital. Some hospitals employ physicians to provide primary care in competition with other physicians who are attending physicians or local nonhospital-affiliated practitioners. Other hospitals contract with physician groups to provide emergency care or subspecialist services on hospital premises or in satellite centers. There are some attending physicians who maintain their own practices distinct from the hospital but who also receive a part-time salary from the hospital for administrative work.

When physicians admit patients to the hospital, in most instances they are free to order whatever tests or treatments they deem necessary. Thus the physician basically determines the amount of services used and the consequent costs of patient care. Physicians have every reason to want the best possible hospital setting in which to practice medicine, especially when it is provided at little personal cost to them.

Although the physician is technically a guest in the hospital, the hospital is responsible for the care its staff renders patients on a physician's orders. Once, hospitals could not be held liable for the wrongful conduct of a physician, but this principle has changed as a result of a series of judicial decisions (Southwick, 1978). Changing legal doctrines regarding negligence and corporate liability of hospitals have established that hospitals are legally responsible, and to the extent that hospital negligence is involved, financially responsible for the care provided by their entire professional staff, including physicians (Showalter, 1999).

Physicians are primarily organized along the lines of the medical specialties. The larger the hospital and hospital network, and the more specialized the medical services, the greater the number of separate medical departments. There is no universal logic to the way in which medical departments are categorized. Some are separated from others by type of skill involved, some by the age or sex of their main patient group, and some by the organ or organ system that they primarily diagnose and treat. Departments found in most hospitals include

1. *Internal medicine:* general diagnosis and therapy of adults for problems involving one or more internal organs or the skin, in which the principal tools do not involve a physical alteration of the patient's body by the physician.
2. *Surgery:* diagnosis and therapy in which the principal tools involve a physical alteration of a part of the patient's body by the physician.
3. *Pediatrics:* general diagnosis and therapy for children, primarily but not entirely with nonsurgical techniques.
4. *Obstetrics/gynecology:* diagnosis and therapy relating to the sexual and reproductive system of women, using both surgical and nonsurgical techniques.
5. *Psychiatry/neurology:* diagnosis and therapy for people of all ages with mental, emotional, and nervous system problems, using primarily nonsurgical techniques.
6. *Radiology/diagnostic imaging:* diagnosis and therapy, primarily through the use of X-ray and other internal imaging techniques.
7. *Pathology:* diagnosis, both before and after treatment.
8. *Anesthesiology:* principally concerned with preparing patients so that they may be surgically operated on with no pain or discomfort during the procedure.

Other general medical departments include family and emergency medicine. More subspecialized medical departments tend to be organized around organs and organ systems, for example, ophthalmology (eye); otolaryngology (ear, nose, and throat); urology (male sexual/reproductive system and the renal system for both males and females); orthopedics (bones and joints); and so on.

There are 23 medical specializations for which professional certification may be attained by passing a medical specialty board examination. Specialties other than the ones previously mentioned include allergy and immunology, proctology, dermatology, neurosurgery, nuclear medicine, physical medicine and rehabilitation, plastic surgery, preventive medicine, and thoracic surgery. There are clinicians other than physicians who also may be granted admitting privileges to a hospital; these include dentists and podiatrists.

Physicians and other clinicians practicing in hospitals have their own staff organization, with bylaws, rules, and regulations that must be approved by the hospital's governing board. Medical staff bylaws specify procedures for election of medical staff officers by membership. The officers are given authority under the bylaws to enforce rules and regulations. The officers delineate privileges and recommend disciplinary action when necessary, through the committee structure. They enforce the bylaws and must oversee the committee structure and submit reports of medical staff activities to the governing board.

There are numerous medical staff committees in the hospital, some of which may include nonphysicians, particularly nurses, as members. The executive committee, if there is one, coordinates all activity, sets general policies for the medical staff, and accepts and acts upon recommendations from the other medical staff committees. The joint conference committee, if there is one, acts as a liaison between the medical staff and the governing board in deliberations over matters involving medical and nonmedical considerations. The credentials committee reviews applications by physicians to join the medical staff and considers the qualifications of education, experience, and interests before making recommendations for appointment to the executive committee, which will then make recommendations for appointment to the governing board. In some hospitals the joint conference committee is also involved in the process.

Through the initiative of the Joint Commission on the Accreditation of Healthcare Organizations, the medical staff (and the board) are increasingly structured to place higher priority on clinical quality improvement and patient care outcomes. Medical staff committees can be structured in various ways to accomplish this purpose. Commonly, there is an overall medical staff committee concerned with clinical quality improvement, as well as various subcommittees such as infections control and quality improvement. In some cases what were formerly medical staff committees have become hospital-wide committees, as physicians and others have realized that improvement of clinical performance rests increasingly on teamwork of physicians and other clinicians and support staff and not on physicians alone.

The infections control committee is responsible for preventing infections in the hospital, through routine preventive surveillance, tracking down of outbreaks of infection, and education of hospital personnel. The pharmacy and therapeutics committee reviews pharmacological agents for inclusion in the list of drugs approved for use in the hospital. The tissue committee is responsible for ensuring quality control of surgery, principally by examining and evaluating bodily tissues removed during operations.

The medical records committee is responsible for certifying complete and clinically accurate documentation of the care given to patients. This committee also acts as a judge of clinical care, based on the written record. The utilization review committee evaluates the appropriateness of admissions and length of stay in the hospital and may review use of services and facilities for patients whose hospital care is paid by third parties.

The tissue, quality improvement, and utilization review committees provide for review of each physician's professional work by other physicians. As the hospital has become more complex, and medical practice more hospital-based and team-based, the practices of physicians have been subjected to more scrutiny. In many hospitals, the medical chain of authority exists side by side with an administrative chain. There are many areas of confused jurisdiction and overlapping or conflicting powers. Managers and physicians working together can attempt to integrate these hierarchies. Physicians are becoming more involved in hospital governing boards; boards of trustees are reviewing more closely the methods used to appoint physicians to hospital staff; and more full-time salaried physicians have been hired by hospitals, resulting in more direct physician-hospital reporting lines.

Because of the vested interests of various medical departments in a hospital, the addition of a full-time or part-time salaried chief of the medical staff and of medical departments can create latent or open conflict with trustees or management. To lessen controversy, in some hospitals appointments of chiefs are made for a specified time rather than for indefinite or lifetime tenure. As full-time chiefs of service become more common, many functions formerly handled by volunteer committees—such as quality improvement review, medical records, and continuing medical education—have been taken over by full-time paid employees.

Many hospitals have hired salaried medical directors and quality improvement review teams. As hospitals are made more accountable for alleged misconduct of attending physicians, much attention has been focused on the concept of due process. If a physician is to be deprived of his medical staff privileges, the process by which the decision is made must be able to stand up to the scrutiny of the courts (Southwick, 1978). Furthermore, many hospitals require physicians to have malpractice insurance as a condition of staff membership (Hollowell, 1978).

There were 92,992 resident physicians in training in American hospitals in 1998 (American Medical Association [AMA], 2000). The number of hospital-salaried physicians other than resident physicians has more than quadrupled, from 10,000 in 1963 to 59,956 in 1998 (AMA, 2000). Salaried physicians are employed by hospitals as chiefs of services, to supervise medical care in intensive care units, as hospitalists who manage the care of inpatients with specific diseases such as heart failure, as emergency department physicians, and in primary care. Attending physicians are affected by such hiring, as hospital-employed physicians may compete with them for patients, deny them medical staff privileges (particularly to physicians new to the community), more closely supervise their practices, and change a strictly clinical patient care orientation to more emphasis on teaching and research.

Models of Medical Services Organization

Shortell (1985) has conceptualized four different models of organization among physicians: traditional (departmental), divisional, independent-corporate, and parallel. Under the traditional model, while each department retains relevant medical specialists, it does not contain the support services required by the physician to provide care. These include nursing, housekeeping, dietary, and clerical staff. Figure 6.1 depicts a traditional hospital organizational chart, in which support services are organized separately from medical services. The medical staff's relationship to the hospital is indirect, as shown by the dotted line. Physicians are not a part of the hospital chain of command, as are nurses or assistant administrators. In hospitals this is referred to as a *dual authority structure* (Smith, 1955). Most physicians are not hospital employees. Many physicians do not see themselves as primarily responsible to hospital administration, but functioning rather as independent medical practitioners who must practice according to medical staff bylaws, rules, and regulations.

Shortell's second model of medical services organization, the divisional model, is characterized by the placement of functional support services within medical divisions, which are organized along departmental lines. Each division, such as medicine or physical medicine, includes many of the support services, like nursing and clerical (and sometimes dietary and medical records and other services), that it needs to do its tasks. Each medical division leader is responsible for management, including financial management, of both medical and support services. The Johns Hopkins Hospital in Baltimore, Maryland is organized along these lines (Heyssel, Gaintner, Kues, Jones, & Lipstein, 1984).

Under Shortell's third model, the independent-corporate model, the medical staff becomes a separate legal entity that negotiates with the hospital for its services in return for receiving support services. An independent group of physicians provides medical services to the hospital, under contract. A version of this type of organization is carried out by the Permanente medical groups, which have contractual relationships with the Kaiser Health Plan to form the Kaiser-Permanente medical care program, the nation's largest staff model health maintenance program.

Shortell's fourth model, the parallel model, involves the creation of a separate organization in order to conduct certain activities that are not handled well by the formal hospital organization. Certain physicians are selected to participate in a parallel organization for some percentage of their time, to work on important problems and report back to the formal structure. Some of these physicians would have positions in the formal

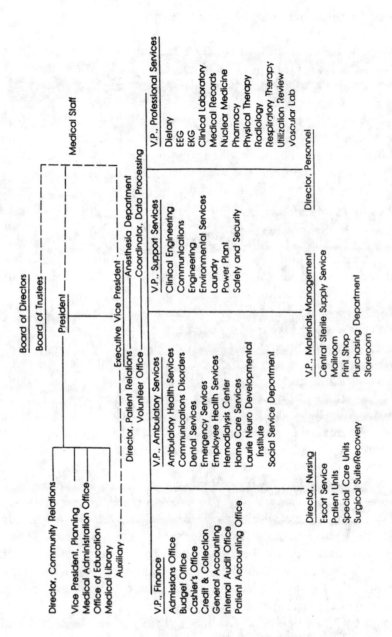

FIGURE 6.1   Traditional (departmental) organizational structure for hospital medical services.

structure as well. Shortell reports that parallel structures have been implemented at Saint Johns Hospital in Santa Monica, California, and at Fairfax Hospital in Virginia.

Other Patient Care Services

The functional divisions of the nursing service follow the patterns discussed in chapter 4. Hospital diagnostic and therapeutic services, which may or may not be attached to one of the medical departments, include laboratory, usually under the direction of the department of pathology; electrocardiography, usually a part of internal medicine; electroencephalography, part of neurology; radiography, part of radiology; pharmacy; clinical psychology; social service; inhalation therapy, often part of anesthesiology or pulmonary medicine; nutrition as therapy; physical, occupational, and speech therapy, often part of the department of rehabilitation medicine, if there is one; home care; and medical records, among others.

Hospital Administrative Structure

The nonclinical services that the hospital provides can be categorized into four subsystems: finance, facilities and equipment, human resources, and management. The financial subsystem includes capital, operating costs, and cash budgeting; pricing and cost allocation; long-range financial planning; and collection policies. In addition, some hospitals also have endowments to invest and grants to prepare and manage.

The facilities and equipment subsystem includes dietary, engineering, and environmental services; clinical engineering; power plant; grounds; housekeeping, communications and purchasing services; and storeroom, among others. The human resources system includes job analysis and description, job evaluation, wage and salary administration, recruitment, screening and selection, communication to employees, training and development, organizational development, collective bargaining, and labor contract administration. Finally, the management subsystem includes planning and marketing; community, patient, and public relations; data processing and management information systems; legal services; and compliance with regulations, among others.

Many of the services above, such as legal, or dietary, housekeeping or even information systems may be contracted out to large corporations such as national law firms, ServiceMaster, Aramark, and 3M Health Information Systems. The organizational structure for a multihospital system is more complex and comprises a central headquarters, sometimes an intermediate divisional organization, as well as the hospitals and other health care organizations, as shown in Figure 6.2.

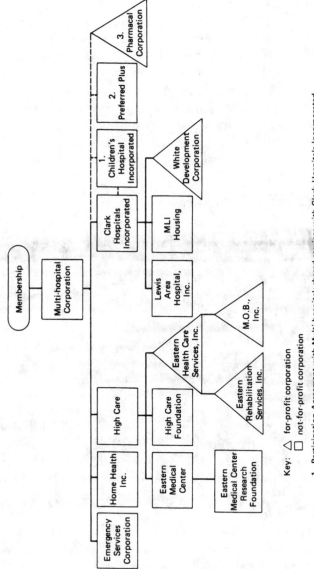

FIGURE 6.2 Multihospital system organizational chart.

Key: △ for-profit corporation
      ☐ not-for-profit corporation

1. Participation Agreement with Multi-hospital; shared services with Clark Hospitals Incorporated
2. Management Contract
3. Joint Venture with Bliss Corporation (Multi-hospital owns ½ of the stock).

New Developments in Hospital Organization

Over the last 5 years, there has been continued pressure on hospitals to contain costs, improve quality, and to justify resources used relative to contribution to community health. Hospitals have adapted to these pressures in many ways. In the 1990s, this includes multiunit organizations, clinical quality improvement, patient-focused care reorganization, and community health benefit programs.

Multiunit Organizations

There were 142 hospital mergers and acquisitions in 1999, involving 142 hospitals. There has been a steady decline in mergers and acquisitions since 1996, when there were 235 deals involving 768 hospitals (Bellandi, 2000). One of the most noteworthy mergers in 1999 was that of St. Louis-based Daughters of Charity National Health System and Sisters of St. Joseph Health System of Ann Arbor, Michigan, to create St. Louis-based Ascension Health. It is the nation's largest not-for-profit healthcare system, with more than $6 billion in revenues and 73 owned or affiliated hospitals (Bellandi, 2000). In 1999, 19 not-for-profit hospitals were purchased by for-profit hospitals. Columbia/HCA Healthcare Corporation, the largest for-profit, spun off 56 hospitals to two new companies, leaving Columbia with 207 hospitals (Bellandi, 2000).

According to Griffith (1999) there are two major forms of multiunit organization. His definition of "alliance" differs from that of the AHA. He defines alliances as separately owned organizations entering into inter-organizational relations primarily for strategic purposes, such as referring patients to each other for services the respective parties do not provide themselves. The participants remain under separate ownership. Multi-corporate organizations are merged organizations with unified ownership. Griffith distinguishes three types of multi-corporate organizations: *parent-subsidiary*, such as an owned foundation dedicated to a specific activity; *holding company*, which retains certain central control but encourages flexibility to companies owned such as hospitals with protected assets and tax advantages; and *joint venture*, which is two or more parent corporations invest in a subsidiary, such as a physician-hospital organization.

Mount Sinai NYU Health is an example of a vertically integrated not-for-profit holding company serving the greater New York City area. It includes ambulatory care, hospitals, and employed and affiliated physician groups. It is centralized, as mission, plans, and CEO financial and acquisition powers are reserved as the parent company's. Local units have separate boards but their strategic authority is limited.

There is a lot of controversy concerning the advantages and disadvantages of large multi-corporate organizations. The advantages behind their formation—to increase volume, cost savings, and greater leverage in bargaining with managed care organizations—have as yet not been proven. Another advantage is said to be improved quality of care resulting from standardization and specialized expertise. Those hospitals remaining independent can argue with some justification that when the advocates of merged multicorporate organizations have not achieved the success that they had argued would occur, the advocates have changed the criteria for success. When mergers occur among for-profit corporations they are usually accompanied by considerable downsizing, on the order of thousands of employees. This has largely not occurred, for whatever reasons, in health care.

Continuous Quality Improvement

Continuous quality improvement (CQI), also called total quality management (TQM), is a concept which has been applied for many years in American business, particularly in response to widespread Japanese implementation of CQI ideas developed by such Americans as Deming (1986), Juran (1964), and Crosby (1979). The basic approach is to measure variation in a work process in relation to a standard, and then to implement programs to decrease process variation and improve performance results.

CQI begins with a definition of what the quality standard is for a particular process, such as a hospital infection rate. Focus is on the consumer of the product or service, where this is a doctor who wishes quick turnaround in X-ray reports, or a patient or a potential patient seeking a diagnosis or a cure. Everyone who provides the product or service becomes involved in understanding how quality is measured and in discussing how to improve quality. Rather than focusing on poor quality outcomes and how to avoid them, the work team becomes involved in setting continuously improving standards for better performance and in finding ways to meet those standards. (See chapter 14 for a further discussion of what is done in hospitals to improve quality.)

The benefits of CQI can perhaps best be understood by comparing CQI with traditional organizations, in which managers are in charge, focus is on production and slogans, and emphasis is placed on getting the work done in the cheapest way, assuming given levels of quality, rather than on meeting or exceeding consumer or user expectations. The steps of the CQI process are as follows:

1. Find a process to improve;
2. Organize a team that knows the process;
3. Clarify current knowledge of the process;
4. Understand the causes of variation in the process;
5. Select the process improvement and continue data collection;
6. Do the improvement, data collection, and analysis;
7. Check the results and lessons learned from the team effort; and
8. Act to hold the gains and to continue to improve the process.

Examples of hospital processes that can be improved are increasing the preadmission rate for diagnostic tests to reduce turnaround time in the operating room; making maximum use of registered nurse skills, employing fewer agency nurses, and improving the recruitment and retention of staff nurses; and, lowering the hospital cesarean rate.

Highlights for this last process, implemented at the West Paces Ferry Hospital, a Hospital Corporation of America hospital in Florida (McEachern & Neuhauser, 1987) are described in the following example. Twelve physicians were taught how CQI works on two evenings and a Saturday from 8:00 a.m. to 2:00 p.m. The C-section rate nationally was 25%, at West Paces Ferry Hospital the rate was 21%; at competitor hospitals the rate was 17%. An 11-person cross-functional team was organized. They saw an opportunity to improve clinical outcomes and patient satisfaction by having fewer cesarean deliveries. A variation among physicians was noted of C-section rates from 15%–26% of all births, and among physicians with over 44 patients per year, from 16%–44%. Forty percent of the C-sections were caused by the baby's failure to progress in the birth canal. A mother's previous C-section accounted for 13% of the cases (27% of these were at the patient's request). The cross-functional group then changed their CQI opportunity statement, focusing on the education of physicians and mothers that a prior C-section was not a necessary reason for another C-section. Lowering the rate of the repeat C-sections was subsequently accomplished.

According to Deming (1986), there are 14 points that must be followed to successfully implement CQI. These are as follows:

1. Create constancy of purpose for improvement of product and service;
2. Adopt the new philosophy;
3. Cease dependence on inspection to achieve quality;
4. Don't award business on the basis of price tag alone;
5. Improve constantly every process for planning, production, and service;
6. Institute training on the job;
7. Institute leadership;
8. Drive out fear;
9. Break down the barriers between staff areas;
10. Eliminate slogans, exhortation, and targets for the workforce;
11. Eliminate numerical quotas for the workforce and numerical goals for management;
12. Remove barriers that rob people of pride in workmanship;
13. Institute a vigorous program of education and self-improvement for everyone; and
14. Put everyone in the organization to work to accomplish the transformation.

The Patient-Focused Hospital

Patient-focused care is an attempt to improve quality and contain hospital inpatient costs by restructuring services so that more of them take place on nursing units rather than in specialized units. Another method of implementing patient-focused care is to cross-train staff so that they can perform several jobs for the same small number of patients in a nursing unit, rather than focusing on performing particular functions in a unit for a much larger number of patients. Thus, for example, X-ray, pharmacy, and admitting services can all be done in the nursing unit by staff who can do more than one function. The same staff can, for example, serve the patient food, clean the patient's room, and assist in the patient's nursing care.

As services have been customarily organized in hospitals, to get a routine X-ray for an inpatient can require 40 separate steps and consume 140 minutes of personnel time. Up to 24 hours of time may elapse from the doctor's initial request to receipt of the report, and it can involve 15–20 employees. Moreover, most of the steps are not medical nor clinical activities. According to Smith (1990) hospital staff spend most of their time on nine activity categories: medical, technical, and clinical; hotel and patient services; medical documentation; institutional documentation; scheduling and coordination; patient and staff transportation; management and supervision; and being "ready for action" (i.e., standing by in the emergency department whether or not patients are there requiring services). In a study in Lakeland Regional Medical Center, a 750-bed hospital in central Florida, Smith and his colleagues found that only one sixth of personnel-related costs were consumed by medical, technical, and clinical activity, and that almost twice that amount of time was spent on writing things down. Scheduling and coordination took as much time as medical activity, and being ready-for-action (in case patients should arrive) consumed more time than those.

Smith (1990) suggests that restructuring services at Lakeland can result in reducing the number of staff required for patient care activities from 2,200 to between 1,200 and 1,300, and that this can actually improve the quality of care and service levels. The hospital would be divided into five 125-bed operating units. The area allotted to each unit would be sufficient to contain: a mini-lab, diagnostic radiology rooms, linen and general supply, stock rooms, and so on. Medical documentation could be reduced by almost two thirds, scheduling and coordination by more than two thirds, and ready-for-action time by two thirds.

If the patient-focused hospital is such a good idea, why haven't more hospitals already implemented it? We can only speculate on the reasons: (a) because hospitals have, traditionally, never had to improve productivity in order to receive adequate reimbursement; (b) because hospital interest groups such as doctors and nurses may oppose changing the status quo and there are no effective champions who see benefit from implementing what are costly and expensive processes; (c) because in many hospitals such changes will require extensive renovations in the physical plant.

Hospital Community Benefit Programs

Rising public concern about the high cost and inaccessibility of quality health services has focused on the acute care hospital as one of the major causes of the problem, rather than as a catalyst for reform. Increasingly, the hospital is viewed as being more concerned with generating income for survival than with improving the health of the community; as competing to offer the latest application of high technology rather than meeting community need and avoiding unnecessary duplication of facilities; as meeting the needs of professionals rather than serving the poor and disadvantaged; and, as filling beds with inpatients rather than responding to community problems affecting the health status of population groups.

The Hospital Community Benefit Standards Program (Hudson, 1992) was funded by the W. K. Kellogg Foundation to demonstrate that new credible standards could assist and encourage leading hospitals to manage highly effective community benefit standard programs. It also demonstrates that community benefit programs based on these standards could put hospitals in the forefront of efforts to reform the health care system and help to provide better access to care for those without health insurance.

This Program adopted four standards (Kovner & Hattis, 1990a): (a) there is evidence of the hospital's formal commitment to a community benefit program for a designated community; (b) the scope of the program includes hospital-sponsored projects for the designated community to improve health status, access to care, and contain the growth of community health care costs; (c) the hospital's program includes activities designed to stimulate other organizations and individuals to join in carrying out a broad health agenda in the designated community; and, (d) the hospital fosters an internal environment that encourages hospital-wide involvement in the program.

Forty-nine hospitals participated in a national demonstration, many of which made substantial movement toward local reform of health services. Community benefit can be viewed as an extension of continuous quality improvement and of patient-focused care beyond the hospital walls and into the community. Focus is on problems of health status, access to care, and containment of community health care costs, about which the hospital, other health care providers, and community leaders can do something meaningful. Initiatives are based on national standards that can be adapted locally, that will alter local resource distribution patterns. Examples of such demonstration site programs include the following: providing more prenatal care, especially to at-risk mothers, thereby improving the health status of mother and child; improving access to care and reducing the number of low-weight babies; closing duplicative facilities and services; and establishing special programs to reach groups lacking access to health care for economic, social, linguistic, and cultural reasons.

Why would hospitals want to spend time or money on community benefit programs for which they are neither reimbursed nor required by government to implement? Obviously, there is no "mission without margin" (provision of services without payment for services) over the long run, particularly given that opportunities for cross-subsidization have been curtailed by managed care and government payers. But there are often opportunities for hospitals to reallocate current expenditures, or raise charitable funds, in ways that lead to improved community health outcomes.

Other possible reasons for a lack of involvement by many hospitals in more active community benefit programs include the following: (a) other priorities such as acquiring new technology are seen as more important; (b) a lack of support for community health priorities by specialist physicians and others who see their vital interests threatened by such initiatives; and, (c) because hospital leadership lacks the skills and experience in working with community leaders to obtain needed data to justify programs, and to integrate and coordinate resources locally to improve health outcomes at current levels of expenditures.

ORGANIZATIONAL CHALLENGES AND RESPONSE

Thirty-five years after the passage of Medicare and Medicaid, hospitals are going through another period of consolidation. Despite acknowledged overcapacity, there is an unwillingness in communities served to let the free market drive failing hospitals into bankruptcy. Hospitals are valued locally, especially by the people who work in them. Pressures for change in hospitals include the following: purchaser pressure on operating margins, regulatory pressure for quality improvement, competition for the premium dollar with health plans and physician groups and for market share with other delivery systems, the cost of rapidly changing new technology, the aging of the population, and changing customer expectations for service. Hospitals have responded and continue to respond by becoming part of larger systems, changing the scope of the services they provide, and by specializing in what services they provide to whom.

There is a vast variance in hospital operating margins depending in large part on where they are located and whom they serve. But because of purchaser pressure hospital margins are decreasing at the same time that cross-subsidization opportunities are being restricted. For example, HMOs do not want to subsidize nonpaying patients nor the cost of medical education; this will force some hospitals to close or become part of larger systems.

There is increasing standardization of clinical protocols in hospitals and of medical processes in delivering care. This followed the publication of the Institute of Medicine's *Report on Errors in Medicine,* and was also a result of the initiatives of the Joint Commission on the Accreditation of Healthcare Organizations for clinical improvement. It was a result as well of the enabling acquisition of information technology and specialized workforce by larger health multiunit organizations.

Hospitals are competing with insurance companies and physician groups to maintain their share of the health plan dollar, and with other delivery systems for market share in their main lines of businesses such as heart, cancer, rehabilitation medicine, women's health, emergency care, and general and orthopedic surgery. Although most hospitals are members of most health plan networks, this may change as health plans work out arrangements with some hospitals and not others to steer volume to network hospitals in exchange for lower prices and assured quality.

Hospital care is the site of rapidly changing new technology ranging from improvements in the care of patients such as laser surgery, organ transplants, intensive care, and burn units, to improvements in medical care support such as optical scanning, information systems, and telemedicine. Only certain hospitals, particularly those in multiunit organizations, are expected to be able to make the necessary investments and risk the higher short-run costs in return for better information, quicker response time, and fewer recording errors.

Partly as a result of improved medical care, life expectancy of Americans continues to increase. Those over 65 and those over 75 are making up an increasing proportion of the total population. The aged use more hospital services per capita. They also use more of other types of health services, which hospitals can also provide and increasingly are providing, such as home care, hospice care, and adult day care. This will increase the demand for hospital care, although there may not be an exact fit between where current facilities that are underutilized are and where the demand actually occurs. If health insurance is extended to nursing home care, this may increase pressure to limit payments to hospitals.

In response to purchaser pressure, certain hospitals will compete primarily on price, while other hospitals will seek a niche in the marketplace by responding to the needs of those who are willing to pay more for customized services. For example, certain obstetrical hospitals can be marketed directly to women, as a combination luxury hotel with beauty treatment and health education, rather than as a workshop for physicians delivering babies. Entire hospitals or important divisions within them will increasingly focus principally on provision of cancer or heart services. Certain general hospitals may be preferred, even though their costs are higher, because their food and nursing services are preferred.

CONCLUSIONS

In this chapter we have reviewed the historical development of hospitals, key hospital statistics and characteristics, concerns about costs and quality, organizational structure, and challenges and responses. I foresee continuation of the following trends for hospitals in the first decade of the 21st century:

- Growth and integration of large multiunit organizations.
- Continuing high costs of hospital care.
- Increasingly differentiated hospitals or larger units within hospitals for patients requiring similar treatments.
- Increasing standardization of treatment for patients with similar medical conditions and demographic characteristics.

The reasons for these changes have to do with the formation of larger hospital systems in response to the competitive demands of large purchasers for adequate quality and contained costs. New technology, information systems, and professional workforce are increasingly expensive, increases in reimbursement are capped, and all hospitals cannot generate sufficient volume to provide a full range of services. So hospitals will increasingly specialize in the types of patients they can best care for. This is less true in sparsely populated, large, rural areas, but even in rural America hospitals will increasingly share services with out-of-area hospitals and partition services between periphery and central hospitals.

CASE STUDY

St. George Hospital has an inpatient capacity of 60% and lost $6 million last year on annual revenues of $200 million. St. George is located in a large eastern city and competes with four other hospitals, two of which are having merger discussions. Most of St. George's medical staff is in private practice, and many physicians admit to other hospitals as well. Managed care companies have 20% of the market in town; St. George's has contracts with most of these companies.

You are Charlie Sweat, Board Chair. You've been approached by Glenn Morris, Board Chair of Victory Hospital (which made $100,000 last year). He has asked you to persuade your board to merge your hospital with his. Victory Hospital is 20% smaller than St. George and is not religiously sponsored. Morris is suggesting a full merger, with 50% of the board from each hospital. He believes that the resulting entity will be better able to compete and have greater bargaining power with managed care plans and government regulators.

What are some of the factors that St. George's should consider before continuing discussions with Victory?

DISCUSSION QUESTIONS

1. Explain how hospitals have developed in the United States.
2. Why are costs so high and quality so uneven in American hospitals?

3. In what ways can hospitals be influenced to play a more appropriate role in the American health care delivery system?
4. How should physicians relate to hospitals and why?
5. To what extent should hospitals be regulated and by whom?

REFERENCES

American Hospital Association. (2000). *Hospital Statistics.* Chicago: Author.

American Hospital Association. (1999). *AHA Guide 1999–2000.* Chicago: Author.

American Hospital Association. (1992). *Environmental assessment for rural hospitals.* Chicago: Author.

American Hospital Association. (1998). *Environmental assessment for rural hospitals.* Chicago: Author.

American Medical Association. (2000). *Physician characteristics and distribution in the United States: 2000–2001 edition.* Chicago: Author.

Bellandi, D. (2000). Spinoffs, big deals dominate in '99. *Modern Healthcare, 30,* 36–44.

Berwick, D. M. (1989). Continuous improvement as an ideal in health care. *The New England Journal of Medicine, 320*(1), 53–56.

Chassin, M. R. (1998). Is health care ready for six sigma quality? *The Milbank Quarterly, 76*(4), 565–591.

Crosby, P. B. (1979). *Quality is free.* New York: New American Library.

Deming, W. E. (1986). *Out of crisis.* Cambridge, MA: MIT-CAES.

Freymann, J. G. (1974). *The American health care system: Its genesis and trajectory.* New York: Medcom Press.

Griffith, J. R. (1999). *The well-managed healthcare organization* (4th ed., pp. 173–186). Chicago: Health Administration Press.

Henry Ford Health System. (2001). *Henry Ford News* [On-line]. Available: www.henryfordhealth.org.

Heyssel, R. M., Gaintner, R., Kues, I. W., Jones, A. A., & Lipstein, S. H. (1984). Decentralized management in a teaching hospital: Ten years later at Johns Hopkins. *New England Journal of Medicine, 310,* 1477.

Hollowell, E. (1978). No insurance—no privileges. *Legal Aspects of Medical Practice, 6*(4), 16–19.

Hudson, T. (1992). Hospitals strive to provide communities with benefits. *Hospitals, 66*(13), 102–110.

Juran, J. M. (1964). *Managerial breakthrough.* New York: McGraw-Hill.

Kohn, L., Corrigan, J., & Donaldson, M. (Eds.) *To err is human: Building a safer health system.* Washington, DC: Institute of Medicine.

Kovner, A. R., & Hattis, P. A. (1990). Benefitting communities. *HMQ,* 4th Quarter, 6–10.

Kenagy, J. W., Berwick, D. M., & Shore, M. L. (1999). Service quality in health care. *Journal of the American Medical Association, 281*(7), 661–665.

Leape, L. L. (1994). Error in medicine. *Journal of the American Medical Association, 272*(23), 1851–1857.

Levit, K., Cowden, C., Lozenby, H., Semsenig, A., McDonnell, P., Stuller, J., Martin, A., & the Health Accounts Team. (2000). Trends: Health spending: Signals of change. *Health Affairs, 19*(1), 124–132.

McEachern, J. E., & Neuhauser, D. (1987). The continuous improvement of quality at the Hospital Corporation of America. *Health Matrix, 7*(3), 5–11.

Premier. (2001). *Public Newsroom* [On-line]. Available: www.premierinc.com.

Rosenberg, C. E. (1987). *The care of strangers.* New York: Basic Books.

Shortell, S. M. (1985). The medical staff of the future: Replanting the garden. *Frontiers of Health Services Management, 1*(3), 3.

Showalter, J. S. (1999). *Southwick's the law of healthcare administration.* Chicago: Health Administration Press.

Smith, D. B., & Kaluzny, A. D. (1986). *The white labyrinth* (2nd ed.). Ann Arbor, MI: Health Administration Press.

Smith, H. L. (1955). Two lines of authority are one too many. *Modern Hospital,* March, 59–64.

Smith, J. (1990). The patient-focused hospital. *Hospital Management International,* (pp. 185–187).

Southwick, A. (1978). *The law of hospital and health administration.* Ann Arbor, MI: Health Administration Press.

Starr, P. (1982). *The social transformation of American medicine.* New York: Basic Books.

Stevens, R. (1971). *American medicine and the public interest.* New Haven, CT: Yale University Press.

U.S. Department of Veterans Affairs. (2001). *Today's VA* [On-line]. Available: www.va.gov.

7

Ambulatory Care

Andrew P. Mezey

LEARNING OBJECTIVES

- ☐ Explain what is meant by ambulatory care.
- ☐ Explain what is meant by primary care.
- ☐ Describe where and how primary care is delivered.
- ☐ Describe how the delivery of primary care is changing due to managed care.
- ☐ Describe the role of emergency services in the spectrum of ambulatory care.

TOPICAL OUTLINE

Ambulatory care
Primary care
Emergency care
Subspecialty care
Home health care
Complementary and alternative medical care
Patient networks and support groups
Summary and current issues in ambulatory care

KEY WORDS

ambulatory care, primary care, primary care provider, emergency care, specialty ambulatory care, home health care, complementary and alternative care, patient networks, support groups

AMBULATORY CARE

Ambulatory care is personal health care provided to individuals, or a population of individuals, who are not occupying a bed in a health care institution or at home. It encompasses all health services provided to individual patients, including community services, such as general information about the hazards of smoking or substance abuse, and some of the services delivered by public health departments, such as information about immunizations and sexually transmitted diseases. Primary care, emergency care, and ambulatory subspecialty care, including ambulatory surgery, are all subsets of ambulatory care. They are provided in a variety of settings—freestanding provider offices, hospital-based clinics, school-based clinics, public health clinics, and neighborhood and community health centers.

Current practice is to attempt to provide health care services in the least costly setting available. This has led to a decrease in hospital admissions, hospital length of stay, and hospital days, and increased utilization of non-emergent ambulatory facilities. There has not been, however, decreased utilization of emergency services; in fact there was no change in emergency department utilization between 1995 and 1998 (U.S. Department of Health and Human Services [USDHHS], 2000, Table 83). The types and severity of those illnesses that physicians and other providers are able and willing to treat in ambulatory settings have also increased. Patients admitted to hospitals are therefore sicker on admission and stay for shorter periods than they did formerly. At discharge they often require support services for variable lengths of time after they leave the hospital. Some of these services are provided in the home, others in ambulatory care settings. This has changed the principal locus of care for certain services, such as rehabilitation services (physical therapy, etc.), and invasive diagnostic and surgical procedures from the hospital to ambulatory facilities and to the home.

What has been the standard of practice, but is now beginning to change, is the single episodic encounter, usually between a physician and a patient, driven by the patient's perceived need for medical care. For example, an individual with a rash that has not responded to usual remedies sees a dermatologist to whom he has been referred by a friend, not by the patient's personal physician. No record of the encounter is communicated by the dermatologist to another physician. The rash recurs, and the patient seeks advice from another dermatologist, with the same result—improvement followed by recurrence. The third physician encounter may be with the personal physician, who may recognize the cause of the rash as related to a condition that the patient has but that was not communicated to the previous two dermatologists. Though the patient has had the luxury of ultimate choice, it may not have been in the patient's best interests to exercise that choice. On the other hand, care by a subspecialist for such conditions such as chronic illnesses may be associated with improved outcomes and decreased costs.

A major problem facing us in this rapidly changing health care delivery system is how to maintain an individual's ability to choose while containing costs, providing quality care, and maintaining satisfaction with the care received. In this latter regard, an aspect of these changes deals with the need to preserve the pleasure that both providers of care and patients derive from establishing long-term relationships. It is similar to the pleasure one gets from maintaining long-term friendships, friendships that are full of shared experiences that allow people to connect easily even after long absences. Long-term relationships between patients and their physicians are involuntarily ruptured when a patient changes jobs and the new employer has a health insurance contract that does not include the patient's physician. This has the effect of diminishing the effort both physicians and patients will make in building trusting relationships.

The need to reduce the costs of health care has had a number of other effects. Primary care providers have taken on patient responsibilities previously referred to specialists. This, in turn, has decreased the reliance on specialists and is one cause of the apparent oversupply of specialists found in some parts of the United States. Consumers have become concerned that controlling costs leads to a decrease in the quality of care. Abuses of the system in the name of controlling costs are difficult to document, but the health care marketplace is adjusting to the concerns of consumers, either through legislation or through market pressures (Bodenheimer, 1996).

This chapter looks at how ambulatory services are provided—who provides those services and where—with particular emphasis on the characteristics of the provision of primary care. The intent is to give the reader an understanding of how and where individuals receive the great bulk of their health care in the United States. The chapter will not discuss mental health, public health, or rehabilitative services.

Ambulatory Care Statistics

In 1997 close to 960 million visits were made to doctors' offices, emergency departments, and to hospital-based outpatient departments. The average person made 3.6 visits to a physician (Schappert, 1999) and spent 0.72 days in an acute care hospital (American Hospital Association [AHA], 2000, Table 3, p. 9). Thus, there were 5 times more ambulatory care episodes than hospital days of care in 1997. Though this ratio has not changed much since 1980 (4.7 ratio in 1980), the number of hospital days has fallen from 1,163 per 1,000 population in 1980 (USDHHS, 1982, Tables 35, 43), to 796 per 1,000 in 1994 to 708 per 1,000 in 1998 (AHA, 2000, Table 3, p. 9). The shift away from inpatient care of the last 2 decades has had an enormous impact on the organization, staffing, and financing of ambulatory services in the United States. The number of Americans who reported a visit to a physician in the past year increased slightly, from 75% in 1980 to 79.1% in 1996 (Markowitz, 2000, p. 212). Meanwhile, the average length of stay in nonfederal acute care hospitals decreased from 7.3 days in 1980 to 6.0 in 1993 (USDHHS, 1982, Table 42; 1995, Table 85) to 5.3 days in 1998 (AHA, 2000, Table 3, p. 9). Thus, in sum, the shift from the focus on the hospital inpatient encounter to ambulatory patient-physician contact continues.

The rates of visits to physicians vary by age, gender, race, and socioeconomic status (see Figure 7.1). Rates for females are higher than for males (4.2 visits versus 3.0 visits) mainly because of the marked difference in the 15–24-year-old and 25–44-year-old categories (3.1 and 3.9 visits for females versus 1.5 and 2.1 for males, respectively). In most other age categories gender rates are similar. Individuals 75 years and older have the highest visit rate, 7.5 per year. This group also visits emergency departments more frequently—0.62 visits per year. There was little difference between the visit rates for whites (3.7) and blacks (3.4), and the rates by age did not differ either (see Figure 7.2). There was a black/white difference in the sites of visits. Blacks were more likely to go to an emergency department—17.6% of total visits, or to a hospital outpatient department—15.7% of total visits, and only 66.7% of total visits were to a physician's office. For whites 84.1% of visits were to a physician's office, with about 7% to hospital outpatient departments and 9% to emergency departments. The rate for total visits for Asians/Pacific Islanders and American Indians/Eskimos/Aleuts was lower—2.6 per year, with 86% of visits being in a physician's office and the rest split evenly between the emergency department and a hospital outpatient department (Schappert, 1999). The eradication of the gap observed between the races also occurred with differences of physician use by the rich and the poor (see Figure 7.3). In 1964, 58.6% poor families reported seeing a physician within the last year; 73.6% of nonpoor families did so. In 1998 these rates had increased to 79.7% and 86%, respectively

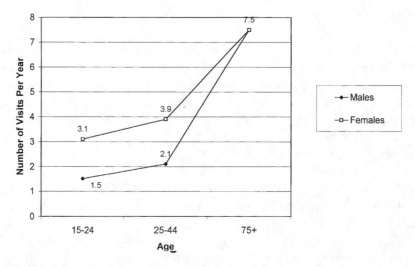

FIGURE 7.1   Physician visit rates by gender.

Source: Schappert, S. M. (1999). Ambulatory Care Visits to Physician Offices, Hospital Outpatient Departments, and Emergency Departments: United States, 1997. *Vital and Health Statistics, 13*(143).

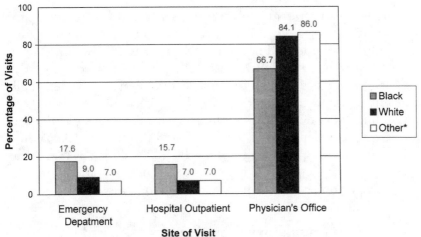

FIGURE 7.2   **Physician visit rates by race.**

Source: Schappert, S. M. (1999). Ambulatory Care Visits to Physician Offices, Hospital Outpatient Departments, and Emergency Departments: United States, 1997. *Vital and Health Statistics, 13*(143).

(USDHHS, 1995, Table 77; 2000, Table 71). The enactment of Medicaid and Medicare accounts for much of the increased use of physicians by lower-income groups.

If, however, one looks at individuals with and without health insurance, similarities disappear. In 1998, 36.8% of the uninsured poor, 35.8% of the near poor, and 29.1% of the nonpoor had no visits to a doctor's office or

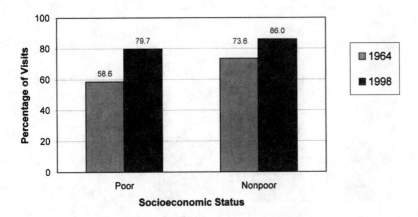

FIGURE 7.3   **Physician visit rates by socioeconomic status.**

Sources: U.S. Department of Health and Human Services. (1995). *Health United States, 1995* (DHHS Publication No. PHS 96-1232). Washington, DC: U.S. Government Printing Office, Table 77; U.S. Department of Health and Human Services. (2000). *Health United States, 2000* (DHHS Publication No. PHS 01-1232). Washington, DC: U.S. Government Printing Office, Table 71.

to an emergency department. For families with health insurance those numbers change drastically; 13.7% of the poor, 15.6% of the near poor, and 13.4% of the nonpoor did not visit either a doctor's office or an emergency department in 1998 (USDHHS, 2000, Table 71) (see Figure 7.4). Lack of health insurance for children under 6 years of age yielded similar disparities in access to care in 1998; 20% of poor children and 16.9% of near poor children under 6 years without health insurance did not see a doctor or emergency department, versus 6.6% of the poor and 3.8% of the near poor with health insurance (USDHHS, 2000, Table 75) (see Figure 7.5). This is the group of children most in need of immunizations and most in need of psychosocial, neurological, and behavioral assessments.

Organization of Ambulatory Care Services

There are two major categories of ambulatory care. The dominant form is provided by private physicians in solo, partnership, or private group practice on a fee-for-service basis or through contracts with managed care organization. The other categories are hospital-based ambulatory services, including clinics, walk-in, and emergency services; hospital-sponsored group practices and health promotion centers; freestanding "surgi-centers" and "urgi-" or "emergi-centers"; health department clinics; neighborhood and community health centers (NHCs and CHCs); organized home care; community mental health centers; school and workplace health services; and prison health services. In 1998 there were a total of 1,005,101,000 ambulatory visits (includes physicians offices and hospital outpatient and

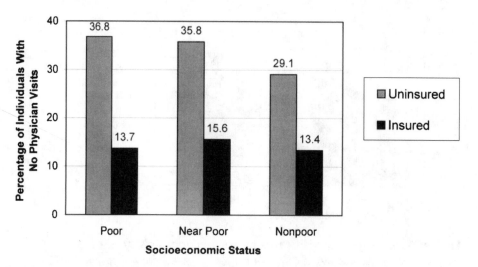

FIGURE 7.4   Physician visit rates based on insurance status.

Source: U.S. Department of Health and Human Services. (2000). *Health United States, 2000* (DHHS Publication No. PHS 01-1232). Washington, DC: U.S. Government Printing Office, Table 71.

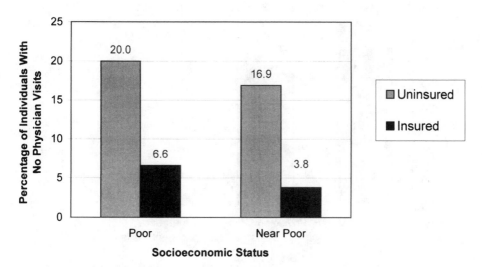

FIGURE 7.5   Physician visit rates of children under 6 years of age based on insurance status.

Source: U.S. Department of Health and Human Services. (2000). *Health United States, 2000* (DHHS Publication No. PHS 01-1232). Washington, DC: U.S. Government Printing Office, Table 75.

emergency departments) (see Figure 7.6). Of these about 83% were to physician offices (829,280,000), about 10% to emergency departments (100,408,000) and about 7% to hospital outpatient departments (75,412,000). The number of ambulatory visits per 100 persons increased from 334 per 100 in 1995 to 378 per 100 in 1998 (see Figure 7.7). Similarly, the number

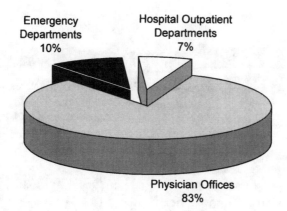

FIGURE 7.6   Composition of total ambulatory visits: 1,005,101,000 visits in 1998.

Source: U.S. Department of Health and Human Services. (2000). *Health United States, 2000* (DHHS Publication No. PHS 01-1232). Washington, DC: U.S. Government Printing Office, Table 83.

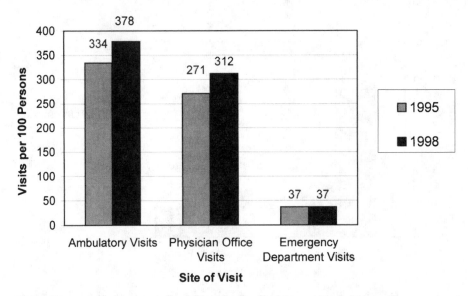

FIGURE 7.7 Increase in ambulatory care services (1995–1998).

Source: U.S. Department of Health and Human Services. (2000). *Health United States, 2000* (DHHS Publication No. PHS 01-1232). Washington, DC: U.S. Government Printing Office, Table 83.

per 100 persons visiting physicians' offices increased from 271 per 100 in 1995 to 312 per 100 in 1998, while the visiting emergency departments remained constant from 1995 to 1998 at 37 per 100 persons (USDHHS, 2000, Table 83). It is apparent from these numbers that while the trend is toward greater ambulatory visits, there has not been a corresponding decrease in the rate of emergency department usage.

PRIMARY CARE

Primary care, as defined by the Institute of Medicine, is "the provision of integrated, accessible care services by clinicians who are accountable for addressing a large majority of the personal health care needs, developing a sustained partnership with patients, and practicing in the context of family and community" (Institute of Medicine, 1996, p. 1). Embedded within this definition is the concept that a primary care clinician should be able to address an individual's health needs over an extended period, that the health needs will vary over time, and that the individual may sometimes need others to care for those health needs (e.g., physician subspecialists, physical therapists, social workers, etc.). It is also implicit in this definition that the primary care provider must act as a coordinator for those health needs. It is obvious that primary care, when defined in this way, is much broader than the provision of the primary health care needs of patients in an ambulatory setting.

Primary care differs from "first contact" care. First contact care occurs when an individual, faced with a new symptom or sign, whether real or perceived, asks some other individual for advice. That person can be a friend or family member who has medical expertise beyond that of the general population—nurses, pharmacists, physical and occupational therapists, respiratory therapists, and the like. It can also be advice sought from someone who has had personal or family experience with an illness that seems to be related to the symptoms or signs at hand. These types of interchange are everyday occurrences. The situation may be as mundane as when the parent of a first child seeks help for what to do about the infant's fever, cold, or diarrhea from a neighbor with several children. It can be as complex as seeking advice from a friend about the possibility of serious heart disease or cancer, when that friend's family member has had a recent experience with cancer or heart disease.

On the other hand, with more and more of the population becoming computer literate, lay access to complex information about health and disease has become commonplace. The Internet is an amazing source of up-to-date information easily available to anyone with access to it. The National Institutes of Health (NIH) maintain a section called "Health Information" (www.nih.gov/health). It lists publications on a variety of subjects but also provides information on a number of special programs, dietary supplements, complementary and alternative medicine, women's health, and rare diseases. The NIH has a quarterly publication, "The NIH Word on Health," that is accessible from the above site.

Hospitals have also entered the consumer information field, offering advice on wellness as well as on illness, and providing information on how to access care at their own institutions. Although clearly a marketing attempt, the information is useful and readily available. Many people use these sources of information on health care prior to calling their primary care provider. Rather than speaking with family members or friends, people can search for health information sites or chat rooms on the Internet to ask questions of experts or to "speak" with others on a variety of subjects dealing with everyday issues, such as ear infections in children, parenting problems, work-related stress, and depression, as well as major life-threatening problems such as cancer.

With increasing numbers of Americans receiving their health insurance through managed care organizations (MCOs), the responsibilities of primary care providers have changed. In a fee-for-service model, the primary care provider is responsible only for those patients who happen to come into his or her office. The provider's practice is viewed as being made up of individual patients, not as a discrete population. In managed care settings, especially when the provider is paid through a capitation system rather than by a modified fee-for-service system, the provider can be held responsible for providing appropriate health services to the entire population of patients assigned to him or her. The MCO can perform an audit of the provider's practice to see if standards of care have been met. Thus, the provider is held responsible for all the patients in his or her panel, even if they have never shown up for a visit. For example, if the standard of care set by the MCO for a pediatric practice requires 90% of children to have received all their immunizations by 2 years of age, the denominator used is the total number of children 2 years of age and older in the provider's panel, not just those that have actually been seen in the office. Standards of care, benchmarks against which the adequacy of care provided by the primary care practitioner is judged, exist for preventive services such as blood pressure screening, breast cancer screening (mammogram, self-breast-exam education), diabetes screening, and colorectal cancer screening, as well as for the appropriateness of illness management. Although quality assurance measures have been required in hospital settings for a long time, it is only since 1991, with the advent of standards for accreditation of MCOs by the National Committee on Quality Assurance (NCQA), the accrediting body for MCOs, that standards of care in ambulatory settings have begun to be monitored.

Primary Care Providers

The providers of primary care fall into four major disciplines: physicians, nurse practitioners (NPs), midwives, and physician assistants (PAs). Although they take very different pathways to become primary care providers, at the completion of their training they are very similar in their capabilities in ambulatory primary care settings. It is estimated that NPs and PAs can typically perform 75% of services that physicians provide in adult practices and 90% in pediatric practices (Scheffler, 1996). Despite this, in 1997 physicians saw 95.2% of all patients presenting to an ambulatory site (physician offices, hospital outpatient departments, and emergency departments), whereas physician assistants saw 2.6%, nurse practitioners saw 1.2%, and midwives saw 0.1% (Schappert, 1999) (see Figure 7.8). In 1998, primary care visits made up 52.7% of all ambulatory care visits, a decrease from 1980 (56.6%) and 1990 (54.9%) (see Figure 7.9). The percentage of visits to general/family practitioners dropped from 33.5% in 1980, to 29.9% in 1990, to 24.2% in 1998. Primary care visits to internists increased from 12.1% in 1980, to 13.8% in 1990, to 17.1% in 1998. Visits to pediatricians increased slightly from 1980 to 1998 (10.9% to 11.4%) (USDHHS, 2000, Table 85).

Sites for the Provision of Primary Care Services

Primary care in the United States is provided in a number of settings, with private physician offices continuing to be the dominant site even in this era of increasing penetration of MCOs. On the other hand, many states have received waivers from the Health Care Financing Administration (HCFA) to introduce mandatory Medicaid managed care. Neighborhood and

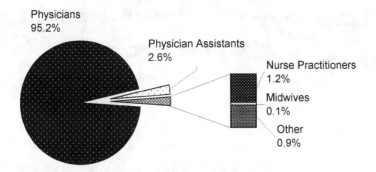

FIGURE 7.8   Percentage of services delivered by primary care providers to patients presenting to an ambulatory site, 1997.

Source: Schappert, S. M. (1999). Ambulatory Care Visits to Physician Offices, Hospital Outpatient Departments, and Emergency Departments: United States, 1997. *Vital and Health Statistics, 13*(143).

community-based organizations, and hospital-based primary care clinics have expanded their primary care capabilities in response to increased numbers of children becoming eligible for subsidized health insurance through the federally funded State Children's Health Insurance Program (S-CHIP), and because of the expansion of mandatory Medicaid managed care waivers (Forrest & Whalen, 2000). These organizations have been the traditional providers of care to patients with Medicaid-financed insurance and wish to continue to be. They have expanded services to cover evening, night, and weekend hours for their patients, and they are to developing the necessary information systems. In the main, however, they have not developed the economic efficiency seen in the private for-profit sector.

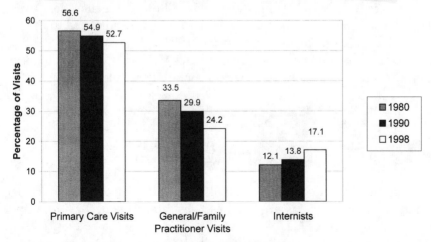

FIGURE 7.9   Change in composition of ambulatory care visits.

Source: U.S. Department of Health and Human Services. (2000). *Health United States, 2000* (DHHS Publication No. PHS 01-1232). Washington, DC: U.S. Government Printing Office, Table 85.

Academic medical centers (AMCs), those teaching hospitals that are closely aligned with medical schools, have also been aggressive in expanding their primary care operations into the community. They have done so in order to maintain their traditional patient base, to educate physicians-in-training and medical students, and to support their clinical research.

EMERGENCY CARE

The United States has developed a complex system of emergency care for its citizens, beginning with the national 911 emergency response system, and continuing with hospital-based emergency services and specialized emergency services such as Level I trauma centers. These centers have 24-hour, 7-day availability of a complete array of medical and surgical specialists, diagnostic imaging, and operating rooms. They are complemented by well-staffed and well-equipped intensive care units.

Most U.S. hospitals provide emergency services; over 92.6 % of community hospitals have emergency departments (AHA, 2000, Table 7, p. 154). These units serve several functions, from caring for the acutely ill or injured patient to providing walk-in services to less acutely ill patients. Many physicians on the hospital staff also use the emergency room as a setting to assess a patient with a problem that either may lead to inpatient admission or require equipment or diagnostic imaging facilities not available in the physician's office. Extended care facilities such as nursing homes and chronic disease hospitals may use the emergency services of an acute care facility for evaluation of a patient with a sudden change in medical status. Emergency services are a major source of admissions to hospitals; in 1997 they constituted about 42% of the close to 31 million admissions to acute care hospitals. Of the almost 95 million emergency department (ED) visits in 1997, about one in seven or 13.5% were admitted to the hospital (AHA, 2000, Table 3, p. 9; Nourjah, 1999, p.11).

The National Center for Health Statistics (Nourjah, 1999) categorizes patients based on the immediacy with which they should be seen:

Nonurgent. Patient should be seen within 2–24 hours.
Semi-urgent. Patient should be seen within 1–2 hours.
Urgent. Patient should be seen within 15–60 minutes.
Emergent. Patient should be seen in less than 15 minutes.

Based on these definitions, Nourjah (1999) found that 21% were categorized as emergent, 32% as urgent, 15.4% as semi-urgent, 9.7% as nonurgent, and 21.9% were listed as "unknown or no triage" (see Figure 7.10).

These terms derive from a professional perspective and are based on medical diagnoses. Most patients cannot make these distinctions and err in both overinterpreting and under-interpreting the gravity of symptoms. Most patients presenting to an emergency service feel that they need immediate

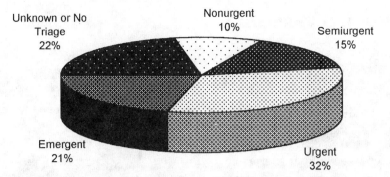

FIGURE 7.10 **Percentage of patients receiving emergency care: Categorized by immediacy of condition, 1999.**

Source: Nourjah, P. (1999, May). National Hospital Ambulatory Medical Care Survey: 1997 Emergency Department Summary. *Advance Data from Vital and Health Statistics,* (No. 304). Hyattsville, MD: National Center for Health Statistics.

attention, regardless of what the professional staff may think. Others know that they do not have an urgent or emergent problem. They simply use the emergency service because it is all that is available to them.

Some hospitals have developed walk-in units to relieve the emergency services of the burden of the nonurgent patients and to respond to the competition from freestanding walk-in services or urgi-centers. By organizing group practices in the outpatient clinics hospitals have been able to provide "add-on" slots in the appointment schedule to accommodate the nonurgent patient demanding urgent attention. Financial incentives are forcing hospitals to make every effort to reduce the costly care of nonurgent patients in the emergency setting. These efforts include evening and weekend hours for walk-in units and after-hours telephone access for clinic patients.

Managed systems of care often require subscribers to get prior approval before authorizing emergency services, and unauthorized use may not be covered. Many states have implemented or are in the process of implementing mandatory Medicaid managed care in an attempt to decrease costs, with emergency room usage being a particular target. To date these efforts have failed to decrease ED usage—the number of ED visits increased from 90.5 million in 1994 to 94.8 million in 1998, a 4.75% increase, while the population as a whole was estimated to have increased by only 3.8%.

Emergency medical services extend beyond the hospital emergency department to include other services provided to accident victims or individuals suffering acute, life-threatening illnesses such as acute myocardial infarction or stroke. The goals of these services are to preserve life and reduce disability by providing prompt treatment and transportation to comprehensive treatment facilities. The intended recipients of care are patients with emergent or urgent problems.

SUBSPECIALTY CARE

Subspecialty care is defined as care given by physicians who are not generalists, and is practiced in ambulatory sites by a large variety of disciplines. Generalists are defined as individuals practicing family medicine, general pediatrics, general internal medicine, geriatric medicine, and general obstetrics and gynecology. All others fall into the categories of subspecialists. Patients can be referred to specialists for conditions that their primary care providers feel they cannot or should not handle. Patients can also choose to bypass the generalist physicians and go directly to a specialist. This route has become less common because of financial penalties associated with self-referral to specialists, imposed by managed care health insurance plans. Despite this, the proportion of ambulatory care visits to other than generalist physicians (about 40%) does not appear to have changed since 1985 (USDHHS, 1995, Table 80; Woodwell, 1999, Table 1). This may be explained by the observation that more services, both medical and surgical, can and are being performed on an ambulatory basis.

Surgical ambulatory care is defined as surgical procedures performed on patients not admitted to an inpatient bed. From 1994 to 1998 ambulatory surgeries rose from 50.5 per 1,000 population to 57.7 per 1,000 population, whereas the rate per 1,000 population of inpatient surgeries fell from 47.8 in 1994 to 36.0 in 1998 (AHA, 2000, Table 3, p. 9) (see Figure 7.11). The percentage of outpatient surgeries (of the total number of surgeries performed) rose from 16.4% in 1980, to 54.9% in 1993 (USDHHS, 1995, Table 90), and 61.7% in 1998 (AHA, 2000, Table 3, p. 9) (see Figure 7.12). This marked

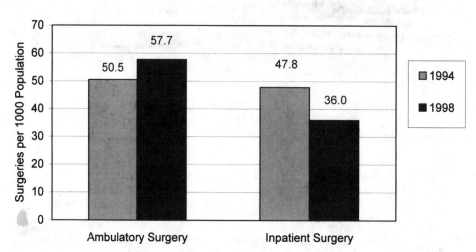

FIGURE 7.11   Changes in surgical ambulatory care procedure rates from 1994 to 1998.

Source: American Hospital Association. (2000). *Hospital Statistics 2000.* Chicago: Health Forum LLC, Table 3, p. 9.

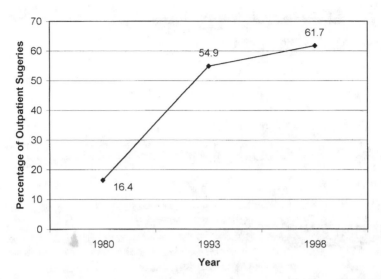

FIGURE 7.12   Growth in percentage of outpatient surgeries (1980–1998).

Sources: U.S. Department of Health and Human Services. (1995). *Health United States, 1995* (DHHS publication No. PHS 96-1232). Washington, DC: U.S. Government Printing Office, Table 90; American Hospital Association. (2000). *Hospital Statistics 2000.* Chicago: Health Forum LLC, Table 3, p. 9.

change can be attributed to improved technology, economic pressures, and the demands of both patients and third-party payers. Patient satisfaction and outcomes appear to be good for all forms of ambulatory surgery.

Imaging procedures can be performed in ambulatory imaging facilities located in hospitals, be part of a large multi-specialty group practice, or be freestanding. All offer similar services, such as standard radiographic studies—X rays, ultrasound, echocardiography, nuclear medicine studies (bone scans, thyroid scans), computed axial tomography (CT scans), and magnetic resonance imaging (MRI). Some of the more esoteric imaging techniques, such as positron emission tomography (PET scans), and most imaging associated with invasive techniques (like cardiac and cerebral angiography), is done in hospitals, the latter as inpatient studies.

Subspecialist physicians in their own offices also do imaging procedures. There are many gastroenterologists, urologists, orthopedists, cardiologists, and radiologists who perform diagnostic imaging in their private offices rather than use the local hospital's facilities. Pulmonary specialists may be set up to perform a whole array of diagnostic tests in their own offices, including radiographic studies.

All this causes competition among the various providers and, although competition may keep costs down in usual markets, it does not necessarily appear to be true of the health marketplace. These facilities require expensive equipment and rely on referrals from other physicians to succeed. Ethical, legal, and financial problems emerge, especially when some of the referring physicians have financial interests in the success of the freestanding imaging centers. On the other hand, this competitive market makes life convenient for patients because some of the centers are open for business 24 hours a day, 7 days a week.

HOME HEALTH CARE

Home health care services were the fastest growing sector of Medicare by percentage of increase in expenditures per year until 1996. In 1997, 1998, and 1999 total expenditures for home-based services fell because of changes in Medicare reimbursement. The primary reason for the initial increase was economic pressure—the need to get patients out of the hospital quicker. This did not cause a general outcry from the public, as did "drive-through" mastectomies and 24-hour hospital stays after delivery. This was likely related to three factors: patients prefer to be cared for in their own homes; most patients, no matter how complex their medical problems, can be cared for as well in the home as in a rehabilitation or skilled nursing facility; and outcomes of home care are similar to other settings for similar conditions (P. Rosenfeld and M. Mezey, personal communication, January 25, 2001).

In addition, in 1989, following a lawsuit, Medicare rules for home care services were clarified, making it easier for Medicare recipients to receive home health services, with expenditures increasing at an average annual rate of 40% between 1988 and 1991, reaching $5.4 billion (Bishop & Skwara, 1993). Overall home health care expenditures in 1993 were estimated to be $23 billion, increasing at an annual rate of 19.1% between 1982 and 1992, and 12.9% between 1992 and 1993 (National Institute for Health Care Management [NIHCM], 1996).

Patients are eligible to receive home health services from a qualified Medicare provider if they are homebound; if they are under the care of a specified physician who will establish a home health plan; and if they need physical or occupational therapy, speech therapy, or intermittent skilled nursing care. Skilled nursing care is defined both as technical procedures, such as tube feedings or catheter care, and as skilled nursing observations. Intermittent is defined as up to 28 hours per week for nursing care and 35 hours per week for home health aide care. Many hospitals have formed their own home health care agencies, finding this a useful way to increase revenues while enabling them to discharge patients from the hospital earlier. In most communities, however, the bulk of home health services are still provided by not-for-profit agencies, such as the Visiting Nurse Service of New York.

COMPLEMENTARY AND ALTERNATIVE MEDICAL CARE

In 1992, Congress established the Office of Alternative Medicine (OAM) at the National Institutes of Health (NIH) with the stated purpose of evaluating complementary and alternative medical treatment modalities to determine their effectiveness and to integrate these treatments into mainstream medical practice. A number of OAM centers were established, including those at the Universities of Minnesota, Texas, and California (Davis), and Stanford and Columbia Universities. The OAM has become the National Center for Complementary and Alternative Medicine (NCCAM). Its home page states "The National Center for Complementary and Alternative Medicine at the National Institutes of Health is dedicated to exploring the complementary and alternative practices in the context of rigorous science; training CAM researchers; and disseminating authoritative information" (NCCAM, 2001b). The NCCAM defines Complementary and Alternative Medicine (CAM) as "those treatments and healthcare practices not taught widely in medical schools, not generally used in hospitals, and not usually reimbursed by medical insurance companies" (NCCAM, 2001a).

The NCCAM has divided CAM practices into five major groups:

1. Alternative Medical Systems (ayurveda, homeopathy, naturopathy).
2. Mind-Body Interventions (certain uses of hypnosis, dance, music and art therapy, prayer, and mental healing).
3. Biological-Based Therapies (herbal, special dietary, orthomolecular, and individual therapies).
4. Manipulative and Body-Based Methods (chiropractic, some osteopathic practices, massage therapy).
5. Energy Therapies (Qi Gong; Reiki; therapeutic touch; bioelectromagnetic-based therapies such as pulsed fields, magnetic fields, AC and DC current).

It appears that there is a growing use of complementary and alternative medicine in the United States, with an estimated 629 million visits to CAM providers in 1997, of which one third were to chiropractors. Eisenberg and colleagues (1993) showed that 34% of 1,539 adults surveyed reported using one or another form of alternative medicine. In two studies of HIV-infected gay or bisexual men, over half stated that they used complementary or alternative treatments (Anderson, 1993; O'Connor, Lazar, & Anderson, 1992). In a more recent study from South Carolina, 44% of adults had used CAM in the year prior to the survey, of which 60% perceived CAM as very effective. Physicians were unaware of CAM use in 57% of their patients (Oldendick, Coker, Wieland, Raymond, Probst, Schell, et al., 2000).

PATIENT NETWORKS AND SUPPORT GROUPS

Patient networks and support groups exist for virtually every illness. They can be accessed in a variety of ways—through the Internet, through the social work department of the local hospital, through community organizations such as the YMCA, or through organizations established for specific diseases or need (e.g., AIDS/HIV disease, diabetes mellitus, blindness, breastfeeding, cancer, colostomies, multiple sclerosis, and cardiovascular diseases). They are a useful adjunct to care, allowing patients to share experiences and concerns. Internet chat rooms allow two or more individuals to "speak" to each other about issues of mutual concern. This method of patient networking and support will likely increase markedly, offering as it does a combination of the convenience of remaining at home, the flexibility of the hours of use, and perhaps the advantage of anonymity.

SUMMARY AND CURRENT ISSUES IN AMBULATORY CARE

In this chapter we have attempted to give the reader a picture of the status of ambulatory care available to the average American. We have emphasized the provision of primary care because we believe that it is through a continuous, mutually trusting relationship between the individual and the provider of primary care that health and emotional needs will best be served. We have tried to show how that continuum starts when an individual, concerned about a specific problem, tries to deal with it. There are a number of options available: asking a knowledgeable relative or friend; using resources available in print or on the Internet, or discussion with a health care provider, either a practitioner of alternative medicine or a traditional practitioner, over the telephone, by email, or in person

The Primary Care Provider of the Future

The definitions of the providers of primary care will expand to include individuals other than those described in the section on primary care. There are, for example, infectious disease specialists—internists with specialty training in infectious disease—who act as primary care practitioners for individuals with infection due to human immunodeficiency virus (HIV). HIV disease was initially recognized as an acute infection but has become a chronic infection with the advent of new and improved therapies. These infectious disease specialists are recognized as the primary care providers for a subset of patients with special needs.

The above is true of diseases such as cancer and of genetic diseases such as cystic fibrosis and sickle cell disease. The list will grow as medical knowledge and effective treatments for many disease entities expand. As the management of patients with mental illness has become more dependent upon the use of psychopharmacological medications, its treatment will become an effort managed by primary care teams that will include psychiatrists, psychologists, social workers, and nurse practitioners or physician assistants, with internists or family practitioners acting as consultants rather than as primary care providers in this setting. The use of primary care provider teams will expand to cover a whole host of diseases now primarily cared for by single practitioners.

Current practice is for patients to access their primary care provider when deciding that they need more information than is available to them through other means. This trend was initially driven by health cost considerations; it has now gone beyond that to the recognition that everyone should have a medical "home," a place one can go to for the full spectrum of care, both for wellness and for sickness, for advice and education about remaining healthy, and for advice about returning to a prior level of health. This primary care medical home will, in the future, consist of teams of individuals with overlapping areas of expertise, offering a spectrum of services—from the management of minor acute illness and advice about diet, exercise, and vitamin supplements to the management of psychosocial issues such as domestic violence, alcoholism, and substance abuse and the coordination of care for serious life-threatening or chronic conditions. Individuals may be referred to health care providers outside their primary care teams, but the responsibility for the coordination and monitoring of their care will continue to rest within their medical homes.

Drivers of Change

This change in how primary care is delivered will be driven by how health care is financed and by the need for efficiency in managing large numbers of patients with changing demands. Thirty years ago husbands were rarely, if ever, allowed into delivery rooms to give comfort to their wives and to witness the birth of their children. Today it is more the rule than the exception. Families drove this change; the health care professions did not drive it. Whether or not capitation payments dominate health care financing, whether or not the capitation is for primary care or full-risk, consumers of health care will demand more health care providers, especially in the areas of health maintenance and health education. They will also demand easier access—same day or next day appointments with their own team of providers—than they currently have (Murray & Tantau, 2000). They will be less likely to accept long waits when arriving at the primary care office. Successful practices will be able to provide health care for a large population of individuals, offering three things: efficient management—prompt appointments, accurate billing; high patient satisfaction—courteous staff, easy telephone access, pleasant surroundings, extended hours; and medical outcomes that meet or exceed expected benchmarks—rare medication errors, adherence to health management guidelines, strict follow-up on medical protocols. To do this, they will need to employ real teamwork and health care managers will have to be trained to function effectively in this new paradigm. Physicians will need to learn to behave as members of a health care team. The culture of medical practice as a cottage industry has already changed in the management of diseases and conditions requiring sophisticated technology and medical protocols. Primary care will be the last frontier.

These changes will occur, but they will occur slowly, driven by changes in the education of primary care physicians. The requirements for the accreditation of primary care residency programs are changing. Experience in the continuity of care of panels of patients in community-based settings, as opposed to hospital-based outpatient clinics, is being developed. Primary care residency programs are required to develop a formal curriculum that documents training in diverse aspects of medicine, such as biomedical ethics, medical legal issues, cost management of health care, and the responsibility of health care providers for an entire population of individuals, as opposed to episodic care. This will become the educational standard for all primary care providers.

Benefits of Change

Care of populations or panels of patients responds to both cost and health concerns. Giving influenza vaccine to an entire population of elderly patients, for example, might save money by decreasing the seasonal number of admissions for pneumonia and other influenza-related complications. Strict adherence to yearly mammograms for women over the age of 40 or 50 might save money by allowing earlier detection of breast cancer and therefore less costly interventions. Early recognition of illness might also decrease the costs of care for prostate cancer, colorectal cancer, and adult-onset diabetes. Emphasis on wellness programs, such as decreasing the incidence of obesity; education on the importance of exercise for weight control; decreasing the risk for the development of, for example, osteoporosis and heart disease; and promotion of smoking cessation to decrease the incidence of lung and heart disease, will become standard features of the care offered by primary care providers, either directly or indirectly, to their populations of patients. Early recognition for conditions that currently have no or minimally effective treatments, for example Alzheimer's disease, will become more important as our ability to treat them improves.

The data on whether or not these practices do save money for specific groups of people insured by a single HMO are not clear, but accrediting organizations like the NCQA are demanding that HMOs adhere to these recommendations. And HMOs, in turn, are demanding that practitioners listed on their panels adhere to these standards as well. In the early 1990s the majority of medical school deans responsible for the oversight of residency education were concerned about the impact that managed care was having on their training programs. That has changed. In the 1997 meeting in Santa Fe, New Mexico, of the Group on Residency Affairs (GRA) of the Association of American Medical Colleges (AAMC), the tone of the discussion changed. There was an emphasis on how to teach the "new medicine" to residents, not based on cost of care concerns but based on the best interests of patients.

Each year approximately 12,000 residents complete training in generalist specialties in the United States. It will be from this group of individuals, trained in a different paradigm of what constitutes primary care that the changes in how ambulatory care is delivered will come. They will be joined by other providers of primary care—nurse practitioners, midwives, physician assistants, and social workers—and formed into primary care teams. They will have profound influences on all aspects of care because these primary care providers/teams have the greatest number of patient contacts. They will demand that their surgical and medical subspecialist colleagues pay attention to their concerns. This will occur irrespective of the way health care is financed.

Current Issues in Ambulatory Care

Ambulatory care issues include: access to care (see chapter 15), cost containment (see chapter 16), and quality improvement (see chapter 14).

Access to Care

There is a lack of access to ambulatory care for the over 40 million Americans who lack health insurance coverage, and for millions of other Americans whose access to care is limited because of where they live, the language they speak, limited insurance coverage, and their inability to read, among other reasons. Regarding the first issue, assuming there are no sizeable improvements in insurance coverage, what should providers of care do about this situation, other than urge the enactment of a national health insurance system or of other coverages leading toward national health insurance? Regarding the second issue, when people can pay for service, what are the responsibilities of provider outreach and for being accessible, for example by providing after hours services or having a system that can handle different languages?

Organizations can respond in several ways. With regard to coverage, they can hold that they are responsible only for paying customers or for providing those services, such as emergency care, where they are required by law to do so. A second approach is to provide medically appropriate services to all who live within the organization's catchment area, or who come for care, and then to attempt to raise money from government or philanthropy or through cross-subsidization from profitable services, to meet the medical needs of those who can not pay for care. A third approach is to bring down the price of health care, either by organizing care in new ways or by recruiting volunteers to provide services at no cost.

Strategies to respond to lack of access among those with more adequate health insurance coverage include more extensive and improved outreach, better health education in the schools and on the job, and enhancing cultural sensitivity and linguistic capability among frontline providers.

Improved technology and better management can result in shortened waiting times for appointments and waiting times in the office. Improved communication (e.g., access through email), between patient and provider, and among patients with the same symptoms or diseases, can result for many. Patients can gain access to comprehensive and targeted information through websites on symptoms, diseases, and treatment. Better protocols for service provision and better information can result in improved case management for patients with chronic conditions, such as for those who have difficulty following different regimens prescribed by multiple specialists at the same time.

Research needs to be done to target individuals who are at health risk if untreated, and on ways to give such individuals better access to appropriate care. How can we predict which individuals are mostly likely to be at risk for conditions that if untreated will have serious health and cost impacts? Once such individuals are identified, how can resources be best allocated so that the people can actually receive needed health care?

Cost Containment

The costs of ambulatory care are rising significantly as more treatment is done outside of hospitals and nursing homes, and the costs of drugs and new technologies continue to rise. Promising ways to contain the costs of ambulatory care include the following: patients leading healthier lives, less costly provision of more primary care through providers other than physicians, and better disease management. Standardized insurance forms and payment protocols can reduce ambulatory care billing costs. So can collecting payments up front rather than billing for care on a per-episode basis.

Costs in the secondary and tertiary sectors of the health care services system can be reduced, thus allowing shifts to greater investment in primary and preventive care. Should hospital-based ambulatory care be phased out and replaced by more efficient alternatives? Less secondary and tertiary care can be provided in the last 12 months of life. Hospital beds can be closed and jobs eliminated through reducing hospital capacity, a process that, of course, has been under way in some parts of the country for the last 20 years.

Research needs to be done, with the best practices disseminated, on the ways to make sure that patients receive certain cost-effective services, such as counseling to stop smoking. Patients must also be helped to follow regimens, for example, through development of computerized systems for patients to enter what behaviors they practice and do not practice daily, for review by providers.

Research needs to be conducted concerning what behavioral practices pay off in improved health outcomes. How can we best help patients and members to improve literacy, eat more balanced diets, exercise more, and consume less alcohol and cigarettes? Research dollars can be reallocated away from measuring how smoking causes cancer, and toward how to prevent persons from beginning to smoke in the first place.

Quality Improvement

There are significant variations in the quality of medical care due to, for example, underuse of known treatments that can improve health outcomes, overuse of treatments that have no predictable positive impact on patient health, and misuse of treatments, such as preventable adverse drug reactions. Improvements can be made regarding the technical quality of ambulatory care and regarding the service amenities provided to patients and members. Care currently ranges widely in quality. The Institute of Medicine has recommended six redesign imperatives in delivering care as follows: redesigning care processes; making more effective use of information technologies; improving knowledge and skills through evidence-based management; developing effective patient care delivery teams; coordinating care across patient conditions, services, and settings over time; and using performance and outcome measurement for continuous quality improvement and accountability (Institute of Medicine, 2001).

Research needs to be conducted regarding the impact on providers and patients of incentives to improve health treatments and healthy behavior. How can we optimize the use of provider time to better communicate with patients? How can patients gain confidence to share information more fully with their providers, not only about disease symptoms, but also about gaining help with the difficulties patients have in leading healthier lives?

Improving access, containing costs, and improving quality will sometimes result in tremendous dislocations for the system and for those it gives care alike. For example, if coverage is improved without lowering costs, this means that health care expenditures will increase and that it will be more difficult to invest in improved schools, environment, and welfare. If hospitals and medical schools are closed, this can result in thousands of health workers losing their jobs, and in patients and students having less access to desired services. Improving quality costs money too. Think of the investment required for better information systems to link all patients electronically with their providers and to educate providers, patients, and members to be able to use systems that will be made available to them. Political leadership is required by government, health care providers, and consumer advocates to facilitate more cost-effective ambulatory care that still allows for some autonomy of providers and some choice for patients and members.

CASE STUDY

You are a health care consultant and Dr. Irving Freedom, the senior partner in a primary care group of six internists and three nurse practitioners
practicing in an affluent suburb of a large eastern U.S. city, has asked for
your advice. His practice has seen a 10% decline in the number of patient
visits and a 12% decline in revenue in the past year. The adult population
of the area has actually seen an increase of 10% in the last 5 years. There
has not been a significant increase in either the number of internists or
family practitioners in the community in the last 5 years. Dr. Freedom
would like to see his practice grow.

You investigate and learn the following: Patient calling for an appointment frequently get a busy signal or are put on hold. When patients do
get through they are always asked whether or not they have been seen in
the office before, told that the next available routine appointment is at
least 4 weeks in the future and may not be with the primary care provider
who is their usual source of care. The practice's information system is set
up only for billing purposes and is not available to either the receptionists
that answer the telephone or to the office nurses that do the bulk of the
triage. The practice has never conducted a patient satisfaction survey.

What should you advise him to do? Include in your answer a discussion of what Dr. Freedom can do in the short and long term to improve
how his practice functions. Include what you believe Dr. Freedom needs
to learn in order to function effectively in this new work environment.

DISCUSSION QUESTIONS

1. What factors are driving the delivery of health care away from emergency
   care and inpatient hospital stays?
2. How has the role of the primary care practitioner expanded?
3. For what groups of patients do medical specialist its primary care
   providers?
4. In the context of this chapter, what is meant by the integrated delivery of
   health care services?
5. What are three factors that have contributed to the increase in patients
   learning to provide more of their own health care?

REFERENCES

American Hospital Association (AHA). (2000). *Hospital statistics 2000*. Chicago:
    Health Forum LLC.
Anderson, W. H. (1993). Patient use and assessment of conventional and alterna-
    tive therapies for HIV infection and AIDS. *AIDS, 74*, 561–564.
Bishop, C., & Skwara, K. C. (1993). Recent growth of Medicare home health.
    Health Affairs, 12, 95–107.

Bodenheimer, T. (1996). Sounding board: The HMO backlash—righteous or reactionary. *New England Journal of Medicine, 335,* 1601–1603.

Eisenberg, D. M., Kessler, R. C. Foster, C., Norlock, F. E., Calkins, D. R., & Delbanco, T. L. (1993). Unconventional medicine in the United States: Prevalence, costs, and patterns of use. *New England Journal of Medicine, 328,* 248–252.

Forrest, C. B., & Whalen, E.-M. (2000). Primary care safety-net delivery sites in the United States: A comparison of community health centers, hospital outpatient departments, and physician offices. *Jounral of the American Medical Association, 284,* 2077–2083.

Institute of Medicine. (1996). *Primary care: America's health in a new era.* Washington, DC: National Academy Press.

Institute of Medicine. (2001). *Crossing the quality chasmi: A new health system for the 21st century.* Washington, DC: National Academy Press.

Markowitz, D. B. (Compiler). (2000). *Health care almanac and yearbook, 2000.* New York: Faulkner and Gray.

Murray, M., & Tantau, C. (2000). Same day appointments: Exploding the access paradigm. *Family Practice Management, 7,* 45–50.

National Center for Complementary and Alternative Medicine (NCCAM). (2001a). *Frequently asked questions* [On-line]. Available: http://nccam.nih.gov/nccam/fcp/faq/index.html

National Center for Complementary and Alternative Medicine (NCCAM). (2001b). *NCCAM home page* [On-line]. Available: http:/nccam.nih.gov

National Institute for Health Care Management. (1996). *Health care system data source.* San Francisco, CA: Institute for Health Policy Studies, University of California.

Nourjah, P. (1999). National Hospital Ambulatory Medical Care survey: 1997 emergency department summary. In *Advance Data from Vital and Health Statistics,* (No. 304). Hyattswville, MD: National Center for Health Statistics.

O'Connor, B. B. Lazar, J. S., & Anderson, W. H. (1992, June). *Ethnographic study of HIV alternative therapies.* Poster presented at the Eighth International Conference on AIDS, Amsterdam.

Oldendick, R, Coker, A. L., Wieland, D., Raymond, J. I., Probst, J. C., Schell, B. J., & Stoskopf, C. H. (2000). Population-based survey of complementary and alternative medicine usage, patient satisfaction, and physician involvement. South Carolina Complementary Medicine Program Baseline Research Team. *Southern Medical Journal, 93,* 375–381.

Schappert, S. M. (1999). Ambulatory care visits to physician offices, hospital outpatient departments, and emergency departments: United States, 1997. *Vital and Health Statistics, Series 13*(143).

Scheffler, R. M. (1996). Life in the kaleidoscope: The impact of managed care on the U.S. health care workforce and a new model for the delivery of primary care. In M. S. Donaldson, F. D. Yordy, K. N. Lohr, & N. A. Vanselow (Eds.), *Primary care: America's health in a new era* (pp. 312–340). Washington, DC: National Academy Press.

U.S. Department of Health and Human Services. (1982). *Health United States, 1982* (DHHS Publication No. PHS 83-1232). Washington, DC: U.S. Government Printing Office.

U.S. Department of Health and Human Services. (1995). *Health United States, 1995* (DHHS Publication No. PHS 96-1232). Washington, DC: U.S. Government Printing Office.

U.S. Department of Health and Human Services. (2000). *Health United States, 2000* (DHHS Publication No. PHS 01-1232). Washington, DC: U.S. Government Printing Office.

Woodwell, D. A. (1999, May). National Ambulatory Medical Care Survey: 1997 summary. In *Advance Data from Vital and Health Statistics,* (No. 305). Hyattsville, MD: National Center for Health Statistics.

8

Long-Term Care

Penny Hollander Feldman, Pamela Nadash, and Michal D. Gursen

LEARNING OBJECTIVES

- ☐ Define the key components of long-term care (LTC) and discuss the factors that contribute to need and demand for service.
- ☐ Describe the principal users and the principal sources of payment for LTC.
- ☐ Discuss the differences and similarities between individual and societal-level goals for the LTC system.
- ☐ Distinguish among the principal paid providers of LTC and the populations they serve.
- ☐ Identify the major cost, quality, and access issues in LTC and discuss the strengths and weaknesses of alternative policy options

TOPICAL OUTLINE

What is long-term care?
Long-term care need and demand
How much does the U.S. spend on long-term care and who pays?
What are the goals of long-term care?
Who supplies long-term care?
Challenging issues
Conclusions

KEY WORDS

long-term care, chronic health conditions, activities of daily living, instrumental activities of daily living, formal and informal services/paid and unpaid caregivers, nursing homes, home- and community-based services (HCBS), home care, home health care, certified home health agency (CHHA), hospice services, adult day care, respite services, assisted living facilities, continuing care retirement communities (CCRCs), public/private financing, integrated long-term and acute care financing, private LTC insurance, access, quality, consumer choice

WHAT IS LONG-TERM CARE?

The senior boom is one of the central challenges of the coming century . . . We must use this time now to do everything in our power, not only to lift the quality of life and the security of the aged and disabled today, and the baby boom aged and disabled, but to make sure that we do not impose that intolerable burden on our children. (Bill Clinton, *Remarks by the President on the Long-Term Health Initiative*, 1/4/99)

The need for long-term care (LTC) is growing. The American population is aging, and the fastest population growth is among the "oldest old"— those people 85 years or older who are most likely to be affected by chronic, disabling conditions. Moreover, technological advances are enabling virtually everyone with a disabling condition—young or old—to live longer. Today, hardly any human being, no matter how handicapped or disabled, is beyond some rehabilitation (Callahan, 1990). As a result, family caregivers, community service providers, health care experts, policymakers, and consumers of care themselves are struggling on a daily basis to identify the kinds of service and supports needed to optimally address the challenges of those who live with disability.

All too often, the public equates long-term care with care in a nursing home or other institution. However, LTC is composed of a broad constellation of services provided in varied settings to a heterogeneous population with diverse needs (Stone, 2000). "Supportive" services form the core of LTC. These services include personal assistance with basic daily functions such as bathing, eating, walking, or going to the toilet. In the LTC literature, such activities are commonly referred to as activities of daily living (ADLs). Supportive services also include help with household chores and related activities such as shopping, cooking, managing money, and paying bills, or traveling to and from one's home. In the LTC literature, these activities are commonly referred to as instrumental activities of daily living (IADLs).

In order to control the symptoms and progression of their disease, millions of individuals with chronic disabling conditions also require ongoing medical monitoring and intervention, in addition to routine help with ADLs or IADLs. Others require rehabilitative services to maintain or at least delay a decline in physical or mental function. Thus, LTC often may have a medical or rehabilitative as well as a supportive component.

In addition, people suffering from chronic disabling disease can benefit from palliative care, defined as the "comprehensive management of physical, social, spiritual, and existential needs of patients" (Kaplan & Urbina, 2000). Although palliative care is most commonly associated with the decision to give up active medical treatment in the last weeks, days, or hours of life, a number of experts are now seeking to incorporate palliative care principles "upstream" in the LTC continuum (Kaplan & Urbina, 2000).

In this chapter we adopt a broad definition of LTC that encompasses a range of supportive, rehabilitative, nursing, and palliative services provided to people—young or old—whose capacity to perform daily activities is restricted due to chronic disease or disability. Table 8.1 outlines the range of services we include in our definition of LTC and provides examples of each. LTC may be provided in institutions, congregate settings, or individual homes or apartments to people of all ages suffering from physical and mental disabilities. Family, friends, neighbors, and other unpaid caregivers provide most LTC. Among paid providers, individual service providers include nurses, aides, therapists, social workers, case managers, physicians, and others. Organized providers include home health agencies, nursing homes, adult day centers, and a variety of community-based residential facilities including board and care homes and assisted living facilities.

TABLE 8.1 Range of Long-Term Care Services

Type of Service	Example
Housekeeping & other IADL support	Cleaning, cooking, laundry, shopping, home maintenance, financial management
Companionship & social support	Visiting, calling, counseling, advising, case management
Transportation	Arranging, accompanying, providing transportation & escort services
Personal care	Hands-on, supervision, or standby assistance with ADLs (bathing, dressing, walking, transferring, feeding, toileting)
Nursing & health care procedures	Assessment, care planning, promotion of optimum health status including recovery from acute illness and relief of symptoms
Rehabilitative services	Exercises and programs to improve or restore functioning (motion, speech, bowel, bladder)
Palliative care	Comfort care, symptom management, and medication management at the end of life
Care management	Planning and arranging appointments, equipment, transportation, and provider communication

Adapted from: Kane, R. A. (1999). Goals of Home Care: Therapeutic, Compensatory, Either, or Both? *Journal of Aging and Health, H*(3), 302–303, Tables 2 and 3.

Service purchasers include individuals and families, as well as third parties such as state Medicaid agencies, area agencies on aging, private insurers, and managed long-term care plans.

LONG-TERM CARE NEED AND DEMAND

Who Needs and Receives Long-Term Care?

In general, people who need help in carrying out one or more ADLs or IADLs due to physical disability, cognitive impairment, or both, are considered candidates for long-term care. However, disabled individuals differ considerably in the severity of their limitations and their need for assistance. Some individuals may require direct, hands-on assistance or supervision in order to meet their basic daily needs, while for others, special equipment or training can enable them to function relatively independently. Disability can be present from birth, as in the case of individuals with developmental disabilities; it may occur as the result of injury or disease; or it may manifest itself as a part of the aging process (General Accounting Office [GAO], 1999a).

Not all older people will need LTC, however. The body of work on "successful aging" shows that the majority of older Americans are generally healthy and that even among the "oldest old"—people aged 85 or older—40% are fully functional (Rowe & Kahn, 1998). Nevertheless, as people age, they do become more dependent. They are at increased risk of the chronic diseases of old age—arthritis, hypertension and heart disease, diabetes, hearing and visual impairments, and Alzheimer's disease. They require help with tasks such as cleaning, shopping, and preparing meals. They also become more reliant on others for transportation and for assistance in activities of daily living, such as bathing, dressing, eating, and moving from bed to chair. At age 65, 10%–20% of a person's remaining years are likely to be spent requiring assistance in one or more activities of daily living. For people 85 years old, the figure is about 50% (Rowe & Kahn, 1998). Table 8.2 illustrates the wide range of conditions and impairments that—regardless of age—may lead to the need for LTC.

Although need for help accelerates with age, it is by no means limited to older persons. Of the 12.8 million Americans who reported need for long-term care services in 1995, approximately 57% were elderly (over 65 years), 40% were working-age adults (18–65 years), and 3% were children (under 18 years) (see Figure 8.1). Four out of five lived in the community, while just under one in five were in institutions (GAO, 1995). Actual use of LTC, either at home or in an institution, also rises with age (see Figure 8.2).

People receiving institutional care differ considerably from people receiving LTC who live in the community. First, they are older: among the elderly, the mean age of those receiving LTC in the community was approximately 79, whereas while the mean age of those receiving nursing

TABLE 8.2 Examples of Conditions and Impairments Requiring Long-Term Care Services

Chronic Illness	*Developmental Disabilities*
Arthritis	Cerebral palsy
Cancer	Genetic or congenital defects
Heart disease	Seizure disorders
Emphysema	
Alzheimer's disease	*Injuries*
Cystic fibrosis	Paralysis from head and spinal cord injuries
	Burns
Impairments	
Blindness	
Hearing loss	
Paralysis	

Source: Richardson, H., Raphael, C., & Barton, B. (1998). Long-Term Care: Health, Social and Housing Services for Those with Chronic Illness. In A. R. Kovner & S. Jonas (Eds.), *Jonas and Kovner's Health Care Delivery in the United States* (6th ed., p. 209). New York: Springer Publishing.

home care was nearly 85. Secondly, they are more likely to be female. Women comprise over two thirds of older persons receiving LTC in the community, but nearly three quarters of those in nursing homes. Thirdly, they are less likely to be black. Black elders constitute nearly 12% of all elderly community-based LTC users but only 8% of nursing home residents. Lastly, nursing home residents are less likely to be married and much more likely to be divorced or separated. Only about 17% of elders in nursing homes are married, while married elders constitute 37% of those receiving LTC in the community. Almost 65% of older nursing home residents are divorced or separated, compared to 7% of older community LTC users. (All figures from Spector, Fleishman, Pezzin, and Spillman, 1998, using data from 1994.)

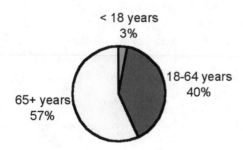

FIGURE 8.1 Long-term care need by age, 1995 (12 million persons).

Source: Spector, W. D., Fleishman, J. A., Pezzin, L. E., & Spillman, B. C. (1998). *The Characteristics of Long-Term Care Users.* Paper prepared for the Institute of Medicine, Committee on Improving Quality in Long-Term Care, Washington, DC.

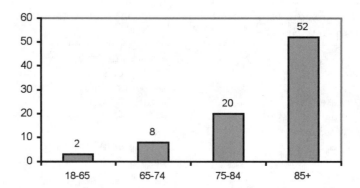

FIGURE 8.2   Percent receiving assistance with one or more ADLs or IADLs.
Source: Spector, W. D., Fleishman, J. A., Pezzin, L. E., & Spillman, B. C. (1998). *The Characteristics of Long-Term Care Users.* Paper prepared for the Institute of Medicine, Committee on Improving Quality in Long-Term Care, Washington, DC.

What Is Likely To Be the Future Demand for Long-Term Care?

The demand for long-term care is expected to grow in the coming years for two main reasons. First, the number of people with functional limitations due to disabling conditions is increasing, as new medical technologies enable people with such conditions to sustain longer lives. The other reason is that both the absolute numbers and the proportion of elderly in the population are expected to increase. Although older people today are less disabled than were people of the same age 10–20 years ago (Manton, Corder, & Stallard, 1997), they are affected by chronic conditions with the greatest frequency and severity. Thus they will account for the majority of the anticipated increase in demand for long-term care services.

In 1997, those 85 and over, who are most at risk for disability and institutionalization, numbered about 3.9 million. By 2030, when the first of the baby boomers reach their 85th birthday, that number will double to approximately 8.5 million, and by 2050 it will more than double again to over 18 million people 85 and older, or nearly 5% of the total population (GAO, 1998). Put in terms of percentage growth, between 1998 and 2050, the under 65-year-old population is projected to grow by 36% (from 236 to 322 million), the total 65+ population by 141% (from 34 to 82 million), and the 85+ population by 363% (from 4 to 18 million) (GAO, 1998; U.S. Census Bureau, 2000).

This exponential growth of the older population will have a dramatic impact on the prevalence of disability and the use of long-term care. For example;

- the number of persons age 65 and older with at least two ADL limitations is projected to increase from 1.8 million in the period 1996–2000 to 2.4 million in 2020–2024 and 3.8 million in 2045–2049;

- the number of nursing home residents and residents of alternative living facilities age 65 and older is projected to increase from 2 million in 2000 to approximately 2.6 million in 2020 and 4.5 million in 2050;
- the number of older users of home-based services is projected to grow from 5.4 million in 2000 to 7.2 million in 2020 and 10.5 million in 2050 (Tilly, Goldenson, Kasten, O'Shaughnessy, Kelly, & Sidor, 2000).

How Much Does the U.S. Spend on Long-Term Care and Who Pays?

In 1998 personal health care spending in the United States stood at more than $1 trillion. Determining how much of this enormous figure went toward long-term care is difficult, because the national chart of health accounts does not clearly separate out long-term care dollars from dollars that may be spent on posthospital, subacute,[1] or end-of-life care. Moreover, the national system of accounting does not take into account the value of unpaid LTC services provided by family, friends, and neighbors.

Many estimates of formal LTC spending in the U.S. simply sum expenditures for nursing home and home health services. In 1998, $117 billion (combined) was spent on nursing home and home health care—75% or $88 billion went to pay for nursing home care and 25% or $29 billion to home health services (Health Care Financing Administration, 2000). Not all care provided by home health agencies and nursing homes, however, is long-term care. Virtually all home health agencies and many nursing homes also serve short-stay patients. Furthermore, long-term care is provided by a wide variety of other organizations, such as local housekeeping agencies, aide registries, and "meals on wheels" programs, as well as community-based residences including board and care homes, assisted living facilities, and many others. Taking these factors into account, one recent study estimated that the U.S. spent $150 billion on long-term care in 1998—$100 billion or two thirds on nursing home care, and $50 billion or one third on home health and other community-based services (Feder, Komisar, & Niefeld, 2000). In addition, it has been estimated that the economic value of unpaid caregiving in the U.S. is close to $200 billion—about one third more than the dollars spent on paid services (Arno & Levine, 1999).

The three major sources of financing for formal (i.e., paid) LTC services are Medicaid, Medicare, and personal, out-of-pocket spending. Medicaid accounted for approximately 40% of all LTC spending in 1998, followed by out-of-pocket expenditures (26%) and Medicare (20%) (Feder et al., 2000). Medicaid covered proportionately more nursing home than home

---

[1] Although postacute care refers to care following a hospital say, subacute refers to "a vague treatment modality that may bypass hospitals altogether or that focuses on longer-term rehabilitation, ventilation care, and the like" (Stone, 2000, p. 4).

care expenses, while Medicare covered proportionately more home health than nursing home care expenses. Although between the two, Medicaid and Medicare cover about 60% of LTC spending, private out-of-pocket payments for LTC are quite substantial. Private health insurance covered only 7–8% of LTC spending in 1998.

Medicaid—the federal-state entitlement program that covers medical and other health-related services for selected low-income families and individuals—is the one national program with a clear mandate to cover long-term care. Within broad federal guidelines, each state determines the type, amount, duration, and scope of services its Medicaid program will cover; sets the rate of payment for services; and administers its own program (U.S. Department of Health and Human Services, 1999). States are free to regulate the supply of nursing home beds in their respective jurisdictions and to determine rates of payment for Medicaid residents. However, federal rules are quite explicit with regard to eligibility for nursing home coverage. These rules stipulate that states must cover nursing home care for disabled individuals 65 and older with income up to three times the limit—$532 per month in 2000—for the federal Supplemental Security Income (SSI) program (Feder et al., 2000). Furthermore, individuals may qualify by "spending down" their income and assets as a result of their institutionalization. In turn, they must contribute all of their income to their nursing home care, except for a small personal needs allowance determined by the state. In 1998, federal and state Medicaid dollars together accounted for 46% of all nursing home expenditures, and Medicaid was the principal source of coverage for more than half of current nursing home residents (Gabrel, 2000b).

Under federal guidelines, state Medicaid programs are also required to cover home health care ordered by a physician for people who are eligible for skilled nursing services. Under the "optional" category, they may choose to cover personal care for all who are eligible. As of 1999, 26 states offered personal care as an optional benefit under their program, spending a total of $3.5 billion. Personal care expenditures per participant per year averaged $6,870 (LeBlanc, Tonner, & Harrington, 2000).

In addition, states may apply for a federal waiver that allows them to provide a broad array of medical and supportive home- and community-based services (HCBS) to selected subgroups of people who would otherwise require nursing home care. Services can include case management, homemaker/chore services, and adult day care, as well as personal care. The waiver option allows states to limit the number receiving HCBS services, thus avoiding the potential liability conferred by an open-ended entitlement.

All states and the District of Columbia offer some type of HCBS waiver. By 1997, 221 approved waivers targeted six eligibility groups, including the frail and disabled elderly, working-age individuals with disabilities, people with developmental disabilities, persons with AIDS, children with a variety of disabling conditions, and individuals with serious mental illness (Miller, Ramsland, & Harrington, 1999). In 1997, spending on HCBS waiver programs was $7.9 billion, of which about three quarters was for persons with development disabilities and about 20% for aged and other disabled persons (Tilly et al., 2000).

The Medicare program, which pays for skilled nursing home care (up to 100 days after a hospitalization for people who need continued nursing or therapy services) and home health services (on a part-time or intermittent basis), was originally intended to provide a finite, post-acute care benefit. Nevertheless, during the 1990s it became an important source of long-term care, especially in states with the least generous home care benefits. Two factors account for this phenomenon. First, settlement of a 1988 federal court case (*Duggan v. Bowen*, 1988) resulted in a relaxation of Medicare rules that had denied home health benefits to beneficiaries who did not show the potential for rehabilitation. Second, once a Medicare beneficiary qualifies for part-time or intermittent skilled nursing or rehabilitation services, a significant amount of personal care provided by a home health aide can also be covered by Medicare payments. Between 1990 and 1997, the combination of these two factors led to increases in both the proportion of Medicare beneficiaries receiving home health care and the number of visits per person. Over that period, the number using home health care rose from 57 to 109 per 1,000 beneficiaries served. Similarly, the average number of visits went from 36 to 73 per user (GAO, 2000).

Although Medicare remains the major governmental payer of home health care, spending about $10 billion in 1999 (down from its peak of $18 billion in 1997) (Health Care Financing Administration, 2000), recent changes in Medicare payment may reduce its role in providing long-term care. The Balanced Budget Act of 1997 (BBA) set forth an Interim Payment System (IPS), effective on October 1, 1997, that imposed an annual per beneficiary cap on the amount of money a home health agency could be reimbursed by Medicare. This was followed by a prospective payment system (PPS), effective on October 1, 2000, that introduced a fixed case-mix adjusted payment rate for each 60-day episode of home health care. Because both IPS and PPS eliminated fee-for-service payment and with it the incentive for home health agencies to provide as many visits as needed over as a long a time period as necessary, LTC experts predicted that the likely "losers" under the new systems would be long-term users of home health care—those who were older, less healthy, poorer, more dependent in ADLs, and higher users of home health aide services (Komisar & Feder, 1998).

Given the limits of both Medicaid and Medicare LTC coverage, it is not surprising that out-of-pocket payments constitute a significant share of spending for both nursing home and HCBS users (Feder et al., 2000). Estimates of such personal expenditures, which do not include premium payments for private LTC insurance, range from $35–$40 billion in 1998, or about 26% of the total $150 billion spent on nursing home and home care combined (Feder et al., 2000; Tilly et al., 2000). The bulk of these payments—about $31 billion—went to cover the costs of nursing home care, as individuals contributed to the high yearly costs of those institutions—

nearly $45,000 on average (Gabrel, 2000a)—often depleting their assets and "spending down," thereby becoming eligible for Medicaid. Other out-of-pocket costs went to cover home-based services that were not covered by Medicare, Medicaid, or private insurance.

Purchase of private LTC insurance policies has grown rapidly over the last 10 years—about 10%–12% annually (Tilly et al., 2000). Nevertheless, private health insurance payments still covered less than 10% of LTC expenditures in 1998. Purchase of these policies tends to be among more affluent individuals who can afford annual premiums of $1,000–$2,300 at age 65 or $4,100–$7,000 at age 79. (These ranges depend on whether or not the policy includes inflation protection or a nonforfeiture benefit (Tilly et al., 2000). Although premiums are significantly lower if policies are purchased at a younger age, younger people are often unaware of the risks of LTC. Moreover, those who are more informed may be skeptical about the value of such policies, given uncertainty about both future service costs and future public LTC coverage policies. Although there is no consensus on the future importance of private insurance as a vehicle for covering LTC costs, some experts have estimated that over the next 20 years, 10%–20% of retirees could have the financial resources sufficient to enable them to purchase such policies (Tilly et al., 2000).

WHAT ARE THE GOALS OF LONG-TERM CARE?

We have discussed what LTC services are, who needs and gets them, and how they are financed. The goals of LTC, however, are less straightforward, primarily because LTC is not an end in itself but rather a means to multiple ends, depending on whose perspective is being considered. Table 8.3 lists some LTC goals expressed from the point of view of the individual consumer, and from a broader, societal perspective (Benjamin, 1999; Feldman, 1999; Kane, 1999).

These goals matter, because it is the balancing of individuals' goals with society's goals that determines the shape of LTC services. Clearly set, consistent goals could better guide providers' practices; they could also facilitate a more rational allocation of public LTC resources. Setting clear goals is difficult, however. Government regulators, for example, aim to balance individuals' goals against societal goals, but they also need to consider providers' needs and interests. Legislators aim to satisfy their constituents by providing more alternatives to institutional care, while also responding to other claims on the public purse, such as education and prisons.

In some cases, societal and individual goals correspond well. For example, both aim to facilitate individual choice. Often, however, individual-level goals expressed as desired outcomes for a single person receiving services or supports conflict with societal goals that define desired outcomes for financing and delivery systems, a step removed from the direct impact on an individual consumer (Benjamin, 1999).

TABLE 8.3   Individual and Societal Goals for LTC

Individual	Societal
Meet needs for care and assistance.	Provide an adequate level of services to meet basic needs.
Ensure comfort, safety, and freedom from pain.	Target those most in need.
Remain "at home" as long as possible, in the face of disability and dependence.	Promote the efficient production of cost-effective services.
Maximize function; prevent or delay deterioration of functional abilities.	Maximize individual responsibility.
Access services readily.	Promote a fair and equitable distribution of services.
Maintain and improve physical, psychological, and social health and well-being.	Provide comprehensive services.
Improve self-knowledge and self-care abilities.	Encourage reliance on "informal" systems of family provided care.
Maximize independence, autonomy, and individual choice.	Facilitate consumer choice.
Receive highest quality care.	Ensure acceptable quality of services.
Find information easily.	Integrate and coordinate services.
Minimize out-of-pocket costs.	Contain costs to government and taxpayers.

In reading Table 8.3, note first that virtually every one of the individual-level goals embodies an element of subjective judgment.[2] For example, the definitions of "comfort," "safety," "function," "health," "well-being," "independence," "autonomy," and "choice" will vary from individual to individual and for any one individual, over time, depending on condition and circumstance. The very subjectivity of individual preferences and tastes suggests that individual choice and service direction will be important in any LTC service system that seeks to maximize goals that are important to consumers.

Note secondly that some of the individual-level goals are therapeutic goals, in that they entail an effort to achieve measurable improvement—or forestall measurable deterioration—in an individual's physical, psychological, or social health. In contrast, others are compensatory goals, in that they aim to compensate for an individual's functional impairments by facilitating comfort, safety, and autonomy in spite of disability. Therapeutic goals are generally associated with "medical models" of care, that tend to rely on professional assessment of clinical problems and clinical guidelines

---

[2] Much of the following discussion of goals is adapted from Feldman (1999).

for treatment of specific conditions. In contrast, compensatory goals are generally associated with "social models" of care, that are more likely to emphasize consumer satisfaction and choice as indicators of success.

Thirdly, note that some of the individual-level goals are contradictory. In recent years, the contradiction between safety and autonomy probably has received the most attention. Family members' concerns about safety often directly contradict their loved ones' desire to remain alone in their own homes. Yet safety concerns often win out over autonomy, particularly when families or public authorities assume legal or financial responsibility. Nevertheless, aging experts and consumer advocates increasingly make the case for informed risk-taking that would allow vulnerable individuals to stay at home with less protection than is judged optimal to prevent harm or injury. In general, the greater priority given to individual autonomy as a goal of care, the greater the possibility that the individual's choice of services or supports to promote his or her well-being will clash with the recommendations of family or the expert judgments of an outside professional.

The list of societal goals also contains much subjectivity and many potential contradictions. For example, "adequate," "equitable," "acceptable," and even "cost-effective" are all subject to widely different interpretations depending upon the discipline, philosophy, politics, socioeconomic status, or institutional vantage point of those defining the terms. Furthermore, potential contradictions among goals abound. For example, depending on how "adequacy" and "basic" are defined, providing an adequate level of services to meet basic needs may imply providing services to a population different from those "most in need." Promoting a "fair and equitable" distribution of services may run counter to relying on informal, family-provided care, while the latter may conflict with facilitating consumer choice. Facilitating consumer choice could raise system costs, depending on the range of choices provided, and thereby conflict with the goal of containing costs to government and taxpayers. Similarly, ensuring adequate quality of care across a diversity of settings and services may require increased government spending. These examples illustrate the challenges facing policymakers who struggle to finance long-term care that is distributed equitably, with quality standards and proven efficiency, while promoting consumer choice and controlling costs. We shall return to some of these policy issues at the end of this chapter.

WHO SUPPLIES LONG-TERM CARE?

Unpaid Caregivers

The vast majority of long-term care provided in the U.S. is provided by family, friends, neighbors, and other unpaid caregivers. Unpaid care provided by family, friends, and others is usually referred to as "informal care." Many advocates object to the term "informal," however, because it seems to belie the amount of time, effort, organization, and coordination dedicated to carrying out such activities.

In 1994, approximately 40% (2.2 million) of elderly long-term care users who lived in the community relied solely on unpaid caregivers for assistance with at least one ADL or IADL. Over a quarter (1.4 million) relied on a mix of unpaid caregivers and paid services, while only 5% (256,000) relied solely on paid help. Among the 5.9 million unpaid caregivers, approximately two thirds were the spouses or children of care recipients. Furthermore, approximately 30% were over 65 years old themselves. Nearly two thirds of unpaid caregivers were female, and a bit more than half were married. Although they were more likely to assist persons limited in IADLs only, 32% cared for persons with at least three ADL limitations (Spector et al., 1998).

Most experts would agree that family care has been undervalued in our society. First, there has been no official, governmental effort—comparable, for example, to the national health accounting system—to calculate the dollar value of unpaid services. Second, despite an abundant literature on caregiver burden and stress, efforts to provide information, training, support, and respite to family caregivers are neither systematic nor well funded. The range of short-term respite services—which may be supplied at home, in adult day centers or in institutions (e.g., nursing homes, hospitals, or foster care homes)—varies across states (Kane & Kane, 1987; Meltzer, 1982; Richardson et al., 1998) and suffers from limited funding dispersed among a wide variety of sources.

The undervaluing of family care is all the more remarkable given nearly universal acknowledgment that the availability of families willing to care for their loved ones is probably the pivotal factor in preventing or postponing nursing home placement, thus limiting government's financial responsibility for the institutional care of indigent elders. In the year preceding the 2000 election, President Clinton, presidential candidates, and members of Congress from both parties put forth a variety of proposals for tax deductions, tax credits, and federal appropriations designed to support informal caregiving. Although none of these proposals was enacted, the 106th Congress did renew the Older Americans Act of 1965, which included provisions for a National Family Caregiver Support Program. This program was authorized to establish support networks providing (a) information about the availability of support services for family caregivers; (b) assistance in gaining access to these services; (c) individual counseling to help make decisions and solve problems; (d) respite care; and (e) supplemental services.

Paid Caregivers

In the U.S. the supply of LTC services has been heavily influenced by the primary payer of those services—government. Communities generally provided the first public support for LTC in one of two ways. Some established almshouses or "poor farms," where they provided shelter for the "deserving poor"—the retarded, the chronically ill, and the frail elderly. Others established the practice—dating back to colonial times—of boarding out the indigent elderly, for a fee, in private households that came to be known as "rest homes" or "convalescent homes." In the late 19th and early 20th centuries rest homes were joined by charitable private homes for the aged. Later, during the Depression, small, private, proprietary facilities began to multiply, as entrepreneurs whose only capital was their own home began to enter the nursing home business, and as unemployed nurses, individually or in groups, established community residences in their own homes in order to survive financially (Vladeck, 1980).

Over the following decades, federal and state legislation heavily impacted the evolution of LTC (Hawes, Wildfire, Lux, & Clemmer, 1993). In 1935, The Old Age Assistance (OAA) program made federally subsidized means-tested cash grants available for older people, stimulating the growth of community homes—but not nursing homes—that were generally residential and custodial in character but offered some personal care services. Then in 1965, the Medicare and Medicaid programs were signed into law and the Social Security program was expanded to include Supplemental Security Income (SSI). These legislative changes had enormous import for the development of LTC. First, Medicare and Medicaid provided a guaranteed source of funding for LTC providers, which stimulated growth in all forms of LTC, with nursing homes benefiting most; meanwhile, SSI stimulated growth in board and care homes. Second, these programs crucially shaped the industry by tying reimbursement to certification and other requirements. Third, dependence on government reimbursement rendered the supply of LTC acutely sensitive to changes in policy.

The two major types of organizations that evolved to provide LTC in the U.S. were home care agencies and nursing homes. Many more people receive home care than nursing home care, although expenditures for the latter are much higher, due to the more complicated range of services provided and the inclusion of housing costs in the nursing home payment. In addition, a small but growing number of individuals receive LTC services in adult day centers, while many more are being served by a large and growing number of "alternative" community-based residential settings, such as assisted living facilities, board and care or adult family homes, and—for the very affluent—continuing care retirement communities.

Home Care Agencies

The first organized home care agencies were established as voluntary, non-profit Visiting Nurse Associations (VNAs) in the 1890s. Home help "paraprofessional" agencies, providing the services of homemakers, home health aides, home attendants, and the like, began to appear midway through the 20th century (Mundinger, 1983). The number and type of home care agencies multiplied after the 1965 enactment of Medicare, which established a new home health entitlement and a new source of payment for posthospital services in the home.

Agencies are divided into two types: Of the 17,000 agencies providing home care in the United States in 1999, 10,000 of these, known as home *care* agencies, did not directly participate in Medicare,[3] whereas some 7,700 home *health* agencies were certified to provide medically related services to Medicare beneficiaries (National Association for Home Care [NAHC], 2000). Home care agencies are comprised principally of organizations or registries of individuals that provide nonmedical personal care, and house-keeping or chore services (including, for example, "meals on wheels") in individual homes and congregate residential settings. They also include specialized agencies that supply durable medical equipment to home users and agencies that assist people in directing their own arrangements for home-based services. Because these organizations may or may not be licensed by the states in which they operate, much less is known about the services they provide or about their clientele than is known about the licensed, Medicare- and Medicaid-certified home health agencies that will be described.

Agencies certified by Medicare, known as certified home health agencies (CHHAs), provide skilled nursing, rehabilitation, and home health aide services to individuals in their places of residence to promote, maintain, or restore health and/or to maximize independence while minimizing the effects of disease and disability (Haupt, 1998). Individuals receiving Medicare services from CHAAs must be homebound and demonstrate medical necessity for intermittent, part-time, skilled nursing or therapy services ordered by a physician. Medicare requirements often influence states' Medicaid programs, in that states' Medicaid home *health* eligibility rules often match Medicare's, although care recipients must meet a state's definition of *indigence* to be eligible for service. To fund long-term home and community-based services outside the home health rubric, all states also operate some type of Medicaid "home- and community-based waiver" program (as discussed in the section on LTC financing).

Since the introduction of the Medicare program, the home health industry has changed considerably in both composition and in size. CHAAs consist of four main types:

1. private nonprofit,
2. public (government-operated),
3. proprietary, and
4. hospital-based.

Freestanding nonprofit agencies, including VNAs, account for approximately 14% of all CHAAs, while public agencies account for approximately

---

[3] Many noncertified agencies, however, provide aide services to Medicare beneficiaries through subcontracts with Medicare-certified home health agencies.

12%; both have declined steeply as a proportion of CHAAs. Proprietary agencies were nonexistent in 1967 but constituted 41% of all CHAAs in 1999. Hospital-based agencies, which accounted for 7%–8% of CHAAs in 1967, were about 30% of the total in 1999 (NAHC, 2000).

Overall, the number of Medicare-certified agencies increased from 1,753 in 1967 to 5,983 in 1985, to a high of 10,444 in 1997, before declining to 7,700 in 1999 (NAHC, 2000). Multiple and complex reasons are behind the rapid growth, changing composition, and recent decline in the number of CHAAs. The responsiveness of the proprietary sector to changes in Medicare entitlement and payment policy, however, has played a significant role.

Both large, for-profit chains and small, for-profit providers were particularly adept at entering the home health care market, becoming CHAAs, and rapidly increasing visit volume in response to cost-based payments and liberalization of Medicare home health benefits in the late 1980s (GAO, 2000). Similarly, these proprietary providers have been particularly sensitive to payment changes embodied in the Balanced Budget Act of 1997, which established a stringent Medicare Interim Payment System (IPS) leading to the new prospective payment system for home health services, which was implemented in October 2000. As a result of IPS cuts in payment, many CHAAs went out of business in 1998 and 1999. Of these, the decline was greatest among proprietary CHAAs, of which more than 1,800 or 36% closed in 1998 and 1999. In contrast, private nonprofit and hospital-based CHAAs experienced a 14%–15% decline over the same period (NAHC, 2000).

Among the array of LTC services, home health services touch the greatest number of people. In 1996, U.S. home health agencies discharged approximately 7.8 million people. An estimated 2.4 million—most of them Medicare beneficiaries—were receiving home health services at any one time (Haupt, 1998), outnumbering the 1.6 million residents of nursing homes. The typical home health patient is 65 years of age or older (72%), female (67%), white (65%), and married or widowed (64%). Individuals with conditions of the circulatory system—most often some type of heart disease—comprise the single largest share of home health patients (about 20%–25%). Those with cancer, diabetes, chronic obstructive pulmonary disease, fractures, and osteoarthritis and related conditions comprise an additional 35%–40%. The presence of comorbid conditions is common among home health patients—in 1996, 3 out of 4 had two or more diagnoses when they were admitted into care (Haupt, 1998).

Most home health patients enter care after a hospitalization, and approximately one third have just had a surgical or diagnostic procedure. In 1996, half of home health patients were discharged either because they had recovered or their condition had stabilized (29%), or because they had learned how to cope independently with a chronic condition (21%) (Haupt, 1998). Another 28% were discharged because their care was being provided by another source (family or friends, another agency, or a hospital or nursing home).

The increasing availability, use, and costs of home health care over the period of 1986–1996 mirrored reductions in hospital lengths of stay, as well as decreases in nursing home occupancy rates and lengths of stay. Because the average cost of a home health visit ($65 in 1997)[4] is considerably less than a day in a hospital ($1,078 in 1997) or a nursing home ($232 in 1997), home health care has generally been viewed as a way to reduce institutional expenditures (Haupt, 1998). The rapid increase in home health service use can also be attributed to the aging of the population and to older persons' preferences for recovering at home.

Hospice Services

Hospice care is defined as a program of palliative care that provides physical, psychological, social, and spiritual services to terminally ill individuals, as well as support to their families and other loved ones (Haupt, 1998). Hospices are staffed by interdisciplinary teams that include physicians, nurses, medical social workers, therapists, and counselors, complemented by volunteers, who develop and implement a coordinated plan of care sensitive to the personal and cultural values of individual care recipients and their families. The main goals of palliative care, that need not be confined to formal hospice programs, are to sustain the highest quality of life attainable through the control of pain and symptoms, and to maintain care for recipients' independence, comfort, and dignity through the period of terminal illness, be it short- or long-term (Hospice Association of America, 2001; Kaplan & Urbina, 2000; Richardson et al., 1998).

The Medicare program has significantly shaped the hospice industry. Since it began funding hospice services in 1983, it has become their primary source of financing, and providers, patients, and program expenditures have increased dramatically. Medicare increased hospice payment rates by 20% in 1989; meanwhile, Medicare hospice payments rose from $118 million in 1988 to $2 billion in 1997 (U.S. Department of Health and Human Services, 1999). Although hospice payments constitute only 1% of Medicare outlays, Medicare accounts for about two thirds of all revenues received by hospices (Hospice Association of America, 2001). Moreover, approximately 90% of all hospice patients are Medicare beneficiaries (Haupt, 1998).

In 1998, the Medicare program certified nearly 2,300 Medicare-certified hospices in the U.S. The Hospice Association of America estimated that, in addition, approximately 400 volunteer hospices were in operation that year. Little information is available about hospices that do not participate in Medicare or Medicaid, as rules for licensure and regulation vary by state. Among Medicare-certified hospices, nearly 40% are freestanding, mostly

---

[4] The costs quoted in this sentence represent Medicare program payment figures obtained from the Medicare and Medicaid Statistical Supplement, 1999, Tables 48, 23, and 36, respectively.

nonprofit organizations. Approximately 35% are owned and operated by home health agencies (both nonprofit and proprietary), 25% are hospital-based, and fewer than 1% are operated by nursing homes (Hospice Association of America, 2001).

Overall, approximately 393,000 individuals received hospice care in 1996, and about 59,000 were being served at any one time—85% of them by a voluntary, nonprofit hospice organization. Over half of hospice patients were female, 78% were elderly, 84% white, 44% married, and 32% widowed (Haupt, 1998). The most common admission diagnosis for hospice patients was cancer (70%), followed by diseases of the circulatory system (10%), and diseases of the respiratory system (5%). The average hospice patient spent about 50 days in care, and four fifths were discharged due to death. Another 10% were discharged because someone else took over their care.

At approximately $108 per covered day of care in 1997 (U.S. Department of Health and Human Services, 1999)—for a wide range of services, including medications and hospital care if necessary—Medicare hospice services are generally viewed as cost effective, especially if terminally ill patients enroll in hospice early in their illness. Furthermore, *although hospice care is designed primarily for people at the end of life, it embodies principles of support and palliation that should be equally beneficial to chronically ill patients earlier in the disease spectrum.* Nevertheless, several barriers have prevented expansion of palliative care either among the terminally ill or to those who are at an earlier stage of illness. These include: (a) limited third party financing, (b) accreditation programs that painstakingly scrutinize facilities' mortality rates and thus encourage the transfer of patients in acute distress to hospitals where they are least likely to receive good palliation, (c) the lack of systematic medical training in palliative care principles, and (d) the widespread perception on the part of both professionals and lay persons that opting for palliative care means "giving up" (Kaplan & Urbina, 2000). As the end-of-life movement gains momentum, and with it a broader understanding that hospice and hospice-like services are a humane and compassionate way to deliver health care and supportive services, some of these obstacles may give way to wider financing and broader accessibility.

Nursing Homes

Nursing homes in the U.S. vary significantly in ownership, size, services, and the population served. For purposes of classification, the federal government defines nursing homes as facilities with three or more beds that routinely provide nursing care services (Gabrel, 2000a). They may be certified by Medicare or Medicaid, or not certified but licensed by the state as a nursing home. They may be freestanding or a distinct unit of a larger facility or chain. All nursing homes employ paid staff to provide basic medical and personal care to address the long-term needs of frail residents.

In 1996, the U.S. nursing home industry consisted of approximately 17,000 nursing homes with approximately 1.8 million beds, an increase of 19%–20% from 10 years earlier (Rhoades & Krauss, 1999). For-profit nursing homes accounted for two thirds of all facilities and beds, while nonprofit homes comprised 26%, and government homes 8%, of total facilities (Gabrel, 2000a). Forty-two percent of nursing homes functioned independently, while 57% operated as part of a chain (i.e., a group of facilities under one general authority or ownership) (Gabrel, 2000a). The average size of nursing homes was 107 beds. Only 8% of homes had more than 200 beds, while 13% had fewer than 50.

In order to receive payment for services provided to Medicare or Medicaid beneficiaries, nursing homes must meet federal standards that are enforced through annual inspections and complaint investigations conducted by the states. They also must be licensed by the state in which they operate. Although a few nursing homes operate only under state licensure and regulation because they choose not to seek Medicare or Medicaid reimbursement, the overwhelming majority depend on such reimbursement. Thus more than three quarters of homes in 1997 were certified by both Medicare and Medicaid, while another 18% were certified by one of the two programs. Only 4% operated without Medicare or Medicaid certification (Gabrel, 2000a).

Over the last 20 years, U.S. nursing homes have experienced significant changes in the services they provide and the populations they serve. While the sole purpose of many institutions was once to provide a permanent residence for frail individuals, especially elders, to live out the last years of their lives, today many nursing homes serve a more disabled population, providing services that are more medically intensive and rehabilitative, to patients who stay for a short time only. Many have also added special care units. In 1996, almost one fifth of nursing homes had at least one special care unit. About 13% of facilities had an Alzheimer's unit, almost 5% of facilities had a special unit dedicated to rehabilitation and/or subacute care, while another 5% contained other types of special care units (e.g., ventilator, hospice, AIDS, brain injury) (Rhoades & Krauss, 1999).

The shift to providing more medically oriented services to a short-stay population can be seen in nursing home certification and sponsorship trends. When the provision of "permanent" long-term care was their sole purpose, nursing homes more frequently sought Medicaid than Medicare certification. Medicare certification became more common, however, starting in 1988, when a variety of regulatory and legislative changes made it more attractive for skilled nursing facilities to accept Medicare beneficiaries eligible for short-term rehabilitation services (Committee on Ways and Means, 2000). Meanwhile, incentives to provide Medicaid services decreased, as states attempted to strictly control LTC admissions and reduce reimbursement for Medicaid services. The reliability of Medicaid as a payer was further undermined by repeal of the Boren Amendment in 1997, which meant that states no longer had to pay nursing homes "reasonable and adequate" rates. Consequently, although in 1987 half of nursing homes were certified by Medicaid only, another 28% by both Medicaid and Medicare, and only 20% by Medicare only, by 1996 the situation had reversed: just 17% of homes were certified by Medicaid only (Rhoades & Krauss, 1999). Even with increased provision of Medicare-reimbursed services, however, nursing home residents are still covered predominantly by Medicaid payments. Moreover, passage of the Balanced Budget Act of 1997, which transformed Medicare nursing home payment from a retrospective cost-based system to a system of fixed daily rates, may cause some facilities to reevaluate the profitability of serving short-stay, high needs Medicare patients.

Nursing home residents are typically the oldest old, and the average age of the residential population has been rising. From 1987 to 1996, the proportion of nursing home residents who were 85 and over rose from 49% to 56% for women and from 29% to 33% percent for men (Rhoades & Krauss, 1999). On an average day in 1996, nine out of ten residents were 65 years of age or older, and 46% were 85 or older. Relatively few residents were 65–74 years old (12%) or under 65 (9%). Seventy-two percent of nursing home residents were female, while just over a quarter were male. More than eight out of ten residents (87%) were white; only 9%–10% were black and 1%–2% were "other." The under-representation of minorities has been attributed to their greater reliance on informal care, as well as to the discriminatory practices of some nursing homes (Richardson et al., 1998).

Marital status is one of the two most important predictors of whether an individual enters a nursing home. Among those who are disabled, the availability of a spouse to provide supportive help is a key factor in averting or delaying nursing home entry. According to one recent quantitative study, the presence of a spouse more than halved the probability of nursing home entrance during the period of 1970–1991, and other studies have shown that the death of a spouse is the life event most likely to trigger nursing home entrance (Lakdawalla & Philipson, 2000). Thus, it is not surprising that among elderly nursing home residents in 1997, only 17% were married, while the rest were widowed, divorced, or never married (Gabrel, 2000b).

Disability is the major predictor of nursing home entry, and by virtually any measure, nursing home residents are extremely disabled. Moreover, the disability level of the residential population has been increasing. The percentage of residents who needed assistance with three or more ADLs rose from 72% in 1987 to 83% in 1996 (Rhoades & Krauss, 1999). In 1997, three out of five elderly residents used a wheelchair and another quarter used a walker. About one quarter of older residents were visually or hearing impaired. Forty-four percent had difficulty controlling both bowel and bladder. Among those residents discharged from a nursing home between October 1996 and September 1997, only 10% were discharged because they had recovered, while another 19% were discharged after stabilization. More than one third were admitted to a hospital or another nursing home, and 27% died (Gabrel, 2000b).

The future need for nursing home beds in the United States will depend on a number of factors, including demographic changes resulting in a rapidly aging population, patterns of marriage and disability in the aging population, public and private financing policies, and the availability of nursing home alternatives. Although changes in the age composition of the population are fairly straightforward to predict, it is far more difficult to predict marriage and disability patterns, as well as public and private financing and delivery system trends. In particular, projecting future nursing home use from past utilization patterns is likely to produce overestimates of the need for nursing home beds. In the mid-1970s, for example, the resident nursing home population grew at a 4.8% annual rate. By the early 1980s, however, this rate had fallen to 1.7%, and in the late 1980s to early 1990s, the growth rate dropped even further to about 0.4% per year. Furthermore, this drop in the use of nursing home beds occurred even though the average annual increase in the older population—the principal users of nursing home care—remained at a roughly constant annual rate of 2.7%. Improvements in older persons' health almost certainly played a part: first, age-specific disability rates declined for all older people, and second, longer living male spouses were available to support their wives at home (Lakdawalla & Philipson, 2000). In addition, increases in the use of home health and other home- and community-based alternatives suggest that elders' long-term care needs are increasingly being met outside of nursing homes.

Adult Day Services

Adult day services can be a viable community-based alternative for disabled and/or cognitively impaired individuals whose family members must work during the day but are able to provide assistance at night and on weekends. Adult day programs provide health and social services to functionally and/or cognitively impaired adults, and give respite to their family caregivers. In this way they aim to forestall or substitute for institutional care. Most programs provide recreation, social services, and meals. Many also provide transportation, nursing care, personal care, and rehabilitation therapies (National Council on Aging [NCOA], 1997b). A few provide physician care as well. These services are provided in a protected setting and are usually available during normal business hours, five days a week. Fees for adult day services ranged from several dollars to $185 per day in 2000, depending on the services provided and the level of third-party reimbursement available.

Licensure and regulation of adult day care providers varies from state to state, and there is no national repository of data on services and expenditures by year or by state. The National Adult Day Services Association (NADSA) provides some general descriptive information on its Web site. According to NADSA, in 1999 there were approximately 4,000 functioning adult day centers in the U.S.—a number over 12 times greater than were open in 1978. The majority of providers are nonprofit agencies (80%). The remaining are either for-profit (10%) or public (10%). Funding for adult day services comes from participant fees, as well as from public and philanthropic sources. Public funding sources principally include Medicaid and Social Security block grants. Before 2001, use of adult day services rendered individuals ineligible for receipt of Medicare home health services; the lifting of this restriction may make adult day services more attractive in the future.

Data available from one national survey conducted in the mid-1990s indicate that the average adult day care user was a 75–76-year-old woman who was cognitively impaired (NCOA, 1997a). Nearly three fifths of adult day users needed help with at least two ADLs, and two fifths needed help with at least three ADLs (NCOA, 1997a). Three quarters lived with family or friends, while about one quarter lived alone—a distribution that no doubt reflects their relatively high level of dependence.

Community-Based Residential Alternatives to Institutional Care

Many adults experiencing or anticipating some disabling condition are seeking noninstitutional residential settings that will allow them to live independently of family but will provide necessary assistance with personal care, meals, and other household activities. Proponents of community-based residential care maintain that these settings provide a better quality of life compared to nursing homes. Many state policymakers also are hopeful that shifting long-term care spending from nursing homes to residential alternatives will result in a more affordable system.

Responding to the demand for a range of supported housing options, community-based residential care and assisted living facilities (ALFs) provide housing, food, supervision or protective oversight, and personal assistance to individuals who wish to receive LTC services in a setting other than a nursing facility or their own home. These residential nursing home alternatives are marketed, reimbursed, and regulated under various labels and definitions across and within states. Their labels include "board and care," "adult family homes," "personal care homes," "assisted living facilities," and some 20 others. Even the single category "assisted living" can encompass a wide range of residential settings with services, depending on whether or not a state chooses to license these facilities and how it defines their essential features.

Ardent proponents of homelike settings argue that the defining features of an ALF should be private rooms and bathrooms, lockable doors, and individual cooking facilities or appliances. In addition, these proponents argue that ALFs should have available a range of services including assessment and care planning, personal care, medication assistance, the option of three meals per day, and 24-hour staffing and access to nursing services. A recent survey of facilities that self-identified as ALFs, however, suggests that the great majority of these residential settings for older persons do not fit the assisted living model put forward by proponents. When facilities were classified along two dimensions—privacy and services—only a small percentage (11%) were found to offer both a high level of services and a high level of privacy (Hawes, Rose, & Phillips, 1999). Thus, only a small portion of self-identified ALFs nationwide meet the definition of what many consider to be "assisted living."

Depending on the state and the services provided, residential care settings may or may not be licensed. Thus an estimate of their numbers is necessarily imprecise. One recent estimate concluded that there were approximately 51,000 *licensed* residences for older adults in the U.S. in 1998, with approximately 879,000 beds (Harrington, 2000). Another source found that about 11,000 of these residences self-identified as ALFs (Hawes, et al., 1999). Other sources have estimated that more than a million people over 65 reside in some kind of community residential setting (American Association of Homes and Services for the Aging [AAHSA], 2000b). Although current residents of alternative settings are less disabled, on average, than nursing home residents, they often have significant disabilities. Data from a recent national survey indicate that almost one fourth of residents in ALFs[5] receive help with at least three ADLS, and approximately one third have moderate to severe cognitive impairments (Hawes et al., 1999).

The variation among community residential facilities is enormous. Some of these settings are designed to be like small family homes; others may house up to 1,000 individuals in semiprivate rooms; while others, such as some ALFs, are designed as apartment-like residences with private bathrooms, cooking facilities, and lockable doors. The services provided range from light housekeeping to assistance with medications or activities of daily living, to daily nursing care on an "as needed" basis (Hawes et al., 1999). Some facilities provide these services themselves, whereas others arrange for outside service providers, while still others require residents to arrange for services beyond a bare minimum.

The cost of living in a residential care facility ranges from a few hundred dollars to more than $3,000 per month, dependent on the type of services available. Residences usually utilize one of four payment models. Some use an all-inclusive rate model that charges residents a flat fee for housing and all other services. Others use a "basic/enhanced" model that provides a pre-defined group of services (including housing) for a flat fee, and charges residents an additional fee for all other services utilized. A third group of facilities uses a fee-for-service model that charges residents for each service used. Finally, a fourth "service level" model charges residents a fixed fee based on a predetermined level of care (AAHSA, 2000a).

---

[5] The study's three basic eligibility criteria were that a facility had to have more than 10 beds and serve a primarily elderly population. In addition, the facility either had to represent itself as an assisted living facility or offer at least a basic level of services—24-hour staff oversight, housekeeping, at least two meals a day, and personal assistance, defined as help with at least two of the following: medications, bathing, or dressing.

While individuals' monthly SSI or social security payments may be sufficient to cover the housing, room, and board costs in low-price, low-service
facilities, such payments are usually insufficient to cover the costs in facilities located in expensive urban areas or offering a high level of services or
amenities. Acting on the assumption that savings can be realized by diverting individuals in need of LTC services from nursing homes to less costly
residential settings, many states have begun to fund the nonresidential
service component of alternative community care settings through the
Medicaid program. By the end of 1999, 35 states funded at least some long-
term care services in ALFs or other supportive housing settings, primarily
through their Medicaid home- and community-based waiver programs.
Still, public financing of long-term care services in ALFs and other residential settings is relatively modest (Stevenson, Murtaugh, Feldman, &
Oberlink, 2000). The most common source of payment is out-of-pocket
payment by residents or family members. In addition, private long-term
care insurance may be used to cover some costs (AAHSA, 2000a).

State efforts to expand residential long-term care options have been tempered by concerns about quality of care (Stevenson et al., 2000). One particular area of concern is the retention of individuals as they grow more
frail and disabled. Two somewhat contradictory fears about retention policies lead to quality concerns. On the one hand is the concern that residents
will be discharged as soon as their care needs increase, preventing individuals from aging in place. Indeed, available information indicates that many
board and care homes and ALFs reject applicants with wheelchairs, incon-
tinence, cognitive impairments, or who need their medications dispensed
to them. Residents who develop such disabilities may be relocated to
another facility. According to one survey, for example, only one quarter of
ALFs will retain residents who have behavioral problems (e.g., wandering
or mild dementia) (Hawes et al., 1999). On the other hand, those
responsible for monitoring quality are concerned that residents will *not*
be discharged to a more intensive setting if their needs outstrip what a
community residence can provide. The incentive to hold on to residents
may be strongest in areas where the market for residential alternatives to
nursing homes is relatively saturated, making high occupancy (and profitability) more difficult to maintain. The difficulty of balancing these two
concerns has made it especially difficult for states to develop uniform regulatory policy in this area.

Continuing Care Retirement Communities

Continuing care retirement communities (CCRCs) are a type of community residential care facility that has explicitly addressed the resident retention issue in its model of care, which is designed to meet the changing
health and personal care needs of occupants over the remainder of their lifetime. The model offers within a single community three types of living situations available depending on the individual resident's needs: independent

living in a housing and/or apartment complex, assisted living in the complex, and nursing home care. Among the services offered by CCRCs are meals, transportation, social services, and nursing services, as well as recreational and educational activities. In addition, many CCRCs are equipped with amenities such as banks, barber shops, fitness centers, and gardening facilities.

The Continuing Care Accreditation Commission (CCAC), an industry-sponsored accrediting body, estimated in 2000 that approximately 2,030 CCRCs were in operation in the 50 states and the District of Columbia. However, 40% are situated in just a few states: Pennsylvania, California, Florida, Illinois, and Ohio. The number of CCRCs has increased by about 75% since 1996, with a corresponding increase in the number of residents, from 350,000 to 625,000 (AAHSA, 2000b; Richardson et al., 1998). The average age of CCRC residents is 81 years, and three quarters of residents are female. Thirty percent of residents are married couples living together, a feature that distinguishes CCRCs from other types of residential facilities (AAHSA, 2000b).

CCRCs offer a variety of payment plans. One, known as "life care," covers housing costs along with unlimited LTC. Another covers housing costs and a limited amount of LTC, charging supplemental fees to residents who require more assistance. The third plan, known as a "fee-for-service" agreement, covers only housing, but guarantees access to LTC at prevailing nursing home rates. In addition, some CCRCs charge residents both an entrance fee and a monthly fee, while others charge only a monthly fee. Least common is an equity plan in which residents own a condominium or cooperative apartment with a membership agreement that requires procurement of services (AAHSA, 2000b).

Despite variation in rates based on region, size, and amenities, most CCRCs are costly and not widely affordable. In the year 2000, entrance fees, which may be fully or partially refundable, ranged from $45,000 to $108,000, depending on the size of the living unit. Monthly rates ranged from approximately $1,100 for a studio to $1,800 for a two-bedroom dwelling, although additional fees could be required, depending on the payment plan (AAHSA, 2000b). Moreover, there has been concern about their financial viability and capacity to provide heavy nursing care to those residents who will eventually require it. Thus they are not viewed as a mainstream solution to the demand for affordable community-based residential care facilities.

CHALLENGING ISSUES

Containing costs, promoting access, and assuring quality of needed services—the classic triumvirate of U.S. health care policy problems—pose a set of challenges for current and future long-term care policymakers. On the cost side, LTC looms as a large and growing component of health care expenditures. Although the rapid growth of LTC spending in the early to mid-1990s resulted in part from large increases in Medicare home health expenditures, the continuing institutional bias of the LTC system has also been a significant contributor, limiting development of and access to affordable community-based LTC alternatives. On the access side, reliance on Medicaid and personal savings as the two main sources of LTC financing means that many people, who risk impoverishment if they avail themselves of long-term care, forgo necessary or beneficial services until the need becomes urgent. Meanwhile, their need for paid services will increase as access to unpaid care (usually from family members) is projected to decrease (Stone, 2000). Finally, on the quality side, increased regulation has yielded some measurable improvements in nursing home care—the principal target of improvement efforts. Nevertheless, serious quality issues remain for all service settings. Clearly, innovative payment, quality, and financing policies—drawing on a mix of public and private responsibility—will be needed to sustain and expand a viable LTC system that can meet the needs of a rapidly growing older population.

Containing Costs While Improving Access

For many years policymakers—particularly state policymakers—have been concerned about the rising costs of LTC, a concern that can only intensify as the disabled and elderly population grows in size. LTC expenditures constituted nearly 15% of U.S. personal health care spending in 1998,[6] and the burden on state and local governments was far greater. Nursing home and home health care alone accounted for 30% of all state and local personal health care expenditures that year, a percentage that did not take into account additional spending on HCBS waiver programs.

In general, states have employed three broad strategies to control their LTC expenditures:

1. substituting private or federal dollars for state dollars,
2. shifting the cost control burden to providers by controlling nursing home bed supply or cutting provider payment rates, and
3. attempting to reform the health care delivery system, through some combination of integrating acute and LTC services and/or increasing the availability of HCBS alternatives to institutional care (Wiener & Stevenson, 1998).

The first strategy includes the creation of incentives for individuals to purchase private LTC insurance—for example, by allowing purchasers of such insurance to keep more assets than generally required to qualify for

---

[6] This percentage was calculated by dividing $150 billion in LTC costs estimated by Feder, Komisar, and Niefeld, 2000, by $1.019 trillion in personal health care expenditures (Levit, Cowan, Lazenby, Sensenig, McDonnell, Stiller, & Martin, 2000).

Medicaid coverage when their insurance benefits run out. It also includes "musical chairs" initiatives designed to shift as many LTC costs as possible from state Medicaid budgets to the federal Medicare program. The second, "provider burden" strategy, based on the assumption that "a bed built is a bed filled," includes the use of state "certificate of need" laws to control the building of nursing beds. It also includes tight reimbursement controls on Medicaid nursing home rates, a practice made possible by repeal of a federal law that required states to pay nursing homes "reasonable costs."

The third strategy, system reform, has two variants. One involves experimenting with ways of consolidating Medicare and Medicaid funding streams, and capitating payments to managed care entities that assume responsibility for providing long-term care, as well as acute and primary care services, to dually eligible Medicare/Medicaid beneficiaries. The second variant involves using a host of state incentives to foster the growth of HCBS and community-based residential care options, which can then be used to divert individuals from nursing homes.

None of the three strategies has produced unmitigated, resounding success; however, several show promise. Efforts to increase private resources going toward LTC by encouraging individuals to purchase LTC insurance policies have been associated with increased private purchase of LTC insurance policies, which have grown at the rate of about 10%–12% per year over the last decade (Cohen, 2000). Much of this growth is probably attributable to forces other than state initiatives per se. Nevertheless, states can benefit if purchasers are drawn from the group of middle income elders with few informal supports who might otherwise divest themselves of assets or spend down to qualify for Medicaid coverage.

It is unclear whether systems reforms that focus on pooling financing for long-term, primary, and acute care can be replicated on a large scale. Advocates of this approach argue that integrated funding for dual eligibles not only will be less expensive due to reductions in cost shifting, but also will lead to gains in service effectiveness and efficiency through better care management. Uncertainty on integration's cost-saving potential stems from the difficulty of implementing integrated care, which has limited the amount of experimentation. Difficulties arise from both the need for states to strike agreements with the federal government and the need for managed care entities to work with unfamiliar patient populations, providers, and services.

Three models have received widespread attention. The first is the Arizona Long Term Care System (ALTCS), which enrolled over 25,000 individuals in 1998, and has capitated its LTC services, but has not necessarily integrated LTC provision into Medicare HMOs. While outside evaluators agree that ALTCS saves money, there is some disagreement about the extent to which savings are attributable to the effective management of LTC services or to the program's restrictive eligibility requirements (Sparer, 1999; Weissert, 1997). The second is the Social HMO, or SHMO, in which a limited LTC benefit is included in a traditional Medicare

HMO's capitated rate and service package. SHMOs had difficulty, however, encouraging physicians to work cooperatively with social workers and LTC providers to create a coordinated system of care (Harrington, Lynch, & Newcomer, 1993), resulting in a second generation of SHMOs that has attempted to address these problems more fully. Meanwhile, evidence on the model's cost-effectiveness is still being awaited. The third model is PACE, the Program of All-Inclusive Care for the Elderly, in which Medicare and Medicaid premiums are pooled to finance a staff-model HMO that focuses on elderly health issues and relies heavily on multidisciplinary care management teams to coordinate and provide services, including a rich package of LTC benefits. While the PACE sites provide excellent care and do appear to save money (White, 1998), they have so far been successful only on a very small scale. In 1999, 25 sites across the country cared for 6,025 individuals (National PACE Association, 2000). Questions have been raised, therefore, about the model's potential to lead to widespread LTC systems reform. Difficulties in implementing large-scale, easily replicable models that involve integrated acute and LTC financing have motivated a number of states, including Minnesota, Wisconsin, and New York, to experiment with less comprehensive but nevertheless ambitious models that capitate Medicaid-financed LTC services only. The jury is still out on their care coordination and cost savings potential.

Meanwhile, a growing body of evidence suggests that state-initiated system reforms aimed at increasing the availability of HCBS resources can serve more individuals without significantly raising total LTC costs. For 20 years or more, the LTC literature has been replete with articles debating whether or not increasing the availability of HCBS resources will result in lowering total LTC costs. Many researchers have argued that it will not, for the simple reason that expanding HCBS options can result in a "woodwork" effect, by which community-residing individuals with unmet LTC needs emerge to increase the total demand for LTC (Weissert & Hedrick, 1994). The result can then be large increases in the use of HCBS, which more than offset the cost of small decreases in nursing home use. Nevertheless, recent experience in Oregon, Washington, and Colorado suggests that the woodwork effect need not result in increasing total LTC costs if entry to nursing homes is tightly controlled and a variety of lower-cost residential care and home-based service options are targeted to those most in need of supportive care (Alecxih, Lutzky, Corea, & Coleman, 1996; GAO, 1994).

Accordingly, states are increasingly focusing on developing home- and community-based alternatives to nursing homes. Spending on HCBS has increased much faster than spending on nursing home care, with much of the growth in HCBS spending due to the implementation and/or expansion of Medicaid HCBS waiver programs serving elders. During the 1992–1997 time period, the median annual rate of growth for home- and community-based services (including both HCBS waiver services for elders and the optional personal care benefit) was 18.7%, whereas the median annual rate of growth for nursing homes was only 4% (Murtaugh, Sparer, Feldman, Lee, Basch, Sherlock, & Clark, 1999) (see Figure 8.3).

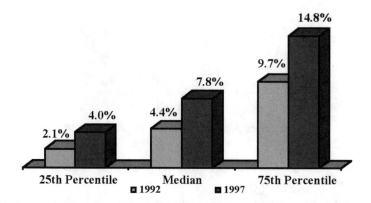

FIGURE 8.3   Share of expenditures going to HCBS[1] still small in most states.

[1] HCBS means spending on waiver programs serving disabled elders plus spending on the personal care benefit.

Despite increasing investment in HCBS services overall, the trend is not uniform across all states, and in most, the share of Medicaid LTC resources going to HCBS is still small. Most public financing for long-term care continues to go to nursing homes (Wiener, Illston, & Hanley, 1994). Half the states spent less than 7.8% of their total Medicaid LTC resources (i.e., nursing home dollars plus HCBS dollars) on HCBS in 1997 (Murtaugh et al., 1999; see Figure 8.3). Half also spent less than $525 per year per Medicaid enrollee on HCBS (see Figure 8.4). A small but growing number, however, are spending a substantial share of LTC resources on HCBS. Five states (North Carolina, New York, Oregon, Texas, and Washington) spent more than 20% of their Medicaid LTC resources on HCBS in 1997. New York was the only state to do so in 1992.

None of the three strategies discussed (the substitution of private or federal dollars for state dollars; cost-control mechanisms; or systems reform) appears to offer by itself a sustainable solution to the problem of how to finance LTC. More ambitious strategies have been proposed for LTC reform in the United States, but the near term political prospects for their enactment seem dim. Wiener and colleagues, for example, recommend a social insurance model that would provide long-term care coverage for all who need services, regardless of income. The insurance would pay for home- and community-based care options, along with nursing home care. As social insurance programs are costly, financing would derive from several sources including recipients (i.e., the elderly), state sources, and taxes (Wiener et al., 1994). Chen proposes an alternative system modeled on a "three-legged stool," consisting of social insurance, private insurance, and personal savings. In this model, the social insurance component would be funded by diverting a small portion of Social Security benefits and would provide a basic level of coverage only. Private insurance—or Medicaid, in the case of indigent individuals in need of LTC—would then supplement

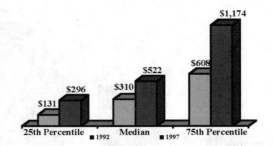

FIGURE 8.4   Large differences among states in HCBS[1] spending per Medicaid enrollee age 65+.

[1] HCBS means spending on waiver programs serving disabled elders plus spending on the personal care benefit.

this basic provision (Chen, 2000). Most observers agree with these authors that the government will need to take a strong role to ensure that future cohorts of older people have access to LTC.

Financing reforms in other countries have proved more successful than in the U.S. For example, in 1994 Germany instituted mandatory, universal social insurance for LTC that covers both community-based and institutional care. Benefits, which people can choose to receive in the form of either cash or services, are financed by a premium set at 1.7% of salary, paid jointly by employees and employers (Cuellar & Wiener, 2000). Similarly, in 2000 Japan introduced a universal LTC insurance program that covers both institutional and community-based care, half of which is paid through general revenue and the other half through premiums levied on those over the age of 40 (Campbell & Ikegami, 2000). Japan's move is surprising for a country with strong social norms regarding family care and the reputation as a "welfare laggard" (ibid), but its experience may show how major demographic shifts can move policy.

Assuring Quality in Long-Term Care

Assuring quality in LTC is an inexact science. On the one hand, the attempt to assure quality in nursing homes has resulted in a welter of monitoring requirements and complicated regulations, that address everything from the width of hallways to the length of time between residents' meals. Despite these efforts and recent improvements, there is general agreement that many nursing homes still deliver substandard care. On the other hand, alternatives to this highly regulated approach are comparatively untested. In particular, systems to ensure quality in LTC settings other than nursing homes are still in their infancy. Although it is hoped that the mistakes of nursing home regulators can be avoided, little consensus exists as to how this can be done.

Historically, nursing homes have been the overwhelming focus of concerns about LTC quality, a fact that reflects their position as the primary providers of care and their extremely vulnerable population. Occasional events such as nursing home fires and patient deaths or other patient care scandals are the targets of media attention when they occur, while the general problems of an institutionalized population have been the subject of consumer advocates and scholars alike. For example, the period between 1970 and 1980 saw a spate of public concern, beginning with Ralph Nader's Consumers' Union book, *Old Age: The Last Segregation* (Townsend, 1970), followed by books with titles such as *Too Old, Too Sick, Too Bad* (Halamandaris, 1977), and *Unloving Care* (Vladeck, 1980).

Although the Nursing Home Reform Act of 1987 constituted a major step forward in quality assurance, with its institution of a wide variety of quality assurance mechanisms, quality has continued to be a problem. For example, a survey conducted by the Health Care Financing Administration from January 1997 through October 1998 showed that only 31% of 17,683 nursing homes in the United States had no cited deficiencies or were in "substantial compliance" with federal regulations (i.e., deficiencies cited had potential for minimal harm only). At the opposite extreme, 27% had deficiencies that posed actual harm, and 1% had deficiencies that posed "actual or potential death or serious injury" (GAO, 1999b). Some of the most frequently cited shortcomings were insufficient attendance to residents' pressure sores, failure to provide supervision or avert accidents, as well as failure to properly conduct resident assessments and prepare appropriate care plans. Additional deficiencies included inadequate nutrition, improper management of incontinent residents, failure to sustain residents' dignity, inappropriate utilization of physical and chemical restraints, and failure to supply appropriate treatment to residents whose range of motion is restricted (GAO, 1999b).

Monitoring to enforce the standards laid down by law is done jointly by state and federal governments. This includes regular surveys to evaluate compliance with regulations and measures to assure that shortcomings are rectified (GAO, 1999b). Nursing homes found out of compliance may be subject to sanctions that include monetary penalties, state assigned substitute management, staff training in problem areas, and correction of deficiencies in specified time intervals (GAO, 1999b). The ultimate sanction is applied when Medicare or Medicaid withdraws certification and payment from a provider.

The government also supports the Long Term Care Ombudsman Program through the Older Americans Act. In contrast to regulators, whose role is to apply laws and regulations, ombudsmen are appointed on a local basis to help identify and resolve problems on behalf of residents in order to improve their overall well-being. Ombudsmen's reports provide an additional source of information on the quality of long-term care institutions.

A key element of quality is whether a system of care responds to individuals' preferences. Here the finding is clear: most people prefer care at home. A poll showed that many elders would rather die than live permanently in a nursing home (Mattimore et al., 1997). When staying in one's own home is not feasible because of long-term care needs, people generally prefer moving to places that provide needed supports that are as homelike as possible.

The expansion of alternatives to nursing homes brings with it additional quality issues, however. As the discussion above makes clear, policymakers are by no means certain that they know the most effective tools to use to ensure quality in nursing homes. Quality assurance in other environments brings a host of equally difficult issues.

For example, home care—the preferred setting for receipt of long-term care—presents a series of quality challenges. First, by definition, home care takes place in the home and is therefore difficult to continuously observe and supervise. A wide variety of difficult to control factors enters into the quality equation, such as the physical environment and family circumstances of the person needing care. Second, home care is largely staffed by paraprofessionals, whose training requirements vary by state or county and whose supervision is often the responsibility of professionals who work for an entirely separate agency or organization. In addition, worker injuries, large workloads, and low wages often result in worker burnout and turnover. In turn, this creates a problem for provider agencies and lowers the morale for remaining staff (Feldman, 1994; Richardson et al., 1998; Stone, 2000).

Assisted living facilities—often touted as homelike alternatives to nursing homes—are not without their own quality problems. Lack of federal regulation of residential facilities has resulted in wide variation and lack of uniform definitions, making them difficult to compare and assess. Facilities vary in size, cost, privacy, staff-resident ratio, and available services. States may set their own standards for licensure, staffing, physical design, and resident population characteristics (AAHSA, 2000a; Richardson et al., 2000), and there is little consensus on what constitutes high-quality service. A number of states are currently debating whether to license and how best to regulate these facilities. On one side are providers and some consumer advocates who are concerned about excessive regulation and fear that the homelike atmosphere of these new residential models of care will be diminished if nursing home-like regulations are implemented. On the other side of the debate are policymakers and other consumer advocates who are more concerned about safety and quality of care than innovation (Stevenson et al., 2000).

The quality assurance regimes for nursing homes, on the one hand, and community-based options such as assisted living and home care, on the other, represent very different approaches to quality assurance. The nursing home industry, while highly regulated and well researched, has not always been successful in maintaining minimum quality standards. Community-based options, which are less regulated and less well researched, are characterized by services of largely undetermined quality. Thus the optimum degree of regulation is left open to question.

The difficulty of determining how best to regulate providers to assure high quality services is compounded by the fact that LTC quality is more than processes of care or clinical and functional outcomes. Most would agree that it also encompasses self-reported quality of life, or self-perceived psychological and social well-being. These, in turn, are partly a function of consumers' self-perceived autonomy and choice.

Do Long-Term Care Consumers Have Choices?

Today in the United States there is wide agreement that consumers should have significant choice over their care arrangements. This argument is made on the grounds of ethical, psychological, and quality considerations. First, it is agreed that the ability to exercise autonomy is an important element of most Americans' moral experience and their sense of self (Cohen, 1988). Secondly, a wide psychological literature speaks to the health impacts of self-efficacy and the ability to control one's environment, particularly among older persons (Rodin & Timko, 1992). Lastly, it is argued that enhanced consumer choice will introduce market mechanisms into the long-term care service environment, thus improving the quality of services.

The consumer direction movement in long-term care takes this thinking about the importance of choice one step further. It arose out of resistance to the "medicalization" of everyday life that people with chronic or disabling conditions sometimes experience. First, younger persons with disability argued that the role of medical professionals in their everyday lives should be as limited as possible, particularly given the low-tech nature of many LTC services. Then advocates for older persons joined the cause, arguing that consumers of long-term care services, regardless of age, should be able to take responsibility for and control those aspects of services they feel capable of managing. In this view, the role of professionals is to assist users of LTC services in assessing and managing their own care, not in determining what they need and when.

Consumer choice first requires that the conditions for choice exist. At a minimum, this means that

1. consumers are considered the primary decision makers regarding the services they receive, unless they choose to delegate that responsibility;
2. a range of service options is available to them;
3. information about these options is available to them; and
4. consumers are involved in service allocation and systems design (National Institute on Consumer-Directed Long-Term Services, 1996).

In some cases, *consumer-directed care* can mean that consumers take responsibility for all aspects of their care including hiring, firing, training, supervising, and evaluating their own care. Another model, known as *consumer-centered care,* refers to involving consumers and incorporating their preferences into their care plans. In one form or another, consumer choice is relevant to all long-term care recipients, including those with developmental disabilities, mental illnesses, and cognitive impairments such as Alzheimer's disease.

Inevitably, respecting consumers' choice involves trade-offs with professional judgments and may, in some cases, compromise patients' safety (Benjamin, 1999). However, advocates of consumer choice argue that it is an individual's right—in LTC as it is in other areas of life—to take risks in order to lead a preferred lifestyle. Nevertheless, family members and service providers are often uncomfortable with anything that is seen to threaten the safety of those receiving services. Service providers have an added reason to be concerned, as they may be held legally liable for any adverse events that occur as a result of increased patient risk-taking.

Currently, efforts to increase choice in LTC are hampered by the institutional bias of the long-term care system, that creates a lack of options for people who need care and ignores their preference for care at home. Long-term care specialists report that, "[t]he disabled elderly prefer home care because it allows them to maintain a sense of independence, helps reduce unmet care needs, lessens their feelings of burden on relatives, and increases their confidence that they will receive the care they need" (Wiener et al., 1994, p. 22). Policymakers, however, have been wary of creating choice by providing community-based alternatives to nursing homes. Despite their desire to expand HCBS, controlling spending on LTC is a top priority for most state policymakers (Murtaugh et al., 1999). Consequently, they are often unwilling to expand community-based options that are seen as an "add-on" rather than a substitute for institutional care.

CONCLUSIONS

This chapter has reviewed key facts about LTC: what it is, who receives it, who provides it, and who pays for it. The most important fact, however, is the growing number of people who will need services and the unpreparedness of the current system to meet that demand in ways that consumers would prefer. This chapter has also covered some of the pressing issues around service provision and the challenges involved in financing care—none of which is likely to be resolved soon. Much work needs to be done before there is agreement on both the goals of LTC and the best ways of meeting these goals.

Although LTC is a necessary service, it is one that has been largely ignored by those not directly affected by the need for care. Many reasons for this have been suggested. Some say it is because the health care system is focused on cure rather than care; LTC is ignored because it is a low-status service within health care. Others point to the lack of financing for services and the difficulty of devising more sustainable ways of paying for care in an era of small government. Yet others argue that social attitudes about disability at the end of life prevent us from thinking hard about the need for care and facing up to the problems involved in providing it. All of these arguments doubtless contain a grain of truth. The growing need for services, however, will make confrontation with these tough issues unavoidable.

CASE STUDY

Joe Ambitious has just been sworn in as governor of Heartland, U.S.A. He ran on a ticket of improving the accountability of local school districts, while improving their Internet connectivity and keeping elementary schools open 9 to 5 across the state. Suddenly he finds himself besieged with a host of long-term-care issues that seem to require immediate attention. The incoming state Medicaid director tells him that the state's LTC budget is already overexpended, and next year's budget must be formulated quickly. Nursing homes want higher payment rates and the association of assisted living providers is clamoring for more generous Medicaid payments for assisted living residents who are eligible for Medicaid services. The consumer advocacy community is waging a major campaign to improve regulation of nursing homes as well as assisted living facilities. Consumer advocates also are arguing vociferously for more Medicaid "waiver" slots to open up community-based LTC options to poor citizens, along with a more generous "needs"-based policy to make home care services more readily available to the citizenry at large and more state dollars to expand respite services for unpaid caregivers. It seems likely that LTC "business as usual" will not fly. Governor Ambitious, however, knows next to nothing about LTC. As the governor's chief of staff, you have been asked to give him a short immersion course in LTC.

DISCUSSION QUESTIONS

1. Who are the main users of LTC and who pays for their care?
2. Who are the main providers of care and how do their interests differ?
3. What are his options for containing LTC costs, and what are the risks of a tight cost-containment policy?
4. Why are the consumer advocates "up in arms," and what should he do about their demands?
5. Assuming he is in office for two terms, what should be his larger goals for LTC in the state?

REFERENCES

Alecxih, L. M., Lutzky, S., Corea, J., & Coleman, B. (1996). *Estimated cost savings from the use of home and community-based alternatives to nursing facility care in three states.* Washington, DC: American Association of Retired Persons.

American Association of Homes and Services for the Aging. (2000a). *Assisted living*. Washington, DC: Author.

American Association of Homes and Services for the Aging. (2000b). *Continuing care retirement communities*. Washington, DC: Author.

Arno, P., & Levine, C. (1999). The economic value of informal caregiving. *Health Affairs, 18*(2), 182–188.

Balanced Budget Act of 1997, Pub. L. No. 105-33, 4 U.S.C.A. §1 (1997).

Benjamin, A. E. (1999). A normative analysis of home care goals. *Journal of Aging and Health, 11*(3), 445–468.

Callahan, D. (1990). *What kind of life*. New York: Simon & Schuster.

Campbell, J. C., & Ikegami, N. (2000). Long-term care insurance comes to Japan. *Health Affairs, 19*(3), 26–39.

Chen, Y. (2000). *Funding long-term care: Application of the trade-off principle*. (Commissioned paper). New York: Home Care Research Initiative.

Cohen, E. S. (1988). The elderly mystique: Constraints on the autonomy of the elderly with disabilities. *The Gerontologist, 28*(Suppl), 24–31.

Cohen, M. (2000). *Private long-term care insurance: A look ahead* (commissioned paper). New York: Home Care Research Initiative.

Committee on Ways and Means, U.S. House of Representatives. (2000). *2000 green book*. Washington, DC: U.S. Government Printing Office.

Cuellar, A. E., & Wiener, J. M. (2000). *Can social insurance for long-term care work? The experience of Germany*. Washington, DC: The Urban Institute.

Duggan v. Bowen: U.S. District Court for the District of Columbia, 87-0383 (1988).

Feder, J., Komisar, H., & Niefeld, M. (2000). Long-term care in the United States: An overview. *Health Affairs 19*(3), 40–56.

Feldman, P. (1994). "Dead end" work or motivating job? Prospects for frontline paraprofessional workers in LTC. *Generations, 23* (2), 5–10.

Feldman, P. (1999). Doing more for less: Advancing the conceptual underpinnings of home-based care. *Journal of Aging and Health, 11*(3), 261–276.

Gabrel, C. S. (2000a). An overview of nursing home facilities: Data from the 1997 National Nursing Home Survey. In *Advance Data from Vital and Health Statistics*, (No. 311). Hyattsville, MD: National Center for Health Statistics.

Gabrel, C. S. (2000b). Characteristics of elderly nursing home current residents and discharges: Data from the 1997 National Nursing Home Survey. In *Advance Data from Vital and Health Statistics*, (No. 312). Hyattsville, MD: National Center for Health Statistics.

General Accounting Office. (1994). *Medicaid long-term care, successful state efforts to expand home services while limiting costs* (GAO/HEHS-94-167). Washington, DC: U.S. Government Printing Office.

General Accounting Office. (1995). *Long-term care: Current issues and future directions* (GAO/HEHS-95-109). Washington, DC: U.S. Government Printing Office.

General Accounting Office. (1998). *Long-term care: Baby boom generation presents financing challenges* (GAO/T-HEHS-98-107). Washington, DC: U.S. Government Printing Office.

General Accounting Office. (1999a). *Adults with severe disabilities: Federal and state approaches for personal care and other services* (GAO/HEHS-99-101). Washington, DC: U.S. Government Printing Office.

General Accounting Office. (1999b). *Nursing homes: Additional steps needed to strengthen enforcement of federal quality standards* (GAO/HEHS-99-46). Washington, DC: U.S. Government Printing Office.

General Accounting Office. (2000). *Medicare home health care: Prospective payment could reverse recent declines in spending* (GAO/HEHS-00-176). Washington, DC: U.S. Government Printing Office.

Halamandaris, V. (1977). *Too old, too sick, too bad.* Germantown, MD: Aspen Systems Corporation.

Harrington, C., Lynch, M., & Newcomer, R. J. (1993). Medical services in social health maintenance organizations. *The Gerontologist, 33*(6), 790–800.

Harrington, C. (2000). *1998 state data book on long term care program and market characteristics.* San Francisco, CA: University of California, San Francisco.

Haupt, B. J. (1998). An overview of home health and hospice care patients: 1996 national home and hospice care survey. In *Advance Data from Vital and Health Statistics,* (No. 297). Hyattsville, MD: National Center for Health Statistics.

Hawes C., Wildfire J. B., Lux L. J., & Clemmer, E. (1993). *Regulation of board and care homes: Results of a survey in the 50 states and the District of Columbia, national summary.* Washington, DC: American Association of Retired Persons, Public Policy Institute.

Hawes, C., Rose, M., & Phillips, C. D. (1999). *A national study of assisted living for the frail elderly: Results of a national survey of facilities* (prepared for the U.S. Department of Health and Human Services, Assistant Secretary for Planning and Evaluation). Beachwood, OH: Myers Research Institute.

Health Care Financing Administration. Office of the Actuary, National Health Statistics Group. (2000). *National health expenditures aggregate and per capita amounts.* [On-line]. Available: http://www.hcfa.gov/stats/nhe-oact/tables/Tables.pdf

Hospice Association of America. (2001). *Basic statistics about hospice.* Washington, DC: National Association of Home Care.

Kane, R. A. (1999). Goals of home care: Therapeutic, compensatory, either, or both? *Journal of Aging and Health, 11*(3), 299–321.

Kane, R. A., & Kane, R. L. (1987). *Long-term care: Principles, programs, and policies.* New York: Springer Publishing.

Kaplan, K., & Urbina, J. (2000). *Moving palliative care upstream: Addressing questions, controversies, practicalities and possibilities regarding integrating curing and caring paradigms along the long term care spectrum.* New York: Partnership for Caring: America's Voices for the Dying.

Komisar, H. L., & Feder, J. (1998). *The Balanced Budget Act of 1997: Effects on Medicare's home health benefit and beneficiaries who need long-term care.* New York: The Commonwealth Fund.

Lakdawalla, D., & Philipson, T. (2000, June). Public financing and the market for long-term care in NBER. In A. M. Garber (Ed.), *Frontiers in health policy research, (Volume 4).* (Forthcoming monograph). Cambridge: National Bureau of Economic Research.

LeBlanc, A. J., Tonner, M. C., & Harrington, C. (2000). *State Medicaid programs offering personal care services.* San Francisco, CA: The Institute for Health & Aging, University of California, San Francisco.

Levit, K., Cowan, C., Lazenby, H., Sensenig, A., McDonnell, P., Stiller, J., & Martin, A. (2000). Health spending in 1998: Signals of change. *Health Affairs, 19*(1), 124–132.

Manton, K., Corder, L., & Stallard, E. (1997). Chronic disability trends in elderly United States populations: 1982–1994. *Proceedings of the National Academy of Science, 94,* 2593–2598.

Mattimore, T. J., Wenger, N. S., Desbiens, N. A., Teno, J. M., Hamel, M. B., Liu, H., Califf, R., Connors, A. F., Jr., Lynn, J., & Oye, R. K. (1997). Surrogate and physician understanding of patients' preferences for living permanently in a nursing home. *Journal of the American Geriatrics Society, 45*(7), 818–824.

Meltzer, W. (1982). *Respite care: An emerging family support service.* Washington, DC: Center for the Study of Social Policy.

Miller, N., Ramsland, & Harrington, C. (1999). Trends and issues in the Medicaid 1915(c) Waiver Program. *Health Care Financing Review, 20*(4), 139–160.

Mundinger, M. (1983). *Home care controversy.* Rockville, MD: Aspens Systems Corporation.

Murtaugh, C., Sparer, M. S., Feldman, P. H., Lee, J. S., Basch, A., Sherlock, A., & Clark, A. L. (1999). *State strategies for allocating resources to home and community-based care.* New York: Center for Home Care Policy and Research, Visiting Nurse Service of New York.

National Association for Home Care. (2000). *Basic statistics about home care.* Washington, DC: Author.

National Council on Aging. (1997a). *Centers offering adult day services have doubled since 1989 as demand mushrooms.* [On-line]. Available: http://www.ncoa.org/news/archives/adult_day_numbers.htm

National Council on Aging. (1997b). *National Adult Day Services Association, adult day services fact sheet* [On-line]. Available: http://www.ncoa.org/nadsa/ADS_factsheet.htm

National Institute on Consumer-Directed Long-Term Services. (1996). *Principles of consumer-directed home and community-based services.* Washington, DC: National Council on the Aging.

National PACE Association. (2000). *PACE profile 2000.* San Francisco, CA: Author.

Older Americans Act, 42 U.S.C. 3001 note.

Richardson, H., Raphael, C., & Barton, B. (1998). Long-term care: Health, social, and housing services for those with chronic illness. In A. R. Kovner & S. Jonas (Eds.), *Jonas and Kovner's health care delivery in the United States* (6th ed., pp. 206–242). New York: Springer Publishing Co.

Rhoades, J. A., & Krauss, N. A. (1999). *Nursing home trends, 1987 and 1996.* Rockville, MD: Agency for Health Care Policy and Research. (MEPS Chartbook No. 3. AHCPR Pub. No. 99-0032.)

Rodin, J., & Timko, C. (1992). Sense of control, aging, and health. In M. G. Ory, R. P. Abeles, & P. D. Lipman (Eds.), *Aging, health and behavior* (pp. 174–206). Newbury Park, CA: Sage.

Rowe, J. W., & Kahn, R. L. (1998). *Successful aging.* New York: Random House.

Sparer, M. S. (1999). *Health policy for low-income people in Arizona.* Washington, DC: The Urban Institute.

Spector, W. D., Fleishman, J. A., Pezzin, L. E., & Spillman, B. C. (1998). *The characteristics of long-term care users.* Paper prepared for the Institute of Medicine, Committee on Improving Quality in Long-Term Care, Washington, DC.

Stevenson, D. G., Murtaugh, C. M., Feldman, P. H., & Oberlink, M. R. (2000). *Expanding publicly financed assisted living and other residential alternatives for disabled older persons: Issues and options.* New York: Center for Home Care Policy and Research, Visiting Nurse Service of New York.

Stone, R. I. (2000). *Long-term care for the disabled elderly: Current policy, emerging trends and implications for the 21st century* [On-line]. Available: http://www.milbank.org/sea/jan2000/index.html

Tilly, J., Goldenson, S., Kasten, J., O'Shaughnessy, C., Kelly, R., & Sidor, G. (2000). *Long-term care chart book: Persons served, payors, and spending.* Congressional Research Service.

Townsend, C. (1970). *Old age: The last segregation.* New York: Bantam Books.

U.S. Census Bureau. (2000). *Projections of the total resident population by 5-year age groups, and sex with special age categories: Middle series, 1999 to 2000.* Washington, DC: Population Projections Program, Population Division.

U.S. Department of Health and Human Services. (1999). *Health care financing review: Medicare and Medicaid statistical supplement, 1999.* Baltimore, MD: Author.

Vladeck, B. (1980). *Unloving care.* New York: Basic Books.

Weissert, W. G. (1997). Cost savings from home and community-based services: Arizona's capitated Medicaid long term care program. *The Journal of Health Politics, Policy, and Law, 22*(6), 1329–1357.

Weissert, W. G., & Hedrick, S. C. (1994). Lessons learned from research on effects of community-based long-term care. *Journal of the American Geriatrics Society, 42*(3), 348–353.

White, A. J. (1998). *The effect of PACE on costs to Medicare.* Cambridge, MA: Abt Associates.

Wiener, J. M., & Stevenson, D. G. (1998). State policy on long-term care for the elderly. *Health Affairs, 17*(3), 81–100.

Wiener, J. M., Illston, L. H., & Hanley, R. J. (1994). *Sharing the burden: Strategies for public and private long-term care insurance.* Washington, DC: The Brookings Institution.

9

Mental Health Services

Steven S. Sharfstein, Anne M. Stoline, and Lorrin M. Koran

LEARNING OBJECTIVES

- ☐ Describe general types of mental disorders.
- ☐ Describe types of treatment for mental disorders.
- ☐ Identify highlights in the development of the U.S. mental health care system.
- ☐ Identify key mental health professionals and their roles in the system.
- ☐ Analyze trends in use over time of the various settings for mental health care.
- ☐ Identify financing differences between general medical and mental health care.

TOPICAL OUTLINE

KEY WORDS

mental disorder, mental health care, public psychiatric hospital, deinstitutionalization, mental health professional, managed care, involuntary treatment

OVERVIEW

Who is mentally ill? The concept of "mental disorder" is not a simple one,
and is influenced by philosophical, social, and cultural considerations. The
same is true for the concept of "physical disorder" and notions of health
versus disease. Every society includes individuals whose significant behavioral or psychological deviancy qualifies for a diagnosis of mental illness,
although the definition of "significant" can vary widely. These syndromes
can be associated with painful emotional symptoms or can present as
impaired ability to think, remember, or concentrate. The syndromes can
also significantly increase the individual's risk of general medical illness,
pain, disability, and even death. The causes of mental disorders may be
developmental, biological, psychological, environmental, or combinations
of these. The important boundary line encompassing the definition of
mental illness, that is, a clinically significant psychological or behavioral
syndrome, is a culturally determined level of personal distress, or of
increased risk of pain, disability, or death.

In 1997, expenditures for treatment of mental and addictive disorders
were $85.9 billion, including $73.4 billion for mental disorders, and $11.9
billion for addictive disorders. Services for mental disorders accounted for
7.8% of the nation's expenditures for health care (Coffey, Mask, King,
Harwood, Genuardi, Dilonardo, et al., 2000), down from 8.8% of total
expenditures in 1987. Indirect costs of mental disorders (including addictive disorders) are estimated to be twice the direct treatment costs. Indirect
costs result from lost wages due to illness or premature death (including
suicide), the value of time family members spend in caring for those with
psychiatric conditions, and productivity losses for individuals incarcerated
for crime related to a psychiatric disorder. Indirect costs of addictive disorders result from adverse health effects, accident-related injuries and fatali-
ties, homicides, suicides, fetal alcohol syndrome, productivity lost by addicts,
their incarceration due to drug-related crimes, costs incurred by the victims of those crimes, and costs associated with AIDS contracted through
intravenous or prenatal exposures (National Foundation for Brain
Research, 1992; Rupp, Gause, & Regier, 1998).

Mental health and substance abuse spending have grown more slowly
than spending for all health care. Inflation-adjusted mental health and substance abuse spending grew by 3.7% annually between 1987 and 1997,
compared to an average of 5% for all health care. The slower growth in
mental health and substance abuse expenditures was due primarily to
spending less on hospital care as inpatient hospital volumes have declined

dramatically during this decade. In contrast, spending on drugs to treat these disorders was one of the fastest growing components. These expenditures grew annually by 9.3% (inflation-adjusted), while those for all health care grew by 8.3% (Coffey et al., 2000).

Managed care has had a major impact on the mode of payment for both inpatient and outpatient care, particularly in the private sector. Partly as a result, the public sector share of mental health and substance abuse expenditures increased between 1987 and 1997, especially in the Medicaid program. States have been moving public programs to managed care strategies such as health maintenance organizations or managed care "carve outs" in recent years, however. The federal government, while maintaining its exemption of psychiatric hospitals and inpatient units from Medicare's prospective payment system, has proposed that prospective payment methods for psychiatric inpatient care be implemented by 2003 (Coffey et al., 2000).

Despite great scientific progress in the past 40 years, the delivery of mental health care, like the delivery of general medical care, is beset by many difficulties. First, the pluralistic health service delivery system is poorly coordinated with other human service systems (e.g., general medicine, civil and criminal justice, education, and welfare). Among the states, there is an unevenness in planning, evaluation, and regulation of the public sector services. Budgetary constraints limit services, and federal, state, and local financing are fragmented. In both the public and private sectors, insurance coverage is not designed to facilitate continuity of care. Mental health personnel and community-based treatment programs are in short supply. The social stigma attached to mental patients (Domenici, 1993) and public apathy toward their suffering also hamper care. These factors lead to inequities in access to care determined by geography, class, and diagnosis.

Like physical disorder counterparts, many mental disorders can only be ameliorated, not cured, and to maintain symptom control, they require long-term management by experienced clinicians. When people with mental illness are also affected by poverty and discrimination, delivering adequate services to them becomes a most formidable task. All of these factors contribute to the major public health problem of how to effectively deliver continuous care to the chronically mentally ill, many of whom have been discharged over the past 3 decades from long-term psychiatric institutions to ill-prepared communities. The public health problems of the homeless and of criminally incarcerated people with schizophrenia and/or substance abuse rivals, in human costs, the major medical crisis of the AIDS epidemic.

At the dawn of a new century, the challenge is to find ways to diminish these difficulties. To help the reader analyze this challenge and develop responses to it, this chapter will discuss the common forms of mental disorder, the kinds of mental health care commonly available, the history of that care in the United States, the prevalence of mental disorders, the mental health labor force, the principal service delivery modes, and financing.

FORMS OF MENTAL DISORDERS

The American Psychiatric Association published its first edition of the *Diagnostic and Statistical Manual of Mental Disorders* in 1952. In late 1993, the fourth edition of the *Diagnostic and Statistical Manual of Mental Disorders (DSM-IV)* was released (American Psychiatric Association, 1994). The manual currently includes more than 450 conditions and their subtypes, grouped in 17 categories. The culmination of more than 4 years of effort, *DSM-IV* included newly-recognized diagnostic entities and reorganized former diagnostic categories to take into account new discoveries of the causes, natural histories, and treatment responsiveness of many forms of mental disorder. This diagnostic manual undoubtedly will be revised again as the research that informs practice brings new understanding and the diagnostic classification is further improved. The 17 major diagnostic classes in *DSM-IV* are as follows:

1. Disorders usually first diagnosed in infancy, childhood, or adolescence (including intellectual, behavioral, emotional, physical, and developmental disorders).
2. Delirium, dementia, amnestic, and other cognitive disorders.
3. Mental disorders due to a general medical condition not elsewhere classified (including catatonic disorder and personality change when due to a general medical condition).
4. Substance-related disorders (including those secondary to alcohol, drug, and tobacco use).
5. Schizophrenia and other psychotic disorders.
6. Mood disorders (conditions with manic, depressive, or mixed symptomatology).
7. Anxiety disorders (including phobias, posttraumatic stress disorder, and obsessive-compulsive disorder).
8. Somatoform disorders (physical symptoms suggesting physical disorders but without organic findings).
9. Factitious disorders (disorders deliberately simulated by the individual for psychological gain).
10. Dissociative disorders (including psychogenic amnesia).
11. Sexual and gender identity disorders (including desire and arousal disorders).
12. Eating disorders.
13. Sleep disorders (including insomnia and nightmare disorders).
14. Impulse control disorders not elsewhere classified (including pathological gambling and kleptomania).
15. Adjustment disorders (maladaptive reactions to psychosocial stress).
16. Personality disorders (enduring, maladaptive patterns of relating to, perceiving, and thinking about the environment and oneself that cause significant impairment in social or occupational functioning or subjective distress).

17. Other conditions that may be a focus of clinical attention (including malingering, bereavement, and adult antisocial behavior).

Although a few mental health professionals asserted in the mid-20th century that all conditions described as mental disorders were nothing more than social myths (Szasz, 1961), the reasoning and evidence to the contrary are powerfully convincing. In addition to the observations of disordered thinking and abnormal behavior collected over several centuries, there is biological evidence as well. For example, in a number of diagnosed mental disorders, imaging studies of brain activity have demonstrated abnormal function (Buchsbaum, 1993). Thus it is all the more important to accurately differentiate the constellations of thoughts, feelings, and behaviors that constitute clinical conditions from those that do not.

PREVALENCE OF MENTAL DISORDERS

Epidemiological studies of the prevalence of mental disorders have encountered the same problems as have analogous studies of physical diseases: deciding what constitutes a "case," establishing operational diagnostic criteria, and choosing a method of case finding.

The largest, most carefully conceived and executed study of the epidemiology of mental disorders was carried out from 1980 to 1982 by the National Institute of Mental Health (NIMH) Epidemiological Catchment Area (ECA) Program. A structured interview, the Diagnostic Interview Schedule (DIS), was administered by trained interviewers to a random sample of nearly 20,000 people in five U.S. cities. After the initial interview, when possible, the subjects were interviewed again 1 year later. Extensive analysis of these data suggests that the 1-year total prevalence rate of the mental and addictive disorders included in the DIS is 28.1% for the adult U.S. population (Regier et al., 1993). The 12-month prevalence of the most common disorders recorded were phobias (10.9%), any alcohol disorder (7.4%), and dysthymia (5.4%). (*Dysthymia* is a form of depressive disorder.) More recent data show similar results. A 1996 study found a 12-month prevalence of 28% for a smaller group of mental disorders (Kessler, Zhao, & Leaf, 1996).

People seek care for mental and addictive disorders from many different sources. About two thirds of all persons with diagnosable conditions in a given year are estimated to receive care in the general medical or specialty mental health sectors. Some in the treatment group as well as some of those in the nontreatment group may consult clergy, social welfare agencies, voluntary support networks, or self-help groups as well (Kessler et al., 1996; Narrow, 1993; Regier et al., 1993).

The numbers suggest that only about one in five persons suffering from a mental or addictive disorder receive any treatment from a specialty mental health professional. The percentage does vary by diagnosis. It is reassuring, although not surprising, that a higher percentage of those with severe and persistent mental illnesses receive care more frequently than those persons who are less severely affected. For example, almost two thirds of people with schizophrenia receive treatment each year, as do more than 40% of those with mood disorders, compared to only one fifth of those with anxiety disorders and 15% with other conditions. The absence of treatment likely reflects a variety of factors, including lack of insurance coverage, other financial barriers to treatment, and lack of motivation to seek care. Among the causes of the latter situation are stigma, lack of insight into one's dysfunction (e.g., in dementia or schizophrenia), lack of sufficient distress to motivate help-seeking, hopelessness regarding potential for improvement (e.g., alcohol and drug addiction), and other psychological barriers to treatment. Some diagnosable conditions (e.g., snake phobia) may not warrant treatment (e.g., the person is an urban dweller). Nevertheless, mental health professionals are concerned by the low proportion of people receiving treatment each year compared to apparent need, and continually search for ways to decrease barriers to care (U.S. Department of Health and Human Services, 1999).

The data that follow focus on the mental health sector of the U.S. health care delivery system. As noted, however, only about one in five people afflicted with a mental disorder receive care in this sector. Most prescriptions written in the U.S. for psychotropic medications are written by primary care physicians rather than psychiatrists, as many persons with subtle forms of mental distress or dysfunction present first to a generalist for care. Thus, training primary care physicians to recognize and treat mental disorders and establishing better linkages between the general health sector and the mental health sector are vital to improving the overall quality of mental health care (Kessler et al., 1996; Narrow, 1993).

TREATMENTS AND SERVICES FOR THE MENTALLY ILL

The term *mental health care* encompasses diverse preventive, therapeutic, and rehabilitative activities. Preventive mental health care aims at promoting mental health in general and preventing the occurrence of specific mental disorders. The first objective is difficult to attain because it is vague: few people agree on exactly what *mental health* is. The second preventive aim has met with some success. Certain disorders with a known biological base such as syphilitic or mercury-related dementia and pellagrinous psychosis, for example, now rarely occur. Efforts to prevent childhood mental disorders through prenatal care, neonatal screening, childhood immunization, adequate nutrition, and public education are receiving increased attention. But primary prevention of schizophrenia, mania, depression, and other mental disorders remains beyond our capabilities.

Therapeutic mental health services include individual, family, and group psychotherapies; expressive interventions such as art therapy and psychodrama; medications; and electroconvulsive therapy. Psychotherapies rely primarily on structured conversation aimed at changing a patient's attitudes, feelings, beliefs, and/or behaviors. The therapist's procedures vary across schools of psychotherapy and with the nature of the patient's problem, and evidence of the effectiveness of psychotherapy is abundant (Nathan & Gorman, 1998). Most forms of psychotherapy, however, have much in common (Frank & Frank, 1991). Cognitive therapy focuses on the primacy of thoughts—the patient's cognitive world—in the creation and maintenance of distress and dysfunction. The therapist teaches the patient to examine negative assumptions and to challenge those assumptions to learn new ways of thinking to himself or herself and to practice new patterns of interaction with others. These shifts both within the individual and in his or her relationships create a more realistic and successful outlook and can reduce distress and improve functioning. A behavior therapist helps the patient stop a destructive behavior such as alcohol or drug use, binge eating, other eating disorder symptoms, and symptoms of obsessive-compulsive disorder (OCD) such as repetitive hand washing. The therapist helps the patient to identify triggers to the behavior, find alternative coping strategies for that trigger, and to interrupt the symptom cycle. Behavioral change is emphasized rather than understanding a psychological source or meaning of the symptoms.

Psychoanalytic therapy emphasizes understanding as a precursor to behavioral and attitudinal change. The psychoanalyst uses structured conversation techniques to bring about change, including encouraging the patient to speak aloud all their thoughts ("free association"), and selective interpretations of the patient's verbalizations or associations. Psychoanalysis is a long-term form of therapy requiring 4 to 5 hourly sessions per week, generally with the patient lying on a couch and the therapist out of view. Some therapists from a variety of therapy schools of thought use hypnosis during psychotherapy sessions. Expressive therapies uncover and explore patients' feelings through professionally-guided creative exercises using drama, painting, sculpture, dance, and other modalities.

Medications are used to treat psychotic, mood, anxiety, cognitive, and impulse control disorders. Most drugs effective in treating mental disorders have been available for less than 40 years. These include phenothiazines, butyrophenones, and the new, "atypical" serotonin/dopamine receptor drugs for treating schizophrenia and other psychiatric disorders; tricyclics, heterocyclics, selective serotonin reuptake inhibitors, and certain receptor blocking drugs for treating depression, panic attacks, and obsessive-compulsive disorders; lithium, valproic acid, carbamazepine, and other anticonvulsant drugs for bipolar (formerly termed manic-depressive) and other mood disorders; and benzodiazepines and azaspirone (e.g., buspirone) for treating anxiety states (Schatzberg & Nemeroff, 1998). Electroconvulsive therapy (ECT), which was introduced in 1938, is effective for certain forms of depression, schizophrenia, and mania.

"Psychosurgery" (neurosurgery performed in an effort to treat a mental disorder) was widely used to treat schizophrenia in the late 1940s and early 1950s. The treatments of choice were prefrontal lobotomy and topectomy (removal of large amounts of cortical tissue). Today, neurosurgical approaches are rarely used (e.g., only in refractory cases of obsessive-compulsive disorder), and very rarely for neurological conditions such as chronic severe pain disorder and uncontrolled epilepsy. Modern techniques permit highly controlled localized destruction of tissue in specific brain regions (Grebb, 1995).

Research advances in the basic sciences are elucidating the fundamental roles played by the serotonin, norepinephrine, dopamine, and gabergic neurotransmitter systems (the chemical mechanisms that produce brain functioning) in modulating cognitive, mood, and anxiety symptoms. Such knowledge has paved the way for synthesis of compounds, and thus new drugs, that affect these neurotransmitter receptors. For example, a new class of antidepressants that selectively affects the serotonin system has been developed in recent years. These drugs, including fluoxetine, fluvoxamine, sertraline, paroxetine, and citalopram have favorable side effect profiles and are safe and effective not only for severe to moderate depressions, but also for obsessive-compulsive disorder, panic disorder, social phobia, bulimia, and milder depressions. Preliminary studies suggest that they have some efficacy in the impulse control disorders as well. Newer antipsychotic drugs have been developed that are effective without disabling neurologic side effects of older drugs, such as those that mimic the uncontrolled muscle movements of Parkinsonism. These improve patient adherence to treatment. Similar advances have been made in pharmacologic treatment of the addictive disorders; for example, agents selectively affecting the brain's receptors for heroin and other opiate drugs (Schatzberg & Nemeroff, 1998).

Rehabilitative mental health care includes occupational therapy, social skills training, and re-education aimed at helping the patient return to normal living patterns. It may begin in an inpatient setting with progressively challenging social activities and can progress through transitional settings such as halfway houses, group homes, or supervised apartments. Rehabilitative care is employed primarily with patients recovering from psychoses, drug addiction, or alcoholism (Kuipers, Fowler, Garety, et al., 1998).

In part through the expansion of the NIMH mission in research and neuroscience, our knowledge of brain functional anatomy, pathophysiology, and activity patterns in disease states is increasing rapidly (Buschsbaum, 1993; Schatzberg & Nemeroff, 1998). Private sector research, particularly by pharmaceutical manufacturers, is also adding to the knowledge base. Our growing understanding of the brain and the frequent introduction of new treatments for mental disorders make psychiatry one of the most dynamic and exciting fields in medicine today.

Brief History of Mental Health Care in the United States

The mentally disordered in colonial America were treated slightly better than their European counterparts: fewer were tortured, burned, hanged, or drowned as witches. (The Salem witch trials of 1691–1692, during which 250 persons were tried and 19 executed, were an exception, not the rule.) Throughout the colonial period, most mentally ill people were kept at home or wandered from town, to town where they might be lodged in jails or almshouses (workhouses) from time to time. This remained the general pattern until the 1840s.

In the early 1800s, the Quakers and American physicians exposed to European psychiatry took the position that mental illness was treatable and urged the use of kind and sympathetic methods. Partly as a result, a few mental hospitals were opened where "moral treatment" (combining work, recreation, education, and kind but firm management) predominated. Violent patients, however, were segregated in separate wards and, in most of the country, mentally-disordered paupers and blacks were sent to workhouses and jails. In 1841, an alliance of professionals and reformers began lobbying legislatures for improved care. Reformers, led by Dorothea Dix, encouraged states to build hospitals specifically for the care of the mentally ill. Many mental hospitals were then built, usually in rural areas, because the countryside was believed to provide refuge from noxious urban and familial influences.

Despite the reformers' successes in getting state mental hospitals built, the quality of care in many of these hospitals was suboptimal. Financial incentives to move large numbers of individuals from local almshouses to state asylums led to outright neglect and custodial care. It also led to overcrowding of the mental hospitals with criminals, alcoholics, vagrants, and the poor, and to the establishment of even larger institutions to keep per capita expenditures down, and to an increasing pessimism regarding the curability of mental disorders. Since mental hospitals were located away from population centers, the dismal conditions within them were easily ignored for a time. Although some improvements were made during the late 1800s, significant changes through implementation of standards and accreditation procedures were not achieved until well into the 20th century.

At the beginning of the 20th century, mental health care was primarily hospital based, and biological approaches to mental illness dominated etiological theories and applied treatments. During World War I, however, an understanding of the psychological and social contributions to the cause and treatment of mental disorders were forcibly brought home to professionals and the public alike. Thousands of men were rejected for military service because of what were understood even then to be "psychoneuroses." When, during the conflict, war neuroses ("shell shock") accounted for a large proportion of psychiatric casualties, it became clear that situational stress could precipitate a mental disorder in "normal" individuals as well as in those with "psychopathic constitutions." Military psychiatrists learned to apply psychological and social techniques to treat war neuroses and return soldiers to the front (Strecker, 1947), lessons which psychiatrists carried back into civilian life.

Between 1910 and World War II, Freud's psychoanalytic theory gradually came to dominate psychiatric training, outpatient care, and popular views of the nature of the human mind. Central to Freud's theory was the categorization of childhood development into the oral, anal, phallic, latent, and genital phases. According to this theory, psychological distress and dysfunction in adults is caused by conflicts originating in one or more of these phases of childhood development. Psychoanalysis did little, however, for severely disturbed individuals such as those with schizophrenia. For the most part, they received nothing more than custodial care in poorly funded, sparsely staffed, biologically oriented state institutions. In the 1930s, renewed hope for these severely disturbed patients was raised by the discovery of new biological treatments including insulin coma, drug-induced convulsive treatments, electroconvulsive therapy, and psychosurgery. The Federal Public Works Administration added more than 60,000 beds to state and local mental institutions during this period.

World War II again focused public attention on mental disorders when 1.75 million men were rejected for service because of mental or emotional disturbances, and a large number of veterans returned home with emotional problems. Reflecting this increased awareness, in 1946 Congress passed the National Mental Health Act, which established the National Institute of Mental Health (NIMH) and gave new federal support for mental health services, training, and research. At that time the outpatient service sector was very limited and most inpatient treatment still took place in state institutions marked by deplorable conditions. Partly to compensate for the limited number of professional personnel, institutions and outpatient clinics began to use group psychotherapy that allowed one professional to treat many patients at once.

By the mid-1950s, the number of persons hospitalized in state and county mental hospitals reached its peak of 559,000. At the same time, however, effective drugs for treating schizophrenia and mania were discovered (e.g., reserpine and chlorpromazine). These drugs replaced insulin coma and psychosurgery and allowed many patients to behave more rationally in institutions, to leave them, or to avoid hospitalization entirely. By reducing symptoms sufficiently to permit patients to leave hospitals, effective drug treatment indirectly created the need for halfway houses and other forms of aftercare.

To examine the nation's mental health care, in 1955 Congress established the Joint Commission on Mental Illness and Health. Thirty-six organizations were represented in it. The Commission's 1961 report, *Action for Mental Health,* concluded that half of the patients in the state mental hospitals were not receiving active treatment. The Commission's recommendations set the stage for the emphasis on community mental health care that marked the 1960s. It proposed establishing one fully-staffed community mental health clinic per 50,000 citizens, limiting the bed complement of large psychiatric hospitals to a maximum of 1,000, and encouraging the use of community-based, short-term inpatient care.

In the 1960s Congress, backed by President John F. Kennedy, passed legislation implementing the Commission's recommendations. It also continued to expand financial support to the NIMH for psychiatric and behavioral science research, psychiatric education in medical schools, and residency training of psychiatrists. Additional effective drug treatments for mental disorders were introduced, including benzodiazepines for anxiety disorders, tricyclic and monoamine oxidase-inhibiting drugs for depressions, and lithium for bipolar affective disorders. Behavior therapy became popular for treating certain psychological symptoms as well as behavior disorders, and researchers began to demonstrate the effectiveness of various psychotherapies.

The creation of Medicare and Medicaid (Titles XVIII and XIX of the Social Security Act; see chapter 12) in 1965 helped transfer some of the costs of caring for the chronically mentally ill to the federal treasury. Federal welfare support (Social Security Disability Income) and food stamps provided a minimal level of economic support for patients with chronic mental illness who were discharged from state hospitals, and such patients were discharged, "deinstitutionalized," over the next 15 years. Unfortunately, the necessary networks of community medical, mental health, and human service agencies provided for by congressional legislation were inadequately organized and severely underfunded, leaving large gaps in services and too few professional personnel to care for those who were deinstitutionalized.

The early 1970s saw a decline in federal support for mental health research and training and slow growth in funding for community mental health services. Under President Jimmy Carter, however, presidential interest in mental health was renewed. In 1977 he established a President's Commission on Mental Health, with Mrs. Carter as Honorary Chairperson. The Commission's 1978 report included an extensive review of the magnitude of the nation's mental health problems and of the resources available to meet them. Detailed recommendations were made for increasing outpatient services for chronic patients, improving access to care for underserved groups (e.g., children, minorities, rural citizens, and the aged), improving insurance coverage for mental health services, increasing public understanding of mental disorders, protecting patients' rights, and expanding the knowledge base through increased federal support of research (President's Commission on Mental Health, 1978).

The passage of the Mental Health Systems Act of 1980 was a significant accomplishment designed to implement many of the recommendations of the Carter Commission. With the election of Ronald Reagan in 1980, however, a new mood pervaded political views regarding the role of government, and the Mental Health Systems Act was never implemented (Foley & Sharfstein, 1983). The decade of the 1980s saw very significant reductions in all areas of national domestic spending, especially at the federal level. This led, among other things, to increasing numbers of Americans on the poverty rolls, cutbacks in programs for the poor, and an increase in the number of homeless persons. Indeed, the mentally ill homeless became the major public mental health problem in this country. Thousands of patients were released from state facilities, but the imperfect psychiatric medication technology that ameliorated the acute phase of psychosis did not provide a long-term cure. Many often wandered the streets, hallucinating, rummaging through garbage, and sleeping on grates. This issue, more than others, has received attention through legislative hearings, the media, and public outcry. Patients enrolled in underfunded community mental health programs often discontinue treatment, relapse, and are readmitted to hospitals for short-term stays—a cycle dubbed the "revolving door" syndrome of psychiatric care.

The desire for minimal government prevailed throughout the 1980s and early 1990s until President Bill Clinton's election campaign. The campaign focused on a number of domestic policy issues, health care prominent among them. Clinton's election in 1992 reflected another shift in national mood, as many Americans became dissatisfied enough with the health care system to support major reform. Soon after his inauguration, he assembled a task force on national health reform, appointing his wife, Hillary Rodham Clinton, as Task Force Chairperson. Vice President Al Gore's wife, Mary Elizabeth (Tipper), a strong ally of the mentally ill, rallied behind parity coverage of mental illnesses as did Senator Peter Domenici (Domenici, 1993). Clinton's health care reform proposal was released in September 1993, and generated a stormy congressional debate. The proposal fell victim to political infighting and strong lobbying by many special interest groups, and no reform was ratified. The President himself subsequently moved to the "less government" side of the equation.

Because citizens with major mental illnesses are unable to engage in effective political lobbying, the coalition of former patients, dedicated professionals, and inspired reformers such as Mrs. Gore came together to maintain the momentum of reform. Congress has tended to move incrementally toward creating equal coverage for mental illness treatment; for example, by passing a bill in 1996 requiring parity in lifetime limits. A White House Conference on Mental Health in 1998 recommended equal or parity coverage for federal employees and dependents. Implementation was for January 1, 2001. Although national reform was not implemented and is not likely in the foreseeable future, these efforts have reinvigorated our society's long-standing moral commitment to care for its disabled and vulnerable citizens. Such efforts continue—small regulatory steps signifying a major victory against stigmatizing mental illness.

MENTAL HEALTH PERSONNEL

Many types of professionals serve patients and clients in the mental health sector, including psychiatrists and other physicians (particularly internists and family practitioners), psychologists, social workers, and registered nurses. In addition, services are provided by vocational rehabilitation counselors, occupational therapists, teachers, and other health workers such as licensed practical nurses (Peterson, West, & Pincus, 1996).

Psychiatrists

Psychiatrists are physicians with 4 years of postgraduate training in caring for mental disorders. The American Board of Psychiatry and Neurology (ABPN) develops and maintains criteria and standards for accredited training programs and offers certifying examinations for their graduates. For example, the first (or internship) year after medical school must include at least 6 months of training in internal medicine and neurology. The 3 subsequent years of specialized training in psychiatry form the residency, after completion of which a physician may practice independently in this specialty.

Approximately 10% of all psychiatrists have undergone additional years of education and training to become psychoanalysts. This training includes part-time didactics, a personal psychoanalysis, and supervision of their treatment cases before they can be certified as psychoanalysts by a psychoanalytic institute. (Social workers and psychologists can also become certified as psychoanalysts.) Modern psychoanalysts base their treatment on Freud's psychological model of the mind, which is embedded within psychodynamic theory as it has been developed over time. This theory has been modified and adapted for clinical use by Freud's followers and by practicing psychoanalysts.

Psychiatrists may subspecialize in certain areas within the field. Accredited training is available in several subspecialty areas including forensics, child and adolescent care, geriatrics, and the addictions. Subspecialty training in psychiatry requires additional years of training after completion of the residency (Dorwart, Chartock, Dial, Fenton, Knewper, Koran, et al., 1992).

Psychologists

Psychologists are nonmedical professionals who have either a master's or a doctoral degree in one of many branches of psychology including experimental, social, general, or clinical. Only psychologists trained in clinical psychology programs must have supervised patient contact as part of that training. Yet, because most states license individuals generically as psychologists, any psychologist, regardless of training can open a private psychotherapy practice. All 50 states plus Washington, D.C., and Puerto Rico regulate the scope of practice of psychologists under a licensing law. Psychology licensure applicants in all states are required to have 3–5 years of work experience in addition to either a PhD or a master's degree.

Social Workers

Social work is a broad field of human service that focuses particularly on the impact of the social environment on the individual. Matters of interest include family and other relationships, conditions at home and work, need for financial assistance through government programs, and other life circumstances. Some social workers are clinically trained to diagnose mental disorders and/or provide various types of psychotherapy. Social workers may have a bachelor's, master's, or doctoral degree in social work; for those doing clinical work, an advanced degree is encouraged. Licensure and regulation of the scope of practice for social workers is provided by all 50 states. Psychiatric social workers bring community health and welfare agency resources to bear on their patients' mental problems, providing care in diagnostic and therapeutic roles, offering consultation to human services agencies, and, to a lesser degree, engaging in research, teaching, and administration.

Registered Nurses

Registered nurses (RNs) are the largest group providing professional care in mental health facilities. The role of the psychiatric nurse includes assessing patient health status; supervising patient interactions on the inpatient unit; administering medications; planning; supervising others in somatic treatments (i.e., general medicine); helping patients with activities of daily living; and providing individual, group, or family therapy. There is a growing trend toward independent outpatient practice.

Scope of practice is regulated by the states. Several important classifications include: Certified Clinical Nurse Specialist, Certified Specialist in Psychiatric Mental Health Nursing, and the growing group of the Nurse Practitioner. Use of these titles requires graduate education, clinical practice with supervision, and successful completion of a written examination.

The Mental Health Team

In private office practice, psychiatrists, psychologists, social workers, and nurses compete for patients. "Turf wars" over such matters as prescribing privileges for nonphysicians abound. Yet in many settings, such as hospitals, community mental health centers, and special schools, mental health professionals work as a team with each member contributing their special expertise in caring for patients with very complex problems. In the hospital, for example, the social worker primarily works with the family and on post-discharge treatment. The psychologist administers diagnostic and functional tests and may provide psychotherapy (individual or group). The nurse provides primary overall supervision of treatment and safety while the psychiatrist provides the diagnosis, medical management—including prescribing drugs, and may provide psychotherapy. They *meet* as a team, often with the patient, and plan treatment together. This is also the case in outpatient community mental health settings throughout the country.

SETTINGS FOR MENTAL HEALTH SERVICES

From the mid-19th century to the mid-20th century, psychiatric services in this country were primarily based in long-stay institutions supported by state governments. Patterns of practice were relatively stable. Over the past 45 years, remarkable changes have occurred. These changes include a reversal of the balance between institutional and community care, inpatient and outpatient services, and individual and group practice.

Deinstitutionalization, or the discharge of tens of thousands of individuals from the large state hospital system, has occurred over the last 3 decades and has had a significant impact on the mental health care delivery system. At the peak of public asylum psychiatry in 1955, 559,000 Americans were hospitalized in state and county mental hospitals. Now, long-stay residents in state mental hospitals number well under 60,000, with the population in the United States having almost doubled during the same period. In 1955, three of four patient care episodes took place in state hospitals, one of four in community settings. Today, three of four patient care episodes occur in community settings, and only one of four in inpatient settings (and less than 10% of these involve state hospital beds). The shift of care to community-based settings began in the public sector, and community settings remain dominant in this sector in comparison to the private sector. The bed capacity of private community settings has increased in the past 30 years. These include psychiatric units in nonfederal general hospitals, private psychiatric hospitals, and residential treatment centers for children. The number of substance abuse centers and child and adolescent inpatient psychiatric units grew particularly quickly in the 1980s, as investors recognized their profitability. Growth of the inpatient private mental health sector has recently plateaued, however, while the number of outpatient and partial treatment settings has sharply increased (Redick, Witkin, Atay, & Manderscheid, 1996).

In the past quarter century, the availability of outpatient services has grown dramatically. The rate of additions to outpatient care more than doubled between 1969 and 1992, from 578 to 1,181 units per 100,000 population, and has now leveled off. Most of this service growth occurred in community mental health centers in the 1970s, in nonfederal general hospitals in the 1980s, and in multiservice mental health organizations in the 1990s (Redick et al., 1996). The increased proportion of the population with private insurance coverage for psychiatric services also stimulated utilization.

These changes resulted from a number of forces, not the least of which was a change in the legal environment in the 1960s, when patients' rights suits established the principle of providing treatment in "the least restrictive setting." Furthermore, deleterious effects of long-term institutional care had been identified, namely, the so-called "social breakdown syndrome." The development of effective psychiatric medications ameliorated patients' behavioral symptoms and allowed discharge into the community.

Probably the most significant factor catalyzing the discharge of patients from state hospitals, however, was financing. (See the next section.) With the enactment of federal Social Security entitlements—Medicare, Medicaid, Supplemental Social Security—it became advantageous for states to discharge patients into nursing homes or board and care-type settings and utilize new federal dollars to reduce state fiscal responsibility. Patients in state institutions were not eligible to have their care paid for by federal funds. With the passage of Medicaid (Title XIX) in 1965, patients who moved into the community or into long-term care institutions that were not devoted exclusively to caring for mental illness could be supported by Medicaid, which provided a 50% federal subsidy. In 1972, the creation of the Supplemental Social Security Income System (Title XVI) allowed patients discharged from hospitals to apply for federal subsidy for board and care home service and other group living arrangements and for daily support. They could also receive Medicaid coverage for treatment costs. This cost-shifting from state to federal coffers further encouraged the emptying of state facilities (Foley & Sharfstein, 1983).

Admissions to state mental hospitals and the number of psychiatric beds located in general hospitals increased dramatically during this same period. Most admissions, however, were actually readmissions, as hospitals experienced the revolving door syndrome, admitting the same patients for multiple acute stays with progressively shorter lengths of stay. Further, nursing homes became a substitute for state mental hospitals and assumed a major responsibility for long-term mental illness care. Most of these nursing home patients suffer from behavioral disturbances or inability to care for themselves due to dementia (including Alzheimer's disease), head injury, or other physical illness. Other patients, however, have other psychiatric diagnoses, such as schizophrenia or bipolar disorder, that require extended stays. For example, Epidemiologic Catchment Area (ECA) data suggest that approximately 20,000 patients admitted to nursing homes in 1 year suffered from schizophrenia or a mood disorder (Narrow, 1993). While many of these patients likely also suffer from functional impairments that render them unable to care for themselves independently, it is unfortunate that most such patients receive a custodial level of treatment, even though they would probably benefit from more active treatment.

Decline in the use of state hospitals has had negative effects. Many patients—likely more than a million—have been discharged into communities that are ill-prepared to provide the therapeutic and rehabilitative services they need, such as halfway houses, aftercare programs, sheltered workshops, and psychosocial rehabilitation (Torrey, 1988). Some of these patients have become homeless wanderers, shifted from the back wards to living on the streets.

In 1999 the Department of Justice reported that as many as 16% of the population of state jails and prisons, that is more than 260,000 individuals, suffer from severe mental illnesses. The Los Angeles County Jail with 3,520 mentally ill inmates, and the New York Rikers Island Prison with 800, are the two largest psychiatric inpatient treatment facilities in the country (Ditton, 1999). The criminalization of mental illness is one of the great tragedies, and ironies, of 20th century psychiatry.

The deinstitutionalization of the mentally ill and the criminalization of mental illness present major policy challenges in this era of managed care and effective therapies. With the progress in psychopharmacology, many patients can do well in noninstitutional settings as long as they take their medications and follow through on outpatient psychosocial treatments. Many patients do not comply with either their psychopharmacological or psychosocial regimens, however, leading to relapse and the need for acute interventions. What is left of the health reform movement in the mid-1990s has shifted from the national to the local level.

FINANCING CARE

Private health insurance has always been more restrictive in its coverage of mental illness and substance abuse than for other medical conditions. The presence of the public mental health system led to an understandable reluctance on the part of private payers to pay for longer term inpatient care. Insurers have also feared the cost of outpatient psychotherapy and so have limited the diagnostic categories for which reimbursement will be made, with number of visits for such treatment as well as charging beneficiaries higher co-payments. "Adverse selection" and "moral hazard" have been the traditional laments of private insurers, justifying discriminatory coverage for mental disorders (U.S. Department of Health & Human Services, 1999). As a result, individuals in the private sector pay more out of their own pockets for psychiatric treatment than for other medical care.

Federal financing through Medicare and Medicaid has also imposed limits on coverage, especially for long-term care, since that has traditionally been a responsibility of the states. The state system has always been seen as the "catastrophic" care system or the safety net for individuals with severe and persistent mental illness. Private insurance continues to have lower annual and lifetime limits on days of care and/or reimbursement amounts in addition to other "inside limits" for acute services. Despite these structural limitations, in the last few years a newer element of cost control has emerged: "managed behavioral health care."

In 1999, almost 177 million Americans with health insurance were enrolled in managed behavioral health organizations (whether they knew it or not). These enrollees have the level of "medical necessity" of their care determined by these outside parties even if they are enrolled in classic capitated systems of care. In addition, 15 states are now using such carve-out arrangements to manage mental health services using public funds. These managed care arrangements have been very effective in reducing the amount of money spent on mental health services, but they have also created much controversy on the issues of access and quality (U.S. Department of Health & Human Services, 1990).

TOWARD PARITY IN COVERAGE OF MENTAL HEALTH CARE

Many states and the federal government have passed legislation to increase access to care through a mechanism known as "parity." This is legislation that treats payment for mental health services on the same basis as payment for general health services. Equal coverage for mental and physical conditions under insurance termed "parity" has been a goal of advocates for many decades. A parity mandate requires all insurance offered in a given market to provide the same levels of coverage for mental health services as is provided for all other disorders. This allows for the spreading of risk to decrease "adverse selection" and, combined with utilization management, to decrease "moral hazard" (National Advisory Mental Health Council, 1997). Although states differ in the scope and level of parity legislation, most states have a parity law on the books, as does the federal government. During the process of passage of the "Kennedy-Kassenbaum" Health Care Reform Bill in the spring of 1996, the U.S. Senate approved an amendment to require employer-based health plans providing coverage of mental health services to do so "without imposing treatment limitations or financial requirements if similar limitations or requirements are not imposed on coverage for services of other conditions." The amendment that actually passed prohibits different treatment of mental health care and physical health care only in terms of lifetime caps and annual reimbursement ceilings. The law, however, allows plans to continue to place annual day and visit limitations on covered services and/or to use higher levels of cost-sharing for mental health care than for other services. Yet the bill certainly was a historic first step—a substantial step toward equal coverage (Frank, Koyanagi, & McGuire, 1997).

The introduction of managed care creates a new context for public and private insurance for mental health services and for parity. Managed care uses information systems, control of referrals and other gatekeeping techniques, expert utilization review, and financial incentives to constrain use and costs of care. Managed behavioral health care companies now cover the majority of Americans who have insurance. They have fueled a continued shift of care from more expensive inpatient settings to less expensive outpatient alternatives, and shorter episodes of both inpatient and outpatient care. As managed care reduces expenditures, parity becomes a less expensive proposition for payers (Sharfstein, Stoline, & Goldman, 1993).

MEDICARE AND MENTAL HEALTH SERVICES

The general benefits and costs of Medicare, a federal program that uses the Social Security system to insure some health care costs of individuals age 65 and over and of disabled individuals regardless of age, are described in chapter 3. Under Part A (hospitalization insurance), benefits for inpatient treatment in a psychiatric hospital are limited to 190 days in a lifetime. Only 150 of these days (90 benefit-period days plus 60 lifetime-reserve days) can be used in any one benefit period. Benefits for psychiatric care in a certified general hospital or extended-care facility are the same as for any other form of medical care. This provision has increased the use of general hospitals to provide psychiatric care for the elderly.

Under Part B (supplementary medical insurance), benefits for physicians' inpatient care for mental illness are the same as for other illnesses; that is, they are not limited. One hundred home visits are also covered and may be provided by mental health agencies. Benefits for physician-provided outpatient care for mental illness initially were limited to 50% of the charges or $250, whichever was less. Congress expanded the outpatient psychiatric benefit in Medicare as part of the Budget Deficit Reduction Act of 1987. Outpatient benefits were increased in two stages over a 2-year period to $2,200 annually, with a 50% co-payment; subsequently, benefits were expanded to equal those of general medical conditions; that is, the benefit cap was eliminated. This quadrupling in benefits, in effect, has kept the outpatient psychiatric benefit on a par with inflation since 1965. Benefits were expanded for partial hospitalization, which was established as a reimbursable service. Perhaps most significantly, all limits and special co-payments were removed for "the medical management of psychopharmacologic agents" for Medicare beneficiaries. Thus, "medical management of psychiatric conditions" is now covered on a par with outpatient treatment for other medical illnesses; that is, with a 20% co-payment and no visit or dollar limits.

MEDICAID AND MENTAL HEALTH SERVICES

Medicaid is a combined federal and state program that covers certain health care costs for eligible persons with incomes falling below established minimums. This program is discussed in detail in chapter 3. Eligibility standards and covered health care services vary from state to state. Although no restrictions by diagnosis are permitted, states can and have limited the amounts of covered mental health care using methods similar to those found in the private sector. Professional reimbursement rates usually fall well below prevailing private sector rates, thus discouraging professionals from participating.

In an effort to gain control over the cost of the Medicaid program and to integrate the funding of Medicaid with other public funding, many states have turned to "managed Medicaid." The privatization of public programs has led to a shift in management from state authority to the private, for-profit managed care industry. This experiment has begun in several states, for example, Massachusetts and Tennessee, and its results are as yet to be undetermined.

CURRENT ISSUES

Access to Care in the Continuum from Hospital to the Community

With the extraordinary improvement in the effectiveness of both biological and psychosocial treatments for severe and persistent mental disorders, the need for hospitalization has decreased dramatically (independent of cost-driven deinstitutionalization without the provision of substitutes). Managed care has reinforced a clinical consensus that hospitalization's purpose is to control only the most acute behavioral symptoms considered to be dangerous to the ill person or to others in the community. Hospitalization is limited to stabilization purposes. These can usually be accomplished in a matter of days. Treatment continues outside in a continuum of partial hospital and outpatient treatment, often combining pharmaco- and psychotherapy. The movement of patients very rapidly from hospital to community, however, has not been accompanied by adequate resources to develop alternative services.

Although the situation varies across states and local communities, there is today a great shortage of outpatient alternatives that adequately follow the patient in treatment at a level of intensity that prevents rehospitalization. The revolving door syndrome, that is multiple short admissions for patients inadequately treated in community-based settings, is one important piece of evidence of the lack of necessary outpatient services in the continuum. Managed care has mostly focused on reducing the perceived high costs of both inpatient and outpatient care and has not exerted a commensurate effort to redeploy resources in the community so that care can be effectively managed for people who require a high intensity of treatment even if not needing 24-hour hospitalization (Schreter, Sharfstein, & Schreter, 1997). This lack of services has led to the second major issue confronting mental health service today—the criminalization of mental illness.

Therapeutic Success and Social Policy Failure in the Criminalization of Mental Illness

One result of rapid deinstitutionalization of patients from public hospitals and multiple short-stay admissions has been the growth of the number of homeless mentally ill people and the incarceration of the mentally ill in jails and prisons. These are both serious public health problems. As noted earlier, about 16% of our jail and prison population consists of individuals with serious mental disorders (Ditton, 1999). Many of these patients have committed nonviolent crimes, but because of inadequacies in the mental health services delivery system, jail becomes the only locus of treatment. This opportunity is often then squandered because of the lack of mental health services in jails and prisons and because of lack of follow-through in community treatment when jail sentences are up and these individuals are once again back in the community. We have a "revolving prison door" for the mentally ill, many of whom have comorbid substance abuse and psychiatric disorders. It is tragic and ironic that we have returned in the latter part of the 20th century to the earlier part of the 19th century when Dorothea Dix and the Quakers found so objectionable the incarceration in prisons and poorhouses of so many persons with "insanity."

Managed Care and Clinical Uncertainty

The extraordinary growth of managed care has intruded on the need for individualized treatment planning and the autonomy of clinicians in trying to care for extremely complex illnesses and human problems. In all of medicine, there is a zone of clinical uncertainty that requires the experienced physician to practice his or her "art" for the good of the individual patient. Today, with managed care's emphasis on disease management, practice guidelines, and clinical protocols, there is less latitude to practice this art. This has been especially true in the practice of psychiatry. Mental health care as managed care in its effort to control costs has not tolerated clinical uncertainty. For example, once it is demonstrable that an individual's suicidal thinking may be somewhat improved, "behavioral health" criteria provide for discharge on the next day. If a patient begins to think more clearly and feels less depressed, medication is often approved, but often without the accompanying psychotherapy that is effective for many individuals (Lazar & Gabbard, 1997). Managed care intrusions have demoralized many in the field and have created a backlash among consumers. The struggle to achieve stated goals of cost containment, access, and quality continues.

Biology versus Psychology

An older but continuing debate within the mental health field is the relative contribution of biological or brain dysfunction versus psychology or dysfunction of that entity we call the "mind" in the syndromes that are labeled mental illness. After 70 years of predominance of psychoanalysis in American psychiatry, the discoveries of antipsychotic, antidepressant, and antianxiety medications have led to a more biological dominant paradigm treatment. It is reinforced by the cost-conscious managed care we have today. Although many studies have found that the combination of medication strategies with psychotherapy is often the most effective, there continues to be a great debate between nature and nurture, brain and mind, medications and psychotherapy (Luhrmann, 2000).

CONCLUSIONS

Mental health care has grown and diversified, particularly over the last 40 years, as psychopharmacologic treatment has made possible the shift away from long-term custodial institutions, and psychosocial treatments can continue the process of care and rehabilitation in community settings. Large state hospitals have been supplemented and in many cases supplanted by psychiatric units in general hospitals, new outpatient clinics, community mental health centers, day treatment centers, and halfway houses. Treatment has become more effective and specific, based on our growing understanding of the brain and behavior. Recent advances in the biological and behavioral sciences continue to improve opportunities for diagnosing, treating, and preventing mental disorders (Nathan & Gorman, 1998).

Now that we have many effective treatments with which to manage psychiatric symptoms and to support patients in rehabilitation, the challenge becomes the optimum allocation of resources and effective treatments to those patients. Resources are limited, so priorities for care must be established and choices made. Managed care has come to mental health care and will not soon disappear. More extensive education of general physicians regarding mental disorders and their treatments is needed. We must improve our ability to triage and match patients' needs with appropriate care. Alternatives to inpatient settings—with continued development of a continuum of care as an approach to the care, treatment, and rehabilitation of those with serious and persistent mental illness—deserve better funding. More day treatment programs, home visit services, psychosocial rehabilitation programs, and therapeutic group homes are needed (Schreter, Sharfstein, & Schreter, 1997).

Much progress has been made in recent years in increasing efficiency in the health care system, but legitimate concern exists that the system has been pushed too far toward cost control to the detriment of patient care. We must rethink issues of access, quality, and cost for mental health and substance abuse treatment with an intensive, public debate about the best way to satisfy the myriad mental health care needs of the U.S. population (U.S. Department of Health and Human Services, 1999). A result of this process should be replacement of our two-tiered public/private system with one tier that provides equal access and quality of care to all. This will require concerted effort by policymakers at national, state, and local levels, and is essential if we are to develop an accountable and fair system for all Americans. There is reason to hope for success, if medical professionals, payers, and policymakers can move beyond entrenched partisan positions to reach consensus on approaches that balance reasonable costs with adequate care. The growth in our knowledge base and ongoing opportunities for new discoveries also support continued optimism and hope. Converting the promise of new knowledge into the reality of new practice is the next challenge for mental health professionals at the dawn of the 21st century.

CASE STUDY

You are governor of a small island, population 100,000. There is no mental health care system in place. The inhabitants of this island are U.S. citizens, thus U.S. epidemiologic data regarding prevalence of mental disorders is applicable to your island as well. How might you use the information in this chapter to design a fair, cost-effective mental health system?

DISCUSSION QUESTIONS

1. Why is it important to consider the indirect costs of mental disorders and substance abuse?
2. What are the general criteria for labeling a condition "a mental disorder"?
3. What factors contribute to the discrepancy between prevalence of mental disorders and extent of their treatment?
4. How did the two-tier system of care for the mentally ill develop, and what perpetuates this discrimination today?
6. What factors might create price competition among mental health professionals?
7. How does stigma surrounding mental disorders contribute to the financial pressures facing today's U.S. mental health care system?

REFERENCES

American Psychiatric Association. (1994). *Diagnostic and statistical manual of mental disorders* (4th ed.). Washington, DC: Author.

Buschsbaum, M. S. (1993). Positron-emission tomography and brain activity in psychiatry. In J. M. Oldham, M. B. Riba, & A. Tasman (Eds.), *American Psychiatric Press review of psychiatry* (Vol. 12, pp. 461–485). Washington, DC: American Psychiatric Press.

Coffey, R. M., Mark, T., King, E., Harwood, H., Genuardi, J., Dilonardo, J., & Buck, J. (2000). *National estimates of expenditures for mental health and substance abuse treatment, 1997.* Rockville, MD: U.S. Department of Health and Human Services.

Ditton, P. (1999, July). *U.S. Department of Justice, Statistics: Mental health and treatment of inmates and probationers* (Special report NCJ-174463). Washington, DC: Bureau of Justice.

Domenici, P. V. (1993). Mental health care policy in the 1990s: Discrimination in health care coverage of the seriously mentally ill. *Journal of Clinical Psychiatry, 54* (Suppl.), 5–6.

Dorwart, R. A., Chartock, L. R., Dial, T., Fenton, W., Knewper, D., Koran, L. M., Leaf, P. J., Pincus, H., Smith, R., Weissman, S., & Winkelmayer, R. (1992). A national study of psychiatrists' professional activities. *American Journal of Psychiatry, 149,* 1499–1505.

Foley, H. A., & Sharfstein, S. S. (1983). *Madness and government: Who care for the mentally ill.* Washington, DC: American Psychiatric Press.

Frank, J. D., & Frank, J. B. (1991). *Persuasion and healing: A comparative study of psychotherapy* (3rd ed.). Baltimore, MD: JHU Press.

Frank, R. G., Koyanagi, C., & McGuire, T. G. (1997). The politics and economics of mental health "parity" laws. *Health Affairs, 16*(4), 108–119.

Grebb, J. A. (1995). Psychosurgery. In H. I. Kaplan & B. J. Sadock (Eds.), *Comprehensive textbook of psychiatry* (6th ed., pp. 2140–2144). Baltimore, MD: Williams and Wilkins.

Kessler, R. C., Zhao, S., Leaf, P. J., Berglund, P. A., Kovzis, A. C., Brule, M. C., et al. (1996). The 12-month prevalence and correlates of serious mental illness. *Mental Health, United States, 1996,* 59–70.

Kuipers, E., Fowler, D., Garety, P., Freeman, D., Dunn, G., Bebbington, P., & Audley, C. (1998). London-East Anglia randomized controlled trial of cognitive-behavioral therapy for psychosis, III: Follow-up and economic evaluation at 18 months. *British Journal of Psychiatry, 173,* 61–68.

Lazar, S. G., & Gabbard, G. O. (1997). The cost-effectiveness of psychotherapy. *Journal of Psychotherapy Practice and Research, 6,* 307–314.

Luhrmann, T. M. (2000). *Of two minds: The growing disorder in American psychiatry.* New York: Alfred A. Knopf.

Manderscheid, R. W., & Sonnenschein, M. A. (Eds.). Center for Mental Health Services. (1996). *Mental health, United States, 1996.* (DHHS Pub. No. (SMA) 96-3098). Washington, DC: Supt. of Docs., U.S. Government Printing Office.

Narrow, W. E. (1993). Use of services by persons with mental and addictive disorders: Findings from the National Institute of Mental Health epidemiologic catchment area program. *Archives of General Psychiatry, 50,* 95.

Nathan, P. D., & Gorman, J. M. (1998). *A guide to treatments that work.* New York: Oxford University Press.

National Advisory Mental Health Council. (1997). *Parity in coverage of mental health services in an era of managed care: An interim report to Congress.* Washington, DC: Department of Health and Human Services, National Institutes of Health, National Institute of Mental Health.

National Foundation for Brain Research. (1992). *The cost of disorders of the brain.* Washington, DC: Author.

Peterson, B. D., West, J., Pincus, H. A., Kahout, J., Pion, G. W., Wicherski, M. M., et al. (1996). An update on human resources in mental health. *Mental Health, United States, 1996,* 168–204.

President's Commission on Mental Health. (1978). *Report to the president—1978* (Vols. 1–6). Washington, DC: U.S. Government Printing Office.

Redick, R. W., Witkin, M. J., Atay, J. E., & Manderscheid, R. W. (1996). Highlights of organized mental health services in 1992 and major national and state trends. *Mental Health, United States, 1996,* 90–137.

Regier, D. A., Narrow, W. E., Role, D. S., Manderscheid, R. W., Locke, B. Z., & Goodwin, F. K. (1993). The de facto U.S. mental and addictive disorders service system: Epidemiologic catchment area prospective 1-year prevalence rates of disorders and services. *Archives of General Psychiatry, 50,* 85.

Rupp, A., Gause, E. A., & Regier, D. A. (1998). Research policy implications of cost-of-illness studies for mental disorders. *British Journal of Psychiatry, 173* (Suppl. 36), 19–25.

Schatzberg, A. F., & Nemeroff, C. B. (Eds.). (1998). *American Psychiatric Press textbook of psychopharmacology* (2nd ed.). Washington, DC: American Psychiatric Press.

Schreter, R., Sharfstein, S. S., & Schreter, S. (Eds.). (1997). *Managing care, not dollars: The continuum of mental health services.* Washington, DC: American Psychiatric Press.

Sharfstein, S. S., Stoline, A. M., & Goldman, H. H. (1993). Psychiatric care and health insurance reform. *American Journal of Psychiatry, 150,*1, 7–18.

Strecker, E. A. (1947). Military psychiatry: World War I: 1917–1918. In J. K. Hall, E. Zilboorg, & H. A. Bunker (Eds.), *One hundred years of American psychiatry.* New York: Columbia University Press.

Szasz, T. S. (1961). *The myth of mental illness.* New York: Hocker-Harper.

Torrey, E. F. (1988). *Nowhere to go: The tragic odyssey of the homeless mentally ill.* New York: Harper & Row.

U.S. Department of Health and Human Services. (1999). *Mental health: A report of the surgeon general.* Rockville, MD: U.S. Department of Health and Human Services, Substance Abuse and Mental Health Services Administration, Center for Mental Health Services, National Institutes of Health, National Institute of Mental Health.

10

Drugs

Robin J. Strongin

LEARNING OBJECTIVES

- ☐ Identify the characteristics of the U.S. pharmaceutical industry.
- ☐ Describe the drug approval process.
- ☐ Analyze pharmaceutical marketplace dynamics.
- ☐ Analyze the growth of prescription drug expenditures.
- ☐ Highlight current issues.

TOPICAL OUTLINE

Pharmaceutical industry profile
Drug discovery and development
Research and development: The price of innovation
Patents
Generics
Drug expenditures
Prescription drug pricing: Multiple markets, multiple prices
Cost control tools
Current issues
Summary

KEY WORDS

biotechnology, clinical trials, drug, human genome, pharmacogenomics, pharmaceutical equivalence, bioequivalence, therapeutic equivalence, generics, prescription, patents, research and development, formulary, rebates, pharmacy benefit manager, physician connectivity

Drug products in the early part of the 20th century consisted mainly of patent medicines, home remedies, and quack cures. The sophisticated, science-based pharmaceutical industry that exists today did not start to develop until the 1930s, when the first sulfa drug was introduced. This discovery set the stage for the development of penicillin and ushered in the "Age of Antibiotics" that lasted from the late 1930s until the early 1950s. The biotechnology industry, born in the late 1970s, moved the industry even further along with the advent of monoclonal antibody technology, cell culture technology, and genetic modification technology, among others.

The dawning of the 21st century, which has witnessed the mapping of the human genome, holds great promise as the research intensive pharmaceutical industry enters the next phase of breakthrough discoveries. The study of pharmacogenomics—analyzing genetic variations and how individuals respond to particular drugs or molecular entities—is expected to revolutionize pharmaceutical research. In fact, given the advances in genomics and biotechnology, the actual definition of prescription drug products is blurring.

Prescription drugs are an essential component of medical care. A staggering number of prescription medicines are on the market today. These include drugs that only a short time ago were unavailable—antinausea medications for chemotherapy patients; cholesterol lowering drugs; drugs for the treatment of migraine headaches; nonsedating allergy drugs; drugs for arthritis; and drugs for impotence.

In addition to the availability of new products, patients are noticing other changes and trends. Products once requiring prescriptions, for example, are now being sold over the counter; more and more products are being marketed directly to consumers; and a large number of top-selling products have or are due to come off patent very soon, enabling consumers to purchase the generic version of these products at a greatly reduced cost.

Many of the products available today are both quality enhancing and cost effective. The potential for using prescription drugs to shift much of hospital-based medical care to less intensive and less expensive settings has long been recognized. This is particularly evident in the case of antidepressants and antipsychotics, vaccines, as well as with the H_2 receptor blockers used in the treatment of peptic ulcer disease. While cost-effectiveness is obvious for certain classes of drugs, it is much more difficult to accurately quantify for other product types. In the case of hypertension, for example, factors such as diet, exercise, genetics, and whether or not a person smokes, must all be factored into the equation, in addition to the benefits of antihypertensive medication. Similarly, while it is clear that there is value in nonbreakthrough drug product advances, such as improved side effect profiles and fewer dosing requirements, it is in some instances methodologically difficult to quantify the value. Similarly, not all drugs are lifesaving products. Some are considered lifestyle drugs, and others have been coined nutraceuticals, cosmeceuticals, and recreceuticals. Many of these products fall into a hazy grey zone when health plans and individuals are faced with making value and financial decisions.

As beneficial as prescription drug products may be, those in the pharmaceutical industry have found themselves at the epicenter of a politically charged environment. With the prices of new drugs rising; with prescription drugs consuming increasing percentages of state Medicaid, employer, and health plan budgets; with most insurers now moving to limit or "manage" drug use within benefit plans; and with large numbers of the elderly affected, especially as Congress debates the addition of a new Medicare prescription drug benefit—increasing attention is being focused on the pharmaceutical industry, at both federal and state levels. While most agree that the scientific breakthroughs are beneficial, critics voice concern over the increasing cost and variability of drug prices, as well as the related problem of lack of access to life-sustaining drugs that low-income people face. While drug costs are climbing, company representatives point out that drug discovery and development is risky business.

Over the years, however, the relationship between pharmaceutical research and development (R&D) and profit has ignited heated discussions in and around Capitol Hill. Much of today's political dialogue revolves around the notion of profitability and "public good." How much profit is too much? Who should decide? Profitability and price, patents and promise—all are at the core of today's political debates. Arguments fly around Capitol Hill and among state capitols: On the one hand, many of the elderly upset with the high cost of drugs are delighted when their drug company stock dividends continue to soar; on the other hand, those representing the low-income elderly argue that seniors should not have to choose between necessities to be able to afford life-sustaining medication. Some groups claim that the only way Medicare beneficiaries can afford their drugs is to buy them in Canada or Mexico; others point out that problems are so great in the health care systems in these countries that Canadian and other citizens are coming by busloads into America to purchase care. These arguments hold for the nonelderly as well.

A September 2000 *Public Opinion Update* on the public and prescription drugs, published by the Henry J. Kaiser Family Foundation, summarized key findings from several surveys conducted by the Kaiser Family Foundation along with *The NewsHour with Jim Lehrer,* The Harvard School of Public Health, and *The Washington Post,* and found that

- More than 9 in 10 Americans (91%) report that they take prescription drugs.
- More than half (54%) say they take prescription drugs on a regular basis, and one fourth (24%) say that they take three or more drugs regularly.
- Almost one third (30%) say they currently have more than five prescription drugs in their medicine cabinet.
- Nearly 1 in 10 (8%) estimate that they spent $1,000 or more out-of-pocket on prescription drugs in the past year.
- One quarter (25%) of Americans report that they do not have prescription drug coverage through their health insurance plan.

- Even though older Americans are more likely than younger Americans to use prescription drugs, they are more likely than people under age 65 to report that they do not have any kind of prescription drug coverage (38% vs. 23%).
- Paying for prescription drugs is difficult for some Americans. Almost 3 in 10 (29%) say they have not filled a prescription because of the cost; 25% say they have to give up other things to buy prescription drugs for themselves or their families; and 10% report having to give up basic necessities such as groceries to pay for medicines.

There is no one specific pharmaceutical marketplace. There is no one price for a specific drug product. There are multiple customers, multiple distribution channels, multiple prescription drug reimbursement systems, multiple purchasing arrangements, multiple pricing methodologies, multiple marketing techniques, and multiple cost control tools. Each of these will be discussed in this chapter, which focuses on prescription drugs.

PHARMACEUTICAL INDUSTRY PROFILE

During the 1950s, American pharmaceutical firms surpassed for the first time their European counterparts, taking the lead in sales and in new drug discoveries. The U.S. pharmaceutical industry retains that lead today. According to the Pharmaceutical Research and Manufacturers of America (PhRMA), the United States is the largest market for pharmaceuticals, accounting for approximately one third of global pharmaceutical sales (see Figure 10.1).

Although there are hundreds of U.S. pharmaceutical companies today, including large and small firms producing both branded and generic products, the 100 U.S. companies with the greatest dollar volume of sales make up approximately 96% of the U.S. market. According to PhRMA, the domestic U.S. sales of its members (nearly all of the approximately 100 major research intensive brand-name manufacturers) totaled $134.1 billion in 1999 and are projected to reach $149.1 billion in 2000 (PhRMA, 2000).

The economics of the pharmaceutical marketplace are extremely complex: the companies themselves range in size from newly merged behemoths to very small one-product start-ups; some of the manufacturers are multinational, spanning the globe, while others are domestic, and still others are foreign companies seeking to do business in America.

In recent years, numerous mergers and acquisitions have brought about a major shift in the pharmaceutical landscape. Industry officials argue that, although these newly merged titans are vast, they hold a relatively small share of the total drug market. The flip side, according to critics, is that individual companies dominate specific therapeutic markets, thus minimizing competition. For example, Schering-Plough controls approximately 40% of the allergy market, while Warner-Lambert controls about 48% of

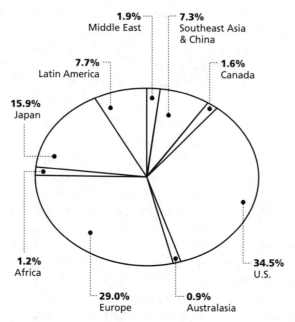

FIGURE 10.1   World pharmaceutical market—1997.

Source: Pharmaceutical Research and Manufacturers of America. (1999). *1999 industry profile.* Washington, DC: Author.

the market for cholesterol drugs. Analysts estimate that Glaxo SmithKline will become the market leader for asthma, AIDS, and migraine drugs, as well as for vaccines. ("Drug mergers change health landscape," 2000).

Consumer advocates are worried that these mergers could lead to fewer drug products and higher prices. Company spokespersons point out, however, that mergers and acquisitions ultimately benefit consumers by increasing their ability to discover and develop new drug products.

DRUG DISCOVERY AND DEVELOPMENT

In 1928, a Scottish bacteriologist inadvertently left a culture of staphylococci uncovered in his London laboratory. A mold grew in the culture. He noticed later that a space had formed between the bacteria and the mold and realized something in the mold was destroying the bacteria. Alexander Fleming eventually named his discovery penicillin. While the process of drug discovery can still be serendipitous today, it is not haphazard. The discovery and subsequent development of new drugs occur within a structural framework and require heavy investments of time and resources.

According to PhRMA, total drug development time has grown from an average of 8.1 years in the 1960s, to 11.6 years in the 1970s, to 14.2 years in the 1980s, to 14.9 years for drugs approved during 1990 through 1996. PhRMA also reports that since 1980, the average number of clinical trials conducted prior to filing a new drug application (discussed below) has more than doubled and the number of patients in clinical trials per new drug approval (NDA) has increased three-fold. The time and expense undertaken by both the industry and the Food and Drug Administration (FDA) is necessary to ensure the safety of patients.

The Preclinical Phase

Drug discovery and development consists of both a preclinical and a clinical phase. A great deal of work must take place before the clinical phase of R&D (research and development) can begin. The scientist, working with the chemists, must learn how to make the drug in quantities larger than a test tube, while insuring that the substance is stable. A company usually files one or more patent applications at this time and begins toxicological tests as well as short- and long-term animal studies.

Depending upon the outcomes of the toxicological tests and other animal studies, a manufacturer must then decide whether or not to move ahead to clinical trials—the beginning of the clinical phase of R&D. Before a company can begin its U.S. clinical trials—testing a new drug in humans to evaluate the safety and effectiveness of a pharmaceutical product—the FDA requires a sponsor to apply to the FDA for permission to initiate human testing with an investigational new drug application, known as an IND.

The Drug Approval Process: Testing for Safety and Appropriateness

The regulatory process begins when an IND is submitted to the FDA. It is important to keep in mind that the FDA itself does not investigate new drugs or conduct any trials. Rather, it reviews the procedures a manufacturer follows and analyzes the data submitted by the company.

Phase I Trials

Once the IND has been approved by the FDA, a manufacturer can proceed with its clinical trials, while at the same time continuing its animal studies. In Phase I trials, initial human safety studies are conducted. This generally involves between 20 and 100 healthy volunteers.

The objective in this phase is to provide information on toxicity and to identify potential side effects. The drug is administered at very low doses, much below the dose that had an effect in the animal studies. If no side effects occur, the dose is gradually increased until a dosage range—establishing toxic levels—is determined.

Regulations issued by the FDA in 1981 require that all research involving FDA-regulated products be reviewed by an Institutional Review Board before human testing can begin. These review boards, known as IRBs, exist in research institutions, academic health centers, and hospitals. They are made up of experts and lay persons whose job it is to make certain that participants are well informed and willing before the studies get under way. A key element in participant protection is informed consent, which the IRB ensures is obtained and documented from each subject.

Phase II Trials

Phase II trials are controlled efficacy studies, that attempt to determine optimal dosage levels and to detect short-term side effects. They tend to be double-blinded, randomized control trials (RCTs). In a randomized control trial, patients are randomly assigned to a treatment group, which receives the experimental drug, or a control group which receives either a placebo, standard treatment, or no treatment. This phase takes approximately 2 years to complete and involves a few hundred patients.

One of the most difficult aspects of clinical trials, which usually occurs during Phase II, involves the selection of clinical endpoints. That is, focusing a study on intermediate endpoints, such as changes in biochemical, physiological, or anatomical parameters, or including clinical endpoints such as effect on mortality, morbidity, or quality of life. These decisions are critical and have enormous impact on the development process. AIDS provides a good example in that a number of drugs being developed today are not necessarily designed to cure this syndrome but rather to target associated symptoms of the disease. The issue of endpoint selection is gaining considerable attention today as more and more drugs are being developed to treat chronic, degenerative diseases.

Phase III Trials

Most of the drugs that make it to Phase III have a very good chance of going to market. During this phase, which takes from 1 to 3 years, the drug is studied in 2,000 to 3,000 human subjects having the disease or condition in order to analyze long-term safety, efficacy, and toxicity effects. Many of the studies in this phase involve multicenter trials. Also occurring at the same time as Phase II and Phase III—although not part of the trials—are efforts by chemists and engineers to "scale up," that is to produce, as efficiently as possible, large quantities of the compound.

Expedited Drug Reviews: Treatment INDs

For patients with serious or immediately life-threatening diseases, the drug approval process presents a difficult dilemma. On the one hand, the process is designed to ensure the safety of investigational new drugs. On the other hand, if a new drug appears promising as a treatment for a terminal illness, time becomes crucial, resulting in a balancing act for the government. The

FDA has responded by developing stopgap mechanisms to provide broader availability of drugs between the time a drug looks promising and its actual approval. One such mechanism is the Treatment IND.

The use of investigational new drugs are usually limited to subjects enrolled in clinical trials. In 1987, new regulations, known as Treatment Use of Investigational New Drugs, changed all that. Known as Treatment INDs, compassionate use approvals, or Group C drugs (in the case of the National Cancer Institute), these regulations enable physicians to use an investigational new drug for desperately ill patients, provided no comparable or satisfactory alternative drug or therapy is available.

New Drug Applications

At the completion of Phase III trials, a sponsor summarizes its study findings, as well as the laboratory formulation and chemistry of the drug, quality control procedures, and manufacturing practices, and submits a new drug application (NDA) to the FDA. Once FDA approval is granted, the manufacturer may market the new drug for the specific indications that are approved. It is important to note that, while the FDA gives permission to market drugs that it believes to be safe and effective, it does not regulate the practice of medicine. Physicians can, therefore, prescribe a drug for "off-label" uses not sanctioned by the FDA.

Phase IV

Phase IV, which takes place after an NDA has been approved, consists of post-marketing studies and occurs over the life of a drug. Its main objective is to examine the long-term safety and effectiveness of a drug and includes the reporting of adverse drug reactions (ADRs) to the FDA. In addition to the submission of ADR reports by manufacturers and health professionals, large-scale randomized controlled trials may also be conducted—often by such agencies as the National Heart, Lung, and Blood Institute, rather than the sponsor—to amass additional data. It is interesting to note that Phase IV activities are a much larger part of the drug approval process in Europe, where the philosophy is to get a product to market sooner and to monitor it more closely than in the United States.

Landmark Legislation: Increasing New Drug Approvals

Analysts studying the pharmaceutical industry follow the FDA's record regarding how long it takes and how many new drugs are approved over a given time period. One of the most meaningful indicators is the number of new molecular entities or NMEs annually approved by the FDA. NMEs are defined as compounds that have never been marketed in the U.S. before. The FDA also approves NDAs or new drug approvals, for those products that are not new molecular entities. Tracking NME approvals provides analysts with a good indication of the pharmaceutical industry's level of innovation.

According to FDA data published on its Web site and taken from the *Comparison of FDA Review Times for NDAs and NMEs, Calendar Year 1994–2000,* "the mean FDA review time (defined as the total approval time minus the time required by the firm to provide information in response to an agency action such as an approvable or not approvable letter) declined from 21.1 months in 1994 to 12.7 months in 2000 for all new drug applications; and from 21.2 months to 13.4 months for applications for new molecular entities."

Accelerated review times have been bolstered by the passage of two key pieces of federal legislation. The first, entitled the Prescription Drug User Fee Act (PDUFA), which Congress passed in 1992, authorized the FDA to collect user fees from pharmaceutical companies to be used to hire more drug reviewers and to improve the computer infrastructure necessary to hasten the review process. In exchange for the money, the FDA was required to meet annual performance targets. In 1997, when the PDUFA legislation was to sunset, Congress passed the Food and Drug Administration Modernization Act (FDAMA). Among other things, FDAMA provided for an additional 5 years of user fee legislation, expanding on PDUFA's emphasis on faster approval times. Faster approval times and access to markets serve to stimulate further pharmaceutical research and development.

RESEARCH AND DEVELOPMENT: THE PRICE OF INNOVATION

In many ways, companies are being forced to rethink their R&D portfolios as the very nature of R&D itself is changing. As the biotechnology revolution advances and as the Human Genome Project is completed, the very essence of our understanding of disease and therapy is undergoing a profound shift. Scientists today now realize that many diseases are actually a collection of several different diseases, each with a unique molecular cause. It is clear that as the secrets of genomics are demystified, promising new miracle products (drugs may no longer be the correct term) will become available.

As a result of sophisticated new tools, such as computer modeling, 3-D computer-visualization techniques, combinational chemistry, and X-ray crystallography, the process of discovery, while still somewhat serendipitous, is much less haphazard than it was 20 years ago. Nevertheless, research and development in the pharmaceutical arena is risky.

Research and development are only part of the risk for a company. The ability to recoup R&D investments is another. Patent protection is the life preserver around the company R&D pipeline. Below are some illustrative statistics about drug development.

- U.S. pharmaceutical companies will spend $26.4 billion this year to discover and develop new medicines, an increase of more than 10% over 1999.
- It costs an average of $500 million to discover and develop just one new medicine.
- It takes nearly 15 years from the time a drug is discovered in the laboratory until it reaches the drugstore.
- The United States leads the world in developing new medicines. Of the 152 major medicines launched worldwide over the last 20 years, U.S. companies developed nearly half.
- Pharmaceutical companies now put back $1 out of every $5 in revenues for R&D. Only 3 out of 10 medicines generate revenues that meet or exceed average R&D costs.
  (PhRMA, 2000)

PATENTS

Patent protection is essential for companies investing in pharmaceutical R&D. Unlike many other technological advances, a drug product, once discovered, is relatively easy to reproduce. Without the period of market exclusivity that patents provide, companies would not have the opportunity to recoup their R&D investments. The 20-year patent "clock" starts ticking immediately, although the effective patent life—that is, the time from FDA marketing approval to loss of patent protection—is actually much shorter, averaging only 11–12 years.

Some argue that patents provide a monopoly, a barrier to market entry for competing products. The other side of that has been articulated by the Congressional Budget Office (CBO):

> Patents do not grant complete monopoly power in the pharmaceutical industry. The reason is that companies can frequently discover and patent several different drugs that use the same basic mechanism to treat an illness. The first drug using the new mechanism to treat that illness—the breakthrough drug—usually has between one and six years on the market before a therapeutically similar patented drug (sometimes called a "me-too" drug) is introduced. (1998, p. xi)

As the future of medical research itself changes, patent policy will face interesting challenges. For example, the area of genetic research has raised significant issues, such as what is patentable (that is, are gene sequences bona fide inventions?). While the future of patenting and biotechnology is still unfolding, past patent legislation and regulation are still affecting today's pharmaceutical market. This is true both domestically and abroad, where patent piracy costs the industry hundreds of millions of dollars every year, despite various provisions agreed to in NAFTA (the North American Free Trade Agreement) and GATT (the General Agreement on Tariffs and Trade).

The 1984 Drug Price Competition and Patent Term Restoration Act

Domestically, the prescription drug market was radically altered with the passage of the 1984 Drug Price Competition and Patent Term Restoration Act (commonly referred to as the Hatch-Waxman Act after its authors, Senator Orrin G. Hatch (R-Utah) and Representative Henry A. Waxman (D-California). The act was intended to strike a balance between promoting innovation (by guaranteeing makers of brand-name drugs a certain number of patent years) and ensuring that consumers have timely access to lower-cost generic medicines (by guaranteeing makers of generic drugs that those patents would eventually end) (Serafini, 2000, p. 548).

GENERICS

Since the 1980s, the use of generics has continued to increase (see Table 10.1). Along with the passage of Hatch-Waxman, the passage of drug-product substitution laws (at the state level) allowing pharmacists to dispense a generic, even in the case of a brand-name prescription, and the active promotion of generic substitution by government health programs and private health plans have all spurred the increase in generic sales.

Some analysts, such as Elliot Wilbur, a securities analyst with CIBC World Markets in Los Angeles, are of the opinion that

> The coming bull market in generics' stocks will be fueled by a never-before-seen combination of surging supply and powerful demand. On the supply side, Wilbur points out that more than $30 billion worth of brand-name drugs will go off patent over the next five years. That's more than six times the dollar level that has been available to the generic industry over the past four years. At the same time, says Wilbur, nearly half of all HMOs now include generic compliance stipulations as part of their financial incentive packages offered to physicians. Wilbur anticipates that number will climb to 75 percent over the next five years. (Menminger, 2000, p. 20)

The opportunity for expansion of generic sales is further illustrated in Figure 10.2.

With a significant number of top-selling prescription drugs coming off patent in the next few years (see Table 10.2), brand-name research pharmaceutical companies are seeking ways to extend their patent protection. One option has been to revise the 1984 Hatch-Waxman Act. While Waxman agrees that the market is different today and recognizes the changing nature of the drug products, he has expressed concern over the motivations of some of the companies seeking legislative revisions. In a recent speech to an industry group, Waxman articulated "the need to stop—once and for all—the numerous efforts to obtain patent extensions benefitting a

TABLE 10.1   Prescription Drugs Facts and Figures

	1993	1998
Rx Sales (in billions of dollars)		
Total	54.3	94.0
Brands	48.5	86.0
Generics	5.8	8.0
% of Total Rx Sales		
Brands	89.4	91.4
Generics	10.6	8.6
No. of Prescriptions Sold (in billions)		
Total	NA	2.6
Brands	NA	1.5
Generics	NA	1.1
% of Total No. of Prescriptions Sold		
Brands	61.4	58.7
Generics	38.6	41.3

Source: Generic Pharmaceutical Industry Association. (2000). Available: [on-line] http://www.gpia.org/edu_facts.html

few at the expense of many. I am talking about efforts to secure special patent extensions and special extensions of market exclusivity, in direct contravention of the Waxman-Hatch Act and its underlying purpose." (Serafini, 2000, p. 548)

Seven companies are seeking legislation that would lengthen patent-term extensions from the Patent and Trademark Office. Companies such as Schering-Plough, which produces Claritin, argue that Food and Drug

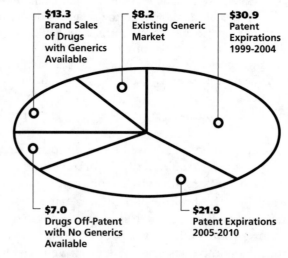

$13.3 Brand Sales of Drugs with Generics Available

$8.2 Existing Generic Market

$30.9 Patent Expirations 1999-2004

$7.0 Drugs Off-Patent with No Generics Available

$21.9 Patent Expirations 2005-2010

FIGURE 10.2   The generic opportunity (in billions of dollars).

Source: Elliot Wilbur, CIBC World Markets. Menninger, B. (2000, Jan/Feb). Can generics turn it around? *Healthcare Business,* p. 20.

TABLE 10.2 Top 20 Prescription Drugs Coming Off Patent by December 31, 2005

Brand Drug	Generic Name	Patent Holder	Indication	Patent Expires	1998 U.S. Sales (in millions of $)
Prilosec	omeprazole	Astra Merck	duodenal ulcers	4/1/01	2,933
Zocor	simvastatin	Merck	hypercholesterolemia	12/24/05	2,170
Claritin	loratadine	Schering-Plough	allergies	12/1/02	1,800
Vasotec	enalapril maleate	Merck	hypertension	2/22/00	1,010
Biaxin	clarithromycin	Abbott	respiratory infection	5/23/03	624
Pravachol	pravastatin	Bristol-Myers Squibb	hypercholestrolemia	10/20/05	1,022
Cipro	ciprofloxacin HCl	Bayer	infection	12/9/03	779
Mevacor	lovastatin	Merck	hypercholesterolemia	6/15/01	595
Zithromax	azithromycin	Pfizer	infection	10/14/05	775
Glucophage	metformin HCl	Bristol-Myers Squibb	diabetes	9/25/01	854
Hytrin	terazosin	Abbott	hypertension	2/17/00	546
Zestril	lisinopril	Zeneca	hypertension	12/30/02	549
Relafen	nabumetone	SmithKline Beecham	arthritis	12/13/01	449
Zofran	ondansetron	Glaxo-Wellcome	nausea	6/25/05	442
Axid	nizatidine	Lilly	duodenal ulcers	4/12/02	301
Ceftin	cefuroxime axetil	Glaxo-Wellcome	infection	5/12/00	365
Diflucan	fluconazole	Pfizer	infection	1/29/04	440

Source: Generic Pharmaceutical, Personal communication, August 2001.

Administration approval delays wasted several years of patent protection. However, as noted in the previously-mentioned CBO study on generics and competition, amending Hatch-Waxman to lengthen patent-term extensions

> . . . would not encourage innovation as much as accelerating the FDA approval process by the same amount would. The reason is that lengthening patent terms increases profits today for drugs whose patents are about to expire, but it does not have as great an impact on the incentive to invest in R&D—that is, on the expected average value of the profits from marketing a drug. CBO calculates that increasing the average patent term by one year would raise the expected value of those profits by about $12 million in 1990 dollars. Accelerating the FDA review period by one year would boost returns by much more—about $22 million in 1990 dollars. (CBO, 1998, p. xiii)

Generic Equivalence: Today and Tomorrow

According to the Generic Pharmaceutical Industry Association (GPIA), the FDA uses three terms to describe generic drug products: pharmaceutical equivalence, bioequivalence, and therapeutic equivalence. Each is defined below.

> *Pharmaceutical equivalence*—drug products are considered pharmaceutical equivalents if they have the same active ingredient(s), the same dosage form and are identical in strength as the brand-name product. Even if a generic has a different color, a different taste, or comes in a different shape or package, the FDA considers the product to be equivalent if it meets the same standards for strength, quality, purity and identity as the branded product.
>
> *Bioequivalence*—a generic drug is considered bioequivalent if it is absorbed in the bloodstream at the "same rate and extent" as the brand drug.
>
> *Therapeutic equivalence*—a generic drug is considered therapeutically equivalent to the comparable brand when the FDA determines the generic is safe and effective, pharmaceutically equivalent, and bioequivalent.
> (GPA, 2000)

Because biologics (for example, human growth hormone) are difficult to produce and because the FDA currently has no mechanism for measuring the equivalency of generic biotech-based drug products, producing generics in the future will become more complicated. The overall effect of this on the market, on competition, and on price, sales, and expenditures remains to be seen.

DRUG EXPENDITURES

According to a new University of Maryland School of Pharmacy study sponsored by the BlueCross BlueShield Association of America, U.S.

pharmaceutical spending in 2004 will reach $212 billion—more than twice the 1999 total of $105 billion. The study also reports that prescription drug spending is expected to rise 15%–18% annually over the next 5 years (Mullins, Palumbo, & Stuart, 2000).

As reported in the March 2000 Kaiser Family Foundation white paper, *Medicare and Prescription Drugs*,

> Pharmaceuticals are the fastest-growing component of national health expenditures. In 2000, national drug spending increased by an estimated 11% compared with 7% for physician services and 6% for hospital care. Since 1990, national spending for prescription drugs has tripled. By 2008, that figure is expected to more than double from an estimated $112 billion today to $243 billion by 2008. (p. 1; see Figure 10.3)

Three factors have contributed to the recent increases in pharmaceutical budgets: *unit cost inflation, utilization* (that is, increases in the absolute number of prescriptions), and *intensity* (that is, availability of new drug technologies and therapeutic mix—substituting newer, higher-cost products for older less expensive products, including generics). The best evidence appears to suggest that while pure price inflation has played a smaller role, especially on existing (older) prescription drug products, utilization growth has played a major role (Brandeis University-Schneider Institute, 2000).

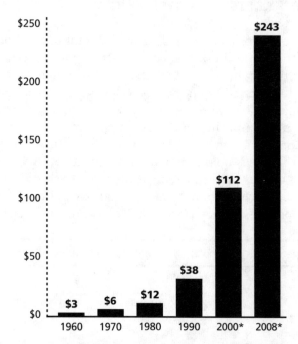

FIGURE 10.3   National spending for prescription drugs (in billions of dollars).
* projected

Source: National Health Expenditure #5. National Health Statistics Group, Health Care Financing Administration, Office of the Actuary. (2000).

Fueling the increase in utilization is the explosion of direct-to-consumer (DTC) advertising by the pharmaceutical companies. The National Institute for Health Care Management's July 1999 study, *Factors Affecting the Growth of Prescription Drug Expenditures,* reported that "the 10 drugs most heavily advertised directly to consumers in 1998 accounted for $9.3 billion or about 22 percent of the total increase in drug spending between 1993 and 1998" (p. iii). The study, citing data from the Scott-Levin Source Prescription Audit Data, found that in 1998, pharmaceutical companies spent $8.3 billion promoting their products in the United States, of which approximately $1.3 billion was spent on DTC advertising and $7.0 billion on advertising and detailing to health care professionals.

Other non-price factors explaining the growth in total drug expenditures include demographic changes (a growing elderly population, changing chronic disease prevalence patterns); the growth in third-party drug coverage, which tends to drive demand; record sales of new products; new product formulations; changing mix of products used; patient noncompliance; and underutilization of prescription drugs and inappropriate prescribing. Another way of looking at total drug expenditures is shown in Figure 10.4.

PRESCRIPTION DRUG PRICING: MULTIPLE MARKETS, MULTIPLE PRICES

As indicated above, pricing alone does not account for the total growth in drug expenditures. But it does, of course, play a role, especially for newer products, many of which are currently working their way through the R&D pipeline. As external market forces change, internal pricing strategies also change.

Defining and comparing pharmaceutical prices is complicated and not always consistent—many terms are used and many methodologies are employed. There is no one way to price a product. A variety of factors are considered in drug pricing, among them: the relative commercial success of the agent; the prices, product features, and past actions of the competition; specific patient characteristics; the economic and social value of the

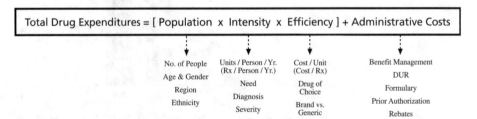

FIGURE 10.4 Factors influencing drug expenditures.

Source: Steven W. Schondelmeyer, PhD, PRIME Institute, University of Minnesota, January 2000.

therapy itself; the decision-making criteria of prescribers and those who influence that decision; company needs in terms of market position, revenue, and other considerations; the current and anticipated insurance reimbursement environment; company abilities, including available budgets and willingness to support the project; and the type of manufacturer supplying the drug (Kolassa, 1997).

Three basic pricing strategies, each chosen to maximize a competitive edge are described below:

> *Skimming*—The product, anticipating little direct competition, is priced above prevailing levels to maximize profits. Prilosec, the first proton pump inhibitor, was priced in this manner, substantially above the price of the H2 antagonists.
>
> *Parity*—The product is viewed internally as being little or no different from current competitors and is priced equivalent to the prevailing levels. The nonsedating antihistamine Claritin and the ACE inhibitor Accupril were priced at parity to the market leaders at the times of their launches.
>
> *Penetration*—A product is viewed as equal to or slightly inferior to current or anticipated offerings and is priced below prevailing levels in hopes of gaining market share with its low price or of erecting a barrier to entry for anticipated future competitors. Lescol appears to be the only pharmaceutical product to have successfully employed a penetration pricing strategy. (Kolassa, 1997, p. 50)

Manufacturers use these various pricing methodologies depending upon internal strategies, external forces, distribution channels, and specific purchasers. The price a manufacturer sets often changes as it makes its way through the distribution chain and onto the negotiating table. It is not unusual for one specific product to be priced differently in different markets, thereby creating a dazzling array of prices paid for the same product. For example, someone with insurance that includes a prescription drug benefit, will almost always pay less for the same drug as someone without insurance, because employers (or their designated representative such as a pharmacy benefit manager, which is described later in this chapter) will negotiate a volume discount on behalf of their beneficiaries. Similarly, different government programs negotiate a variety of prices, based on different legislative and regulatory requirements (see Table 10.3).

Domestically, the pharmaceutical market can be broken down into various segments essentially falling into two broad categories: private markets and government programs. Again, as seen in Table 10.3, tremendous price variation exists across these market segments.

Private Markets

The private marketplace includes retail (which comprises traditional chain drugstores, mass merchandisers, independent pharmacies, supermarket

TABLE 10.3   Illustrative Example of Pricing for Brand-Name Prescription Drugs

	Cash customers (no third-party payment at point of sale)	Insurers and PBMs	HMO[1]	Medicaid	Federal Supply Schedule
List price (AWP[2])			$50		
Manufacturer's price (manufacturer to wholesaler or other entity)	$40 (AWP - 20%)	$40[3] (AWP – 20%)	$34 (AWP – 33%)	$40[3]	$24 (AWP – 52%)
Acquisition price (wholesaler to pharmacy)	$41	$41	n/a[4]	$41	n/a
Retail price at pharmacy (total of amounts paid by customer and reimbursed by 3rd-party payer)	$52 (AWP + 4%)	$46[3] (AWP – 13% + $2.50)	n/a	$41 + $2.50	n/a
Retail price, less typical manufacturer rebate	n/a	$30 to $44 (5% to 35% rebate)	n/a	$30 to $37 (15.1% to 30% rebate)	n/a
Ultimate (net) amount paid by final purchaser and/or consumer	$52	$30 to $44	$34 (avg.)	$30 to $37 $34 (avg.)	$24

Source: Assistant Secretary for Planning and Evaluation. (2000). *Report to the President: Prescription drug coverage, spending, utilization, and prices.* Washington, DC: Department of Health and Human Services, p. 98.

[1] This column refers only to HMOs that buy directly from manufacturers.

[2] Average Wholesale Price

[3] Without rebate

[4] n/a = not applicable

Notes: 1. Prices are based on a composite of several commonly prescribed brand-name drugs for a typical quality of pills. For some cells in the table, the relative relationships have been calculated based on relationships reported in *How Increased Competition from Generic Drugs Has Affected Prices and Returns in the Pharmaceutical Industry* (CBO, 1998) and on other relationships widely reported by industry sources.

2. These prices are used for illustrative purposes only and do not represent any type of overall average.

3. Prices reported in this table include both amounts paid by third-party payers and amounts paid by the consumer as cost-sharing.

pharmacies, and mail-order pharmacies); wholesale; hospital; managed care organizations and providers (such as clinics; long-term care facilities, including nursing homes, outpatient facilities, and physician offices); and the Internet (see Figure 10.5).

Retail, Wholesale, Mail Order, and the Internet

- Nationwide, there are more than 340,000 pharmacies operated by traditional chain pharmacy companies, supermarkets, and mass merchants. In addition, there are another 20,000 independent pharmacies.
- In recent years, the retail prescription drug industry has grown dramatically. The number of retail prescriptions dispensed each year increased from 2.0 billion in 1992 to 2.6 billion in 1997. This represents a 23% increase in just 5 years. In 2001, this number reached 3.15 billion.
- The chain pharmacy is the leading component of this industry. It dispenses more than 71% of these prescriptions.

(National Association of Chain Drug Stores, 2001)

- Over the past few years, the wholesale drug industry has become quite concentrated. While there are still a number of wholesalers in operation, the top five wholesalers account for 90% of the entire wholesale drug market (National Wholesale Druggists' Association, 1999). In 1998, the net sales of prescription drugs by wholesalers were $57 billion.
- Mail order pharmacy accounts for about 12% of the total retail prescription market. Between 1997 and 1998 mail service pharmacy grew by 19% ("Mail order drug sales," 1999). This compares to the total prescription market, which grew by 18.5% (Glaser, 1999). It is interesting to note that Internet pharmacies use mail order to distribute their products and are members of the mail-order pharmacies' professional organization.

(*Prescription Drug Coverage, Spending, Utilization and Prices*, DHHS-ASPE, 2000)

Government Programs

The federal government, which spends billions of dollars on pharmaceutical products annually, encompasses such programs as the Federal Employee Health Benefit program, the Department of Veterans Affairs (VA) and its federal supply schedule (FSS), Medicaid, and various public health service programs, such as the Indian Health Service and the Coast Guard. Various government programs have legislated drug pricing and reimbursement methodologies.

The VA Federal Supply Schedule

In fiscal year 1999, the Department of Veterans Affairs spent more than $1.8 billion or approximately 11% of its health care budget in order to provide pharmacy benefits for U.S. veterans. The VA negotiates FSS contracts with individual manufacturers according to a set statutory and regulation

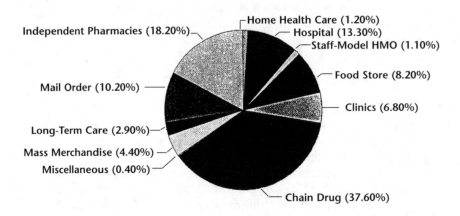

FIGURE 10.5   Prescription sales by outlet, U.S. market, 1999.
Source: IMS Health. (2000).

framework. The Veterans Health Care Act of 1992 established a mandatory federal ceiling price (beyond those of the FSS) on a manufacturer's sales of innovator medicines to four federal agencies: the VA, the Department of Defense, the Public Health Service (including the Indian Health Service), and the Coast Guard. The formula establishes an upper limit on all procurements by any of the four agencies equal to 76% of the weighted average nonfederal selling price for the product, limited to annual increases of no more than the increase in the consumer price index-urban (CPI-U). The FSS generally limits annual increases in any pharmaceutical price over the life of a contract (typically 5 years) to the increase in the CPI-U over the same period.

Medicaid Rebates

The Omnibus Budget Reconciliation Act of 1990 (OBRA) established the Medicaid rebate program. The basic formula requires that, in exchange for having their products reimbursed (that is, on the formulary), pharmaceutical manufacturers rebate to the states the greater of (a) 15.1% of the average manufacturer price (AMP)[1] paid by wholesalers for brand-name drugs that Medicaid beneficiaries purchase as outpatients, or (b) the difference between AMP and the manufacturer's "best price." The best price is the lowest price offered to any other customer, excluding FSS prices and prices to state pharmaceutical assistance programs. Similarly, manufacturers pay a rebate equal to 11% of the AMP on generic and over-the-counter drugs.

---

[1] Average manufacturer price is the weighted average price to wholesalers for product distributed to the retail pharmacy class of trade, where wholesaler is defined as any entity to whom the manufacturer sells (except relabelers) and where retail pharmacy class of trade excludes hospitals and HMOs.

"If a brand-name drug's AMP increases faster than the inflation rate, an additional rebate is imposed so that manufacturers cannot offset the basic rebate by raising their AMP. The additional rebate is equal to the difference between the current AMP and a base-year AMP increased by the inflation rate as measured by the consumer price index" (CBO, 1996, p. xi).

OBRA 93 changed the pricing schedule of single-source and innovator multiple-source drugs approved by the FDA after October 1990. "In general, OBRA 93 had an impact on the computation of the unit rebate amount for covered outpatient drugs. The effective date for implementation of OBRA 93 was October 1, 1993. Presently, more than 500 manufacturers have rebate agreements with the Federal Government which, in turn, address approximately 55,000 drug products" (David, Baugh, Pine, & Blackwell, 1997, p. 80).[2]

International Comparisons

Many cross-national drug pricing comparisons have been made over the years. Although these findings are significant, they merit caution in how the comparisons are made and in how the conclusions are drawn. Because markets, demographics, and values vary, and because medical practices and economic circumstances also vary, it is difficult simply to transfer one country's pricing methods to another. Nevertheless, for many reasons, price differentials between products purchased in the U.S. and other countries are oftentimes substantial.

An October 1999 Alliance for Health Reform document, *Prescription Drugs, A Primer for Policymakers,* reported that

> U.S. Government Accounting Office studies found U.S. drug prices for specific drugs were, on average, one-third higher than in Canada (1991), and 60 percent higher than in the United Kingdom (1992). Patricia Danzon of the University of Pennsylvania finds that drug prices vary by country, some are higher abroad and some are higher in the U.S. (April 1999) (p. 2)

COST-CONTROL TOOLS

Prescription drug benefits, once viewed as a relatively small expenditure by employers, have recently come under tighter cost controls. While the clinical benefits of many of these new products are significant, their high costs place a heavy burden on payers and patients. As new products make their way into the market, the market has responded with new tools to control drug costs. One of the most dramatic responses has been the growth of pharmacy benefit managers, or PBMs.

---

[2] The figures in this quotation that concern the number of manufacturers with rebate agreements with the federal government are derived from a personal communication with S. Gaston, March 11, 1999.

Pharmacy Benefit Managers

By acting as intermediaries between pharmaceutical manufacturers and third-party payers (that is, employers, managed care organizations, labor unions, and state-funded pharmaceutical assistance programs for the elderly), PBMs administer prescription drug benefits. In addition to offering their core services—claims processing, record keeping, and reporting programs—PBMs offer their customers a wide range of services, including drug utilization review, disease management, consultative services, and most recently, Internet fulfillment. PBMs also assist clients with establishing their benefit structure. Options for plan design include developing and maintaining a network of pharmacy providers, providing a mail service component, and developing and maintaining a drug formulary. In an effort to save plan sponsors' money, PBMs negotiate with pharmaceutical manufacturers for rebates on products selected for the formulary (Strongin, 1999).

To counter the rise in prescription drug prices, employers and third-party payers have begun instituting various benefit restrictions and cost control measures, some of which are used more than others. In addition to the more traditional methods—formulary compliance; generic substitution; prior authorization; beneficiary cost-sharing (i.e., the recent move by most third-party plans to triple-tiered co-payments); prescribing and dispensing limits; drug utilization review; disease management; and the use of mail service pharmacies for maintenance drugs—additional cost control tools are being utilized. Some of these are detailed below.

Negotiated Discounts

Negotiating discounts for pharmaceuticals is a common practice (although senior citizens without drug coverage generally do not enjoy the benefits of "preferred pricing"). PBMs and managed care plans, for example, negotiate discounts in exchange for the ability to move market share, while the federal government (for example, the Veterans Health Administration, the Public Health Service, and the Indian Health Service) mandates discounts.

Physician Connectivity

Physician connectivity is a relatively new phenomenon where the physician in his or her office prescribes on-line, from a handheld wireless device. Going from a POS (point of sale) system in the pharmacy to a POP (point of prescribing) system in the physician's office enables the PBM, for example, to intervene more rapidly. A problem message (such as "potential drug interaction" or "nonformulary drug") could immediately flash on the physician's screen, allowing the physician to change the prescription instantly, thus eliminating the need for the pharmacist to telephone the doctor. While this technology exists today, it is not yet widespread. It is thought that within 5 to 10 years, this tool (which has the capacity to decrease prescribing errors) will become commonplace.

Drug Interchange Programs

The use of various drug interchange programs, such as generic substitution, therapeutic substitution (which requires pharmacists to give patients chemically different, less costly drugs that may accomplish the same thing as the ones their doctors prescribe), and step therapy (which requires doctors to begin by prescribing lower-cost drugs whenever possible; if they prove ineffective, physicians can prescribe more expensive medications)—has sparked a good deal of controversy. At issue is the question of whether these programs compromise patients' access to necessary therapies, thereby contributing to negative health outcomes. On the other hand, proponents are of the opinion that these programs hold great promise in slowing the growth rate of drug expenditures by promoting clinically appropriate and cost-effective products.

When analyzing the success—or failure—of these cost control measures, it is important to examine their effect on the overall cost and quality of health care.

CURRENT ISSUES

The question of how best to provide access to prescription drugs for all Medicare beneficiaries has challenged Congress since shortly after the Medicare program was enacted in 1965. Many drugs—when prescribed accurately and taken properly—can be a lifeline for people of all ages, and this is especially true for the elderly. Medicare beneficiaries with one or more chronic conditions, such as heart disease or diabetes, are often particularly reliant on prescription medication. As lawmakers debate how best to reform the Medicare program, outpatient prescription drug coverage has once again become a lightning rod for heated debate. See *Case Study* for further discussion.

SUMMARY

While lawmakers seek to curb drug prices and reduce industry profits, it is difficult to say whether or not Americans pay too much for their prescription drugs. Critics of the pharmaceutical industry maintain that prices and profits are too high and that this is indicative of monopoly power. Abuses, critics contend, include price discrimination (selling the same drugs for less to large purchasers); drugs priced at levels out of proportion to their costs of production; and a lack of price competition among companies.

In response to such accusations, those in the pharmaceutical industry and some in academia point to the extremely expensive costs of research and development, that include costs for the great number of "dry holes" that must be dug before a successful drug therapy is produced as well as the high price of developing drug treatments for the complex diseases—such as cancer—that are still unconquered. Moreover, they note that drugs increase the quality of life by reducing mortality and morbidity and that drugs are less expensive forms of treatment for a number of diseases, such as ulcers and asthma, than are surgery and hospitalization. In order to measure more accurately the *value* of pharmaceutical products, decision makers will need to move away from "silo budgeting"—analyzing prescription drug cost expenditures without accounting for total health care offsets.

CASE STUDY

The political pressure for providing a Medicare outpatient prescription drug benefit has not only gained the attention of Congress but has become a major campaign issue in the 2000 presidential election and in key congressional races. Determining the ultimate program design, however, has proven to be challenging—both administratively as well as politically. As history has shown, legislation, regulation, and market adjustments in one sector of the market often result in a chain reaction of intended and unintended consequences throughout the entire pharmaceutical marketplace.

What impact do you expect such legislation, should it pass, will have on

- Current prescription drug coverage?
- Utilization trends?
- Prescribing patterns?
- Pharmaceutical R&D?
- Total health care costs?
- Quality of care?

Should this legislation be part of a broader reform of the Medicare program?

What design elements should be incorporated into the legislation to protect Medicare beneficiaries from medication errors, from polypharmacy, from noncompliance?

DISCUSSION QUESTIONS

1. How has the nature of pharmaceutical R&D changed over the past 20 years? What effect will biotechnology and the mapping of the human genome have on prescription drug and ultimately on patients? How will the practice of medicine change as R&D continues to change?
2. The FDA must walk a regulatory tightrope, balancing patient safety on the one hand with timely access to needed medications on the other. Is

the FDA meeting its dual objectives? How will the increased pressure from the additional burdens of regulating DTC advertising and Internet pharmacy activity affect the FDA's performance?

3. What effects have generics, patents, PBMs, and formularies had on the pharmaceutical marketplace?
4. Much of today's political dialogue revolves around the notion of profitability and "public good," in the case of drug products. For the pharmaceutical industry, how much profit is too much? Who should decide?
5. What factors drive up prescription drug expenditures?
6. Should the federal government regulate the price of drugs? If so, what marketplace dynamics could be expected?
7. How is the *value* of pharmaceuticals measured? How should it be measured?

REFERENCES

Alliance for Health Reform. (1999, October). *Prescription drugs, a primer for policymakers.* Washington, DC: Author.

Assistant Secretary for Planning and Evaluation. (2000). *Report to the president: Prescription drug coverage, spending, utilization, and prices.* Washington, DC: Department of Health and Human Services.

Barents Group LLC (1999). *Factors affecting the growth of prescription drug expenditures.* Washington, DC: NICM.

Baugh, D. K., Pine, P. L., & Blackwell, S. (1999). Trends in Medicaid prescription drug utilization and payments, 1990–1997. *Health Care Financing Review, 20*(3), 80.

Brandeis University-Schneider Institute for Health Policy Prescription Drug Analysis Group. (2000, May). *Prescription drug policy: Background paper for the Princeton Conference.*

Congressional Budget Office. (1996, January). How the Medicaid rebate on prescription drugs affects pricing in the pharmaceutical industry. *CBO Papers,* xi.

Congressional Budget Office. (1998, July). *How increased competition from generic drugs has affected prices and returns in the pharmaceutical industry.* Washington, DC: Author.

Drug mergers change health landscape. (2000, January). *American Medical News, 4.*

Food and Drug Administration. (2000). *Comparison of FDA review times for NDAs and NMAs, calendar year 1994–2000* [on-line]. Available: http://www.fda.gov/cder/rdmt/NDANME9500.htm.

Generic Pharmaceutical Association. (2000).

Glaser, M. (1999, April). Boom year. *Drug Topics,* 47–53.

Henry J. Kaiser Family Foundation. (2000). *Medicare and prescription drugs.* Washington, DC: Author.

Health Care Financing Administration. (2000). *National health expenditure #5.* Washington, DC: National Health Statistics Group.

Kolassa, E. M. (1997). *Elements of pharmaceutical pricing.* Binghamton, NY: The Pharmaceutical Products Press.

Mail order drug sales leap 10 percent. (1999, July). *American Druggist.*

Menninger, B. (2000, Jan/Feb). Can generics turn it around? *Healthcare Business,* p. 20.

Mullins, C. D., Palumbo, F., & Stuart, B. (2000, April). *The impact of pipeline drugs on pharmaceutical spending.* Presented at a joint BCBSA/HIAA symposium. Washington, DC.

National Association of Chain Drug Stores. (2001). [Accessed October 29, 2001.] Available: NACDS.

National Wholesale Druggists' Association. (1999). *Industry profile and health care fact book.* Reston, VA: Healthcare Distribution Management Association.

Pharmaceutical Research and Manufacturers of America. (1999). *1999 industry profile.* Washington, DC: Author.

Pharmaceutical Research and Manufacturers of America. (2000). *2000 industry profile.* Washington, DC: Author.

Serafini, M. W. (2000, February). No easy prescription on no-name drugs. *National Journal,* p. 548.

Strongin, R. J. (1999, October). *The ABCs of PBMs* (National Health Policy Forum Issue Brief No. 749). Washington, DC: National Health Policy Forum/George Washington University.

11

Managed Care

Helen L. Smits

LEARNING OBJECTIVES

- ☐ Identify the causes of the growth of managed care in the United States.
- ☐ Describe the current impact of managed care on the health insurance marketplace.
- ☐ Distinguish the major organizational types of managed care plans, including group, staff, IPA, and network models.
- ☐ Describe the use of "at risk" subcontractors such as pharmacy benefits managers and managed mental health companies.
- ☐ Describe what large purchasers want and expect from managed care plans.
- ☐ Analyze the current efforts to monitor plan quality.
- ☐ Analyze the issues of public policy and of health care markets that will drive the evolution of HMOs and managed care in the future.

TOPICAL OUTLINE

History of managed care and HMOs
Variations in HMO and MCO organizational structure
Methods of cost control
The growth of specialized subcontractors
Government programs
Measuring quality
Purchaser expectations
Current issues
Summary

KEY WORDS

managed care organizations, health maintenance organizations, Prepaid Group Practice, open and closed panel models, point of service, physician-hospital organization, integrated delivery system, pharmacy benefits managers, carve outs, independent practice association, HEDIS, NCQA

Managed care has become the dominant method of health care financing in the United States. In the process, the term has gained a wide range of meanings, many of them highly emotional: providers denounce "managed care" as the source of all pressure for cost containment; purchasers continue to hope that "managed care" will keep down premium increases; consumers worry that "managed care" will mean that company profits are put ahead of patient benefit. The literal meaning of managed care is simple: it includes any system in which insurance risk is tightly linked to a predefined group of providers and in which data systems are used to identify and modify utilization patterns. Managed care plans are known as managed care organizations (MCOs) or health maintenance organizations (HMOs).

This chapter will introduce the reader to a wide-ranging and complex topic. The chapter begins with a history of the early growth of managed care in this country and reviews briefly the statistics on the industry in the late 1990s. The wide variations in organizational types, and some of the most common terms and acronyms used to describe those types, are then reviewed. The chapter goes on to explore the common methods used by MCOs and HMOs to manage their costs including subcontracting with some of the "hidden" managed care plans—companies that manage specialized areas such as pharmacy benefits. The chapter will then look at the quality measures that are being specifically used to evaluate plan performance and at the ways in which purchasers are using that measurement process to make decisions about plan choice. Finally, the chapter explores some of the current pressures on MCOs including the public "backlash" against tight cost control methods.

History of Managed Care and HMOs

The Early Years

Health maintenance organizations had modest beginnings as "Prepaid Group Practices" that were founded by innovative physicians and supported by interested employers (Fox, 1997). The goal of these organizations was to provide affordable, well-organized health care (Mayer & Mayer, 1985) by allowing patients to prepay on a regular monthly basis for all services provided by the practice. This ensured providers a regular income and also allowed them to plan care around the needs of their enrolled population. The concepts of prepayment and of exclusive relationships between physicians and patients were seen by organized medicine as a threat to the financial independence of the practicing physician. The history of prepaid practice is replete with stories of physicians expelled from their county and state medical societies and threatened with loss of license because of their advocacy of prepaid group practices.

The Western Clinic in Tacoma, Washington, established in 1910, is sometimes cited as the first example of a prepaid group practice. The program, which cost $.50 per person per month, was made available to lumber mill owners and employees. A Dr. Bridge started a similar clinic in Tacoma; this later expanded into sites throughout Oregon and Washington (Kovner, 1998). In 1929, Michael Shadid, MD, began a cooperative for rural farmers in Elk City, Oklahoma, that raised capital for a new hospital through its membership and promised to provide medical care at a discount to those who contributed. Some of the most important of the prototype HMOs are described below:

In 1937, Dr. Sidney Garfield, at the behest of the Kaiser Corporation, developed a fully capitated model of care for employees of the Grand Coulee Dam project in Washington and an aqueduct project in the southern California desert. The experiment was so successful that Kaiser proceeded to establish the Kaiser Foundation Health Plan in California in order to help attract workers to their shipbuilding plants in Oakland during World War II. Long held as the model of successful HMO development, Kaiser Health Plans have extended their reach nationwide. Faced with competition from aggressive for-profit managed care companies, they struggled financially during the 1990s but continue as an important force in many parts of the country. Reported enrollment in 2000 was 8 million covered lives in 11 states (Kaiser Permanente, 2001).

Also in 1937, the Group Health Association (GHA) was founded in Washington, D.C. by a consumer cooperative supported by the Home Owner's Loan Corporation (that wanted to reduce mortgage defaults that resulted from overwhelming medical expenses.) Faced with a well established and well-organized local medical society, GHA struggled to obtain admitting privileges and the right to have its physicians belong to the District of Columbia Medical Society. A bitter antitrust battle resulted, which GHA won at the Supreme Court. Despite its victory, GHA never grew beyond approximately 125,000 members. It experienced severe financial difficulties in the early 1990s and was first sold to the Humana Corporation and then closed down.

In 1947, consumers in Seattle organized the Group Health Cooperative of Puget Sound that was, predictably, opposed by the Kings County Medical Society. Despite the opposition, Group Health has flourished. It remains a consumer cooperative; at most recent report it had 575,000 members and was the largest plan in the state of Washington (Group Health Cooperative, 2001).

The most successful of these early HMOs had a number of characteristics in common. Most of them were originally built on the west coast at times when there was significant in-migration of the labor force. New arrivals in California, Washington, and Oregon were pleased to find an easily accessible, well-organized source of care. The fact that choice was restricted to certain doctors and certain hospitals made less difference to patients who lacked a previous attachment to established local institutions. In addition, these prepaid practices worked to attract young families by offering well-organized and effective care by means such as well-designed reminder programs for childhood immunizations and preventive visits. A second important element in the growth of prepaid practice in the West was the relatively weak position of local medical societies when these practices were initiated. The new doctors who came to work for plans like Kaiser Permanente quickly came to be a significant force in local medical politics, effectively muting the kind of resistance experienced by GHA in Washington, D.C.

The Federal Government Steps In

The combination of cost control and quality of early prepaid practices caught the eye of policy makers, with the result that, in 1973, a federal HMO act was passed. It was in association with the work for this legislation that Dr. Paul Ellwood coined the term "health maintenance organization." The intent of the legislation was to encourage the growth of managed care by three major means:

- A category of *federally qualified HMOs* was created and employers were required to offer the choice of one or two such HMOs when the HMO itself made a request.
- Grants and loans were available for planning and start-up of new not-for-profit HMOs.
- State laws that restricted HMO development were overridden by the new federal legislation.

The effects of this law have always been controversial; some observers believe that HMOs would have grown faster in its absence. The requirements for federal qualification were extensive and sometimes difficult for new plans to meet, diverting resources away from the urgent need to focus on serving customers well and growing quickly. In addition, these regulations were issued only very slowly, leaving many new plans unable to obtain qualification and therefore unable to exercise their right to be offered as a part of "dual choice." Many of the law's requirements, such as member grievance procedures and quality assurance mechanisms, are now commonly accepted as appropriate and necessary; some form of these requirements is built into many state laws governing managed care. At the same time, with the best of intentions, the law forced federally qualified HMOs to engage in some practices, such as open enrollment and community rating, that were not required of competing indemnity plans. As a result, sicker patients who would have difficulty obtaining insurance elsewhere could always purchase it from a qualified HMO. With adverse selection such as this, HMOs had to work even harder to control costs.

Despite its drawbacks, the HMO law had the effect of supporting the development and early growth of many new plans, some of them now considered to be among the country's best. Once the regulations for qualification were issued, rapid growth of HMOs did result, with many plans taking advantage of the dual choice mandate. At the same time, many indemnity plans began to understand and make use of the cost-control measures found in HMOs so that the sharp distinction between plan types began to change.

1985 and Beyond

Growth in managed care from 1982 to 1986 was very rapid both in the numbers of plans available and in their enrolled membership. Although growth in the numbers of plans slowed after 1986, membership continued to increase (see Figure 11.1). Employers were increasingly concerned about the steady and rapid rise in the cost of health insurance. As managed care plans became more experienced at cost-control techniques, they were able to enter markets without need for special federal protections. Managed care premiums were often well below that of competing indemnity plans in the same market.

Beginning in the late 1980s, a pattern of rapid growth in plan size emerged, based in part on mergers and purchases of plans. By July of 1998, the 10 largest plans in the country controlled almost 65% of the entire

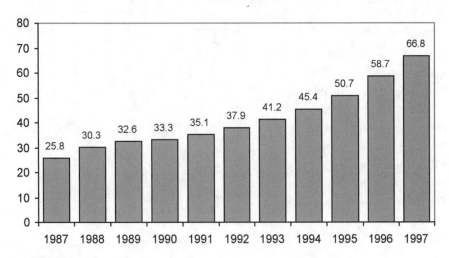

FIGURE 11.1   Total HMO enrollment (millions) 1987–1997.

Source: The Interstudy Competitive Edge: HMO Industry Report 9.1.

market (Table 11.1). For-profit companies became an increasingly important part of the picture; Figure 11.2 demonstrates the very rapid shift
towards membership in for-profit plans. Many of managed care's most
effective techniques are based on statistical analyses of patterns of care that
can be applied as easily on a large scale as on a small; mergers were driven
by the need to spread administrative costs over as wide a base of customers
as possible. The rapid growth of companies such as Oxford Health Plans
created enthusiasm among investment analysts and investors with this sector. As a result, large amounts of equity capital became available for managed care, further sparking rapid growth. A number of HMOs became, at
least temporarily, among the best performing stocks in the market. Not-
for-profit plans also used merger as a means to growth although, as the
financial difficulties experienced by Harvard Community Health Plan
show, merger and growth alone is not enough to guarantee success (Brewster
& Ginsburg, 2000).

One aspect of managed care growth that has received a great deal of
public attention is the shift of both Medicare and Medicaid enrollees into
managed care plans during the 1990s. In Medicare, this shift was entirely
voluntary. Beneficiaries not only have the choice of remaining in traditional
fee-for-service Medicare, they also have the right to leave a plan at any time
if they wish. The very rapid growth of plan participation and enrollment
in the mid-1990s has been followed by an almost equally rapid decrease in
both the numbers of participating plans and in enrollment in 1999, 2000,
and 2001 (Health Care Financing Administration [HCFA], 2001).

**TABLE 11.1   Managed Care Enrollment of the Ten Largest Plans,
July 1, 1998**

National managed care company	Total enrollment	Percent of total total enrollment
Blue Cross and Blue Shield	13,337,328	17
Kaiser Foundation Health Plans, Inc.	8,420,312	11
United Healthcare Corporation	5,554,946	7
Aetna U.S. Healthcare, Inc.	4,306,057	5
Foundation Health Systems	4,178,773	5
Pacificare Health Systems, Inc.	3,736,014	5
CIGNA HealthCare, Inc.	3,406,577	4
Humana, Inc.	2,977,003	4
Prudential Insurance Co. of America	2,871,706	4
Oxford Health Plans	1,712,948	2
All Other	28,294,076	36
Total	78,795,740	100

Source: The Interstudy Competitive Edge: HMO Industry Report 9.1

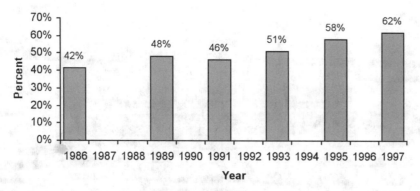

FIGURE 11.2   Percent of total enrollment in for profit HMO.

Source: The Interstudy Competitive Edge: HMO Industry Report 9.1.

Medicaid managed care has also grown, largely through the imposition of managed care mandates by many states (HCFA, 2001). Medicaid managed care has been more controversial than Medicare because of fears that systems aimed at controlling utilization would not be appropriate when applied to underserved individuals. The expectation on the part of many state legislatures that Medicaid managed care can somehow simultaneously cut costs and improve quality does not seem to be entirely realistic. Nevertheless, many Medicaid plans have been able to use their information systems to good purpose to ensure that beneficiaries receive the care they need, and the focus on customer service has changed the ways in which our poorest citizens receive their care.

VARIATIONS IN HMO AND MCO ORGANIZATIONAL STRUCTURE

Managed care has grown and succeeded largely as a result of its ability to adapt to the rapidly changing marketplace. As a result, almost any kind of organizational structure imaginable can now be found somewhere within the managed care arena. For the new student of managed care, one of the most frustrating byproducts of this variety is the bewildering number of new acronyms that are used to describe the field. There is an excellent glossary available (Center for the Health Professions, 2001) from the University of California for anyone who wants to move beyond the few basic terms listed here.

There are three major characteristics to consider in describing the structure of any MCO:

1. Is it organized as a for-profit or not-for-profit company?
2. What individuals or entities control the company?
3. How do the providers relate to the entity that accepts the risk of issuing insurance?

For Profit or Not?

Early prepaid group practices were largely not-for-profit entities. They raised the necessary capital through debt, grants, or contributions from institutional owners. As managed care grew, however, finding sufficient capital through these means became more difficult. Managed care companies provide insurance, and are required by state Departments of Insurance to establish large reserves to meet their potential obligations. In addition, MCOs need capital to build the systems that will support growth. For-profit ownership became an increasingly dominant characteristic of the industry in the 1980s and 1990s, with some large not-for-profit plans actually converting themselves to for-profits in order to access capital markets. One of the earliest, and still the most notable of these is Wellpoint Health Plans, which evolved out of Blue Cross of California. A number of other Blue Cross plans have taken similar steps in recent years. Some observers believe that not-for-profit plans provide higher quality than do for-profits (Himmelstein, 1999), although others argue that the differences are modest at best and that they may be explained by factors other than ownership structure.

Who's in Control?

Ownership of HMOs varies widely from plans owned entirely or almost entirely by providers, to traditional insurance companies whose health insurance lines are strictly managed. The many Medicaid plans owned by Federally Qualified Community Health Centers (FQHCs) are one example of the former type; Aetna-U.S. Healthcare is an example of the latter. As the market has evolved, the mixture of for-profit and not-for-profit ownership has become increasingly complex. HMOs owned by not-for-profit hospitals or FQHCs are often for-profit; even large not-for-profit HMOs such as Tufts Community Health Plan own for-profit subsidiaries. The outside observer interested in learning who actually makes the decisions needs to explore in some detail who exactly controls the board of directors in order to gain insight as to how strategic direction is decided. (See chapter 13 for further information regarding governance of health care organizations.)

How Is It Structured?

It is easiest to think of managed care as a continuum with very tightly structured organizational systems at one end and very loosely structured systems at the other end. At one extreme in the organization of MCOs is the *closed panel staff model.* In this arrangement, all physicians in the plan are either actually salaried by the plan or work in a group practice that contracts exclusively with the plan. Members must see these physicians and only these physicians; a member who leaves the HMO must change physicians. At the other extreme are relatively loose *network model* plans that contract with all or a substantial proportion of all of the providers in a given community.

If these two models are thought of as the extremes, then most of the alternative organizational types now in the market can be seen to fall somewhere in between. *Point-of-service (POS)* plans permit members to go to any provider they choose—but financial incentives are present that encourage the use of those providers most closely affiliated with the plan. Co-payments and deductibles rise considerably when the member receives care "out of network." In recent years the greatest growth in HMOs has been in "mixed" models that incorporate a variety of different methods in their relationships with physicians. A few of the most common acronyms and terms associated with HMO organizational structures are included in Table 11.2.

METHODS OF COST CONTROL

Managed care plans control their costs through two main mechanisms: targeted contracting and utilization controls. Large plans with significant market share have been able to obtain very significant discounts from hospitals, physicians, and other suppliers such as laboratories. Hospitals originally entered into discount arrangements with a few plans in the hopes of increasing their patient base within their own market; the practice is now widespread and few hospitals can avoid it. The contracts between hospitals and managed care plans usually involve a *per diem* or fixed price per day that includes all services and all medications. There might be different rates for different types of care, such as a higher per diem for the intensive care unit, but negotiated contracts no longer permit hospitals to simply add on costs such as supplies and medications. In theory, such an arrangement can serve both the hospital and the plan well; the hospital has an incentive to keep its daily costs under control and the plan has an ability to predict what its costs will be. In practice, however, HMOs have been very aggressive both in their contracting arrangements and in reducing the length of hospital stays. Since the first day of each stay is much more costly than all the rest, this means that hospitals often have experienced difficulty in managing within the per diems they agreed to in their contracts.

Example:

Hospital X negotiates a per diem of $900 per day with Health Plan Y. The hospital's negotiators expect an average length of stay (LOS) of 5 days, which means a revenue of $4,500 per case. The hospital anticipates spending $1,500 on the first day of each patient's stay and $700 on each day thereafter. In a 5-day stay, hospital costs will be $4,300 and each patient will generate a surplus of $200. If the health plan is able to reduce the LOS to 4 days, then revenues will fall to $3,600 per case, the actual cost of the hospitalization will also fall to $3,600 and the surplus will disappear. Any further reductions within this contract period will result in a loss to the hospital.

TABLE 11.2   Terms Associated with HMOs

PPO	Preferred Provider Organization
IDS	Integrated Delivery System
PHO	Physician Hospital Organization
IPA	Independent Practice Association
POS	Point of Service (a plan that offers the patient a choice each time they receive a service)
gatekeeper	A provider, usually a primary care physician, who controls the patient's access to specialists and other services

Plans have also negotiated contracts with independent physicians and physician groups that both reduce the total amounts paid for care and offer various incentives to practice "cost-effective" care. The most common approach to incentive-based contracting is simple *capitation* that pays the doctor, or the group practice, a fixed fee per month for every HMO member who lists that physician as his/her primary care provider. Many health policy makers have long touted capitation as a payment mechanism with good incentives. Providers are, in effect, rewarded for keeping patients satisfied and healthy—if patients are satisfied then more will sign up and capitation payments will increase. If patients stay healthy then the physician reaps any benefit from actually seeing the patient less often. In practice in the United States, capitation is neither as easy as it sounds nor as effective as appears to be the case in other countries.

To begin with, American health plans are required by various oversight agencies to keep a record of every encounter between physician and patient. Capitation in an ordinary office practice means that the plan and the physician must specify a lengthy list of procedural and visit codes that count as part of the capitated obligation. Physicians must submit dummy bills to the plan for which they receive no additional payment. As a result, one of the greatest attractions of capitation—the fact that it is administratively simple—is not true here. In addition, even health plans that claim to be focused on primary care have often placed very tight limits on capitation payments with the result that physicians receive less than they would have under efficient fee-for-service practice, with the result there may be little interest in pleasing patients or building up the capitated side of the practice. Capitation does have one very strong positive aspect: it permits innovation. Many new approaches to managing patients, such as telephone management of complex conditions or having all of the patients with the same condition come to a group meeting for educational purposes, are not reimbursed under fee-for-service but have no restrictions placed on them under capitation.

Primary care physician groups and physician hospital organizations (PHOs) may also accept *global capitation* in which a significant proportion of the entire insurance premium is paid to the group in return for a commitment to provide all care to the members enrolled with that PHO.

These arrangements in effect shift the risk of insurance—as well as the potential profits from insurance—to the providers and away from the managed care company itself. There was considerable enthusiasm for these arrangements among physicians in the early to mid-1990s. Unfortunately, some PHOs greatly underestimated the inherent risks in becoming an insurer and a number of large organizations failed as a result. Several major bankruptcies of physician groups in California and elsewhere have made both plans and providers more cautious in expanding this form of payment.

Managed care plans can, and do, also pay extra for certain types of good performance, such as ensuring that all patients receive screening tests or that all children receive their immunizations. In fact, so many different incentives are now built into managed care contracts that many physicians find it difficult to keep track of either the purpose or the result of the contracts they have accepted (Grumbach et al., 1998).

Utilization Management

In addition to negotiating favorable contracts, MCOs focus considerable effort on managing the care delivered. One of the most basic—and to date most profitable—activities is known as utilization management (UM). Utilization management occurs when the plan focuses on a specific type of service, most notably hospital length of stay, and undertakes a systematic effort to reduce the use of that service, often by substituting a less expensive alternative service. Standard utilization management techniques include steps such as requiring that patients be admitted on the day of surgery—rather than the day before—and requirements that lengths of stay for every case meet certain stringent criteria established in advance. There has been a great deal of public concern about length of stay reductions, so much so that in two specific areas—maternity stays and post-mastectomy stays—a minimum length of stay has actually been built into law. There seems to be no question that some patients, particularly the poor, who have less ability to manage care well at home, have been poorly served by shorter lengths of stay. Taken on the whole, however, most length of stay reductions appear to have worked well without harming the public; for many conditions the earlier ambulation and increased activity associated with early discharge appears to be beneficial, not harmful. In some cases, MCOs have developed innovative approaches to facilitate shorter lengths of stay. For example, some now require physical therapy before rather than after major orthopedic surgery—an arrangement that helps both to facilitate early discharge and to improve outcomes of the surgery itself.

Case Management

Many plans make a sharp distinction between utilization management, which is a routinized and standardized process based on preestablished criteria, and case management, which is more dependent on the clinical judgment of nurses employed by the plans. Few terms in managed care are more confusing than case management, since many providers use the same words to describe a similar, but quite distinct, activity in which they engage. A managed care case manager is involved in approving and over-seeing all of the various services provided to a specific patient with a complex and potentially costly condition. For example, a case manager might work with an individual recovering from major trauma by coordinating their home health care, their need for durable medical equipment in the home, and their various rehabilitation services. At its best, case management can be a useful support to both physician and patient in complex circumstances since the plan case manager knows what benefits are available and can guarantee payment for appropriate services in advance. At its worst, case management can become a confusing and frustrating addition to the insurance process for a patient with an already complex situation. Case management is dependent on the services of experienced nurses and is, as a result, expensive; most plans reserve it for only the most complex, costly, and difficult cases.

Disease Management

Disease management is the term used to describe efforts by health plans and/or specialized subcontractors to establish a prospective approach to managing a complex disease with the aim of reducing unnecessary use of costly services. The term can be a confusing one since physicians have obviously been managing diseases since the profession first evolved. In managed care terms however, disease management means a process that "redirects the intervention efforts toward the outpatient setting for several chronic disorders, often featuring noncompliance with prescription drugs, and captures information from all sites of care for each patient with that disorder into a single longitudinal episode" (Plocher, 1997). The important elements of disease management are

- integration of all components of care using the data available to the managed care plan,
- emphasis on prevention and education, and
- use of guidelines endorsed by expert professionals to guide the process of care.

Disease management began as a way to approach problems such as refractory asthma, diabetes, and congestive heart failure. It has been clear-ly shown in demonstrations to decrease emergency room use, improve the quality of life, and reduce long-term complications (Diabetes Control and Complications Research Group, 1993). The important new element that managed care disease management adds to conventional medical treatment is data. A managed care plan can set its systems to flag the times when asthma patients fail to refill prescriptions and can identify emergency room visits as they occur, in order to intervene effectively before problems escalate. The concept has now been extended to even more complex areas such as cancer treatment. In some cases the organization that offers disease management actually accepts risk for the patients involved. That is, they provide all care associated with cancer (or some other condition) for a fixed, prospective fee.

The next challenge for disease management is the approach to the patient with multiple illnesses. Managed care plans and the integrated delivery systems with which they work should be able to apply the lessons learned from less complex medical situations, such as childhood diabetes or asthma, to the patient with multiple illnesses since the principles are very much the same. Here too, effective information systems that can identify problems such as potential drug-drug interactions can both reduce costs and improve life for the patients in question.

Pharmaceutical manufacturers have attempted to capture the enthusiasm for disease management by offering programs that are, predictably, built around their own medications. Both practicing physicians and many HMO medical directors are skeptical of disease management based in an individual drug company for the simple reason that the protocols will inevitably cut against innovative products from competitors.

THE GROWTH OF SPECIALIZED SUBCONTRACTORS

One aspect of modern managed care that is little understood by outsiders is the importance of specialized subcontractors, organizations that contract to assume the responsibility for management of certain aspects of care. There are essentially two different models for such subcontracting: the specialty organization can accept risk, as is usually the case in mental health or it can operate as a specialized service provider without assuming risk as is the customary case with pharmacy benefits management. These two areas were chosen as good illustrations of the kinds of arrangements currently available; many other examples can be found.

Mental Health

Managed mental health is one of the most controversial areas within managed care (Iglehart, 1996). In the past, the classic method of controlling the costs of mental health benefits was not to offer very much: limits on length of stay and on the number of outpatient visits were common in all types of health insurance contracts until the recent passage of legislation intended to make mental health benefits more "mainstream." Well before this date, managed care plans had turned to tight utilization controls rather than specific limits. The approach is based on a cluster of observed facts about the treatment of mental illness. These are as follows:

- There is, or at least has been in the past, considerable unnecessary hospitalization and many overly long hospitalizations.
- There is wide variation in the patterns of treatment for various types of psychiatric problems.
- There is no evidence that more costly methods, particularly inpatient treatment, are more effective than the alternatives.

During the mid-1980s a number of specialized companies were formed to deliver managed mental health services. A well structured managed mental health benefit requires sophisticated psychiatric input and must involve careful attention to the seriously mentally ill, including methods to ensure that suicidal and violent patients are not denied treatment. Many managed care plans, even those of a reasonable size, found it difficult to offer these arrangements themselves. In addition, a well managed mental health benefit requires a carefully adjusted provider network; one method of cost control is the steering of less acutely ill patients to social workers and psychologists, reserving psychiatric care for only the sickest and the most problematic from a diagnostic point of view. Specialized managed mental health services that contract with a number of different managed care plans assume responsibility for large numbers of patients. This enables them to fine-tune their network by ensuring a steady stream of patients to those providers they accept.

One trend observed within mental health has been the tendency by large purchasers to "carve out" mental health benefits entirely, contracting for them independent of the more general health insurance. A number of large employers now do this as do many states in their Medicaid programs. The problem from the providers' point of view is that this creates a problematic separation between primary care and the treatment of mental illness, making the transfer of valuable information between providers caring for the same patient particularly difficult.

Many mental health professionals, particularly psychiatrists, are adamantly opposed to any management of the care they deliver. They argue that managed mental health violates patient privacy and intrudes very directly into their capacity to make decisions about care. Some observers within the field note that one of the greatest contributors to the development of managed mental health has been the fee-for service providers themselves who have not, until recently, focused on measuring the outcomes of care or documenting the perceived benefits of lengthy and expensive treatment patterns when compared to shorter and less costly ones. Despite this deep unrest within the profession, managed mental health services seem unlikely to disappear; the profession must inevitably evolve to cope with the new payment methods.

Pharmacy Benefits Management

Pharmacy benefits are managed for most health plans by a small group of organizations known as pharmacy benefits managers (PBMs) (Lyles & Palumbo, 1999; National Health Policy Forum, 1999). Twenty years ago payment for newly emerging drug benefits was problematic for most health plans. Pharmacists, unlike many other health care providers, expected immediate payment. Given their very significant investment in the cost of drugs sold and the foundation of their businesses on cash transactions, they were unwilling to adapt to delays in payment. In addition, paying for drugs involves the payment of very large numbers of relatively small claims. The first PBMs developed direct-access information systems that allowed the pharmacist to verify at the time of sale that a given drug was covered and also informed him/her of the size of the co-payment and any limits on the amount to be dispensed.

Over time, this advantage in efficiency has led to the growth of large organizations with lots of capital, many of them publicly traded, that serve multiple health plans. PBMs have been able to moderate the very rapid growth in the cost of medications that has been seen in recent years. The techniques used involve

- the development of specific formularies that limit the medications provided by offering limited choice within a therapeutic class;
- the development of limited pharmacy networks that allow the PBM to negotiate better prices from pharmacies;
- incentives for physicians to increase the prescribing of generic drugs;
- incentives for pharmacists to engage in generic substitution where permitted by law;
- the negotiation of rebates from drug companies in return for inclusion in a formulary and growth in a specific drug's market share;
- preapproval of certain very expensive drugs such as growth hormone, and
- use of complex co-payment structures to encourage the consumer to ask for generics and drugs included on the formulary.

The information systems, which were the PBMs' original competitive edge, remain one of their strongest advantages. The on-line approval systems now used by essentially all pharmacists in the United States serve as the only claim that the pharmacist must submit. Payment for approved claims can take place as quickly as the contract specifies; same day electronic transfers of funds are often used. In addition, the information system can alert the pharmacist to potentially dangerous drug-drug interactions and can prevent inappropriate early refills of a medication. Pharmacy systems can also be used to flag certain kinds of patients, such as asthmatics, when refills are not obtained in time.

The growth of PBMs has not been as controversial as that of managed mental health, but there still are concerns that the systems can be abused. Physicians who belong to multiple health plans are frustrated by the variations in formularies. In addition, there is considerable suspicion of PBMs based on the fact that pharmaceutical companies own some PBMs. In order to prevent abuse of antitrust statutes, PBMs owned by drug companies are required to develop "firewalls" that permit the PBM to operate independently of its parent. Despite the assurance that this is the case, many physicians remain very skeptical of such arrangements. Another aspect of PBMs that worries observers is the vast quantities of information they own on physician prescribing habits and consumer use of medications.

GOVERNMENT PROGRAMS

In the past decade, the beneficiaries of both Medicare and Medicaid have increasingly moved into managed care plans. The two fields are, however, very different. Medicare beneficiaries have joined managed care plans only when they wished to; they have always been guaranteed the right to leave a plan with a month's notice if they become dissatisfied. Medicaid programs, by contrast, have increasingly made use of waivers from the Health Care Financing Administration to create mandatory Medicaid managed care programs, in which all enrollees within certain eligibility categories must join managed care plans. Their only choice is among several different plans.

Medicare

In both programs, there have been underlying difficulties based on the methods that the government uses to set rates for managed care, but the sources and nature of the problems have been different. In Medicare, managed care monthly payments are based on information about the average cost of care in the specific area where a beneficiary receives service. Rates are risk adjusted for a variety of factors including age and gender; the result is a complex formula known as the Area Adjusted Per Capita Cost (AAPCC). Because there are wide variations in the cost and use of services in different parts of the country, AAPCC rates have been very high in high-cost areas such as Florida and much less so in lower-cost areas such as Minnesota. Naturally, managed care companies have moved to offer their services largely in the higher rate areas.

Even though the government sets rates, restrictions have been placed on the amount of profit that plans can earn from those rates. Instead of retaining profits, plans have been required to return part of their savings to the beneficiaries themselves in the form of enhanced services. This arrangement at first worked well for everyone: Plans were happy to offer extra benefits, particular drug benefits, because these led to rapid growth in the numbers of members; beneficiaries were delighted to find increased services for no more than they would have paid for routine Medigap policies, and the Health Care Financing Administration, which was pressured by Congress to encourage the growth of managed care, could point to dramatic rates of increase in voluntary enrollment.

The Balanced Budget Act of 1997 brought this happy arrangement to a halt. The tight restrictions paid on payments to hospitals, home health agencies, and other providers were quickly converted by the formulas into restrictions on the AAPCC. In addition, the AAPCC formulas themselves were altered to move toward a national, rather than a local, rate; the result has been a rapid decrease in the difference between the highest and lowest AAPCCs. Although the rates have not officially been reduced, rates in high-cost AAPCC areas stopped rising, even though health care inflation continued to increase. Managed care companies found that they could no longer generate profits in many parts of the country and many of them, even those with the most experience in Medicare, began to withdraw their services in some areas. Beneficiaries have been greatly distressed by these withdrawals, that in some instances mean the complete loss of supplemental benefits with resulting drastic changes in the individual's cost of care.

Medicaid

Managed care within the Medicaid program has had an even more troubled history. There is no question that the principles of managed care can be put to excellent use in offering care to the underserved: The same data systems that identify costly cases can also identify children who are not getting routine care and the chronic sick who are not getting their prescriptions refilled. Evidence about the benefits of managed care for Medicaid came from two principal sources: the long running "experiment" in Arizona, in which all Medicaid beneficiaries have been required to join managed care plans, and the growth of a number of innovative managed care companies that offered managed care to Medicaid beneficiaries on a voluntary basis. Plans such as the Bronx Health Plan in New York, the Neighborhood Health Plan in Boston, the Wellness Plan in Detroit, and the United Health Plan in Los Angeles have demonstrated both high levels of customer satisfaction and much better than average results in providing the critical preventive services to the women and children who make up the largest number of individuals eligible for Medicaid. During the period from the early 1980s until the mid-1990s, when these voluntary plans were thriving, the usual method of payment was for the state to establish a rate at 95% of the fee-for-service costs.

Encouraged by this evidence and pressed by the need to control the steady growth in Medicaid costs, states began to apply to the HCFA for permission to waive some of the requirements of the Medicaid program and move to mandatory managed care. There have been two effects of this shift: First, the rapid movement of Medicaid beneficiaries into managed care has led to an equally rapid growth in the number of plans offering such services. This meant that state Medicaid agencies, new to the problems of regulating managed care companies, were faced with new entities to regulate. The result at times has appeared to be real confusion about the nature of the critical markers of plan performance. Many plans complain bitterly that state regulation in this area is redundant and excessive and does not contribute to improved quality. In addition, a number of questions have been raised in larger states about how well plans are performing and how well members understand what they are getting into.

Once states had full control of the payment rates, legislatures began to steadily reduce the amounts offered, or at least to strictly limit cost increases. As a result, some of the very long-standing plans have found themselves facing budget crises for the first time in their history. Despite the many concerns, most states have not abandoned managed care and the program appears to be stabilizing in many parts of the country as it did in Arizona.

MEASURING QUALITY

The gold standard for measuring quality in managed care plans has been established by the National Committee for Quality Assurance (NCQA) (NCQA, 2001), which was established in 1990 with a grant from the Robert Wood Johnson Foundation and conducted its first accreditation survey in 1991. The board of NCQA is made up of purchasers, health plan representatives, and experts in the field of quality measurement. Like the Joint Commission on Accreditation of Hospitals (JCAHO), NCQA has a number of requirements that involve the plan's internal processes in areas such as credentialing of physicians. What has made NCQA unique, however, has been its commitment to the development and reporting of actual measures of the quality of care. The Health Plan Employer Data and Information Set (HEDIS) includes a group of measures that accredited plans must report and that nonaccredited plans may report to NCQA. The data are then analyzed and made available to the public.

NCQA has moved the field of quality assurance and quality reporting far ahead. Beginning with simple, easily obtainable information such as mammogram rates and rates of immunizations of children, HEDIS has rapidly become increasingly sophisticated; it now includes measures such as the percentage of post-myocardial infarction patients who receive appropriate treatment. As might be expected, the annual reporting process in HEDIS has begun to show substantial improvements throughout the country in the areas of care that are measured.

Despite these important advances, concerns remain that both corporate purchasers and individual citizens often have difficulty deciding whether or not a given plan is better than another. Since the great majority of hospitals and physicians belong to more than one plan, and since the caregivers themselves are ultimately responsible for improvements in quality, better HEDIS scores for one plan in an area are very likely to mean better HEDIS scores for all. In the long run, NCQA's contribution may be more in putting a very public face on the outcomes of care than in helping purchasers choose between plans.

PURCHASER EXPECTATIONS

A distinguishing characteristic of the American health care system is that services are largely purchased by organizations on behalf of individuals rather than by individuals themselves. These purchasers include private employers as well as Medicare and Medicaid. Purchasers have been dissatisfied for a long time with the value they have been getting for the health benefits they purchase. To a great extent it is this pressure from purchasers that led to the formation of NCQA and the development of HEDIS. Since about 1990, more purchasers are beginning to believe that they can intervene to do something about high costs and uneven quality.

For example, the Xerox company gives its employees standard comparisons of health plan performance to help them choose among a limited number of plans approved by the company. The information provided includes, for instance, years of operation, numbers of HMO members, percentage of eligible Xerox employees enrolled, premium changes over 3 years, and the percentage of HMO total premium revenues spent on medical care. Xerox also informs employees as to whether the NCQA has accredited the HMO and what its most recent HEDIS reports show. Xerox has established a "centers of excellence" program for hospital care, helping to ensure that patients have access to hospitals that have more than the average experience with complex procedures and have documented evidence of better outcomes. As of 1996, 35,846 or 75.9% of Xerox beneficiaries were HMO enrollees.

CURRENT ISSUES

Guaranteeing Quality

Managed care in the beginning of the 21st century faces a variety of challenges. Perhaps most important of these is what is described as the "managed care backlash," a rapid shift in public opinion toward dislike and suspicion of managed care plans. This attitude has relatively little to do with an individual's own experiences or even the type of plan the individual belongs to (Blendon, 1998; Reschovsky & Hargraves, 1999). One result is a growing interest on the part of employers in direct contracting with health care providers such as large integrated delivery systems (IDSs). The concept is that such arrangements would "save" that part of the premium

dollar that traditionally goes for "overhead." As this chapter has attempted to make clear, however, much of plan overhead is the cost of systems
that closely track and monitor care; whether or not IDSs could replicate
plan performance is an interesting—and still open—question.

Another direct result of the backlash has been the interest on the part of
government in increasing the oversight of managed care plans. At the federal level, much of this interest has focused on the questions of how to structure a "patient's bill of rights"—legislation that would require plans that
have denied care to permit external review of the reasons for that denial and
would also, in some versions, permit individuals to sue their plans for poor
results of care. A variety of similar statutes already exist at the state level.

Monitoring the quality of care in plans, though, can go far beyond simply ensuring appeals when providers and patients disagree with the plan's
decision-making. Traditionally, oversight of managed care has been the
responsibility of state insurance departments and has focused primarily on
financial stability and viability. Many states now acknowledge that the
quality of delivered services ought to be as important as the financial health
of the managed care organization. With Medicare and Medicaid, plans are
mandated to report information similar to the voluntary reporting under
NCQA; the same is true for all health plans in many states. All large health
plans, however, show more variation in quality measures within themselves
than they do when compared to other plans. In other words, the real variations in quality of care in this country lie at the level of individual hospitals, group practices, and even individual physicians. As the interest in and
focus on the reporting of health care outcomes increases, MCOs are very
likely to remain a central target for both voluntary and mandatory reporting.

Costs and Payment Methods

Costs of managed care are also rising rapidly in the early 2000s, largely as
a result of the rise in the cost of prescription drugs (Freudenheim, 2000).
In a tight labor market, employers have found themselves unable to relin-
quish health insurance that is, in the United States, often a critical element
in recruiting good staff. Some sort of cost shift toward the consumer seems
likely, however, since employers cannot easily absorb double-digit inflation.

For the large public programs, methods of managed care payment
remain a largely unsolved dilemma. As noted earlier, changes in the rate of
overall inflation within Medicare, as well as changes in the calculation of
the AAPCC have led to reductions in the availability of managed care to
Medicare beneficiaries, and reductions in the kinds and extent of supplementary benefits offered. Innovative approaches, such as rewarding quality
through the payment system or even simply allowing Medicare plans to
retain more of the benefits of efficiency, seem very unlikely to be adopted
given the pressure on Congress to deal with so many other issues in the
Medicare benefit. Medicaid managed care is, potentially, an even more

serious problem. Many states continue to believe that they can simultane-ously "save money and improve quality" by reducing rates paid to Medicaid managed care plans, while simultaneously attempting to vigorously regulate the quality of services delivered. There is, however, clearly a floor below which plans cannot deliver services because they cannot pay providers enough to induce them to participate. Close observers of Medicaid have expressed real concern about the potential fate of some of the best Medicaid managed care plans as states continue to ratchet down payment levels.

From the perspective of the providers, managed care presents a series of problems around the subsidies that were, in the past, hidden from the pub-lic eye but of critical importance to many institutions. Traditionally, med-ical education, medical research, and health care for the uninsured have been financed, in substantial part, out of dollars paid for services. Education and research have come largely from the money paid to hospitals; free care has involved funds paid to all hospitals but particularly to public hospitals and also to Federally Qualified Community Health Centers (FQHCs), that offer primary care to all comers. Managed care plans have no short-term interest in paying for these noncontracted activities out of medical care services dollars. Without replacing these dollars, there will be cuts in medical education and research, and access to care will be further limited for those lacking health insurance. Kassirer argues that market driven care is likely to . . . cripple academic health centers, handicap the research estab-lishment, and expand the population of patients without health care cover-age (1995, p. 51). But is this the responsibility of HMOs, or of government and the general citizenry? There are at least three opinions about expendi-tures in these areas: (a) HMOs should pay their fair share; (b) government or someone else should foot the bill for medical education, research, and health care for the uninsured; (c) less money should be spent on these activities. Again, there is no current consensus on how these issues can best be resolved.

SUMMARY

Managed care has grown rapidly in the past decade, taking advantage of new technology and the information revolution. Managed care plans are making every effort to sell their services in the marketplace based on asser-tions that they can provide medical care of higher quality at lower price meven when paid by PPOs at discounted rates. From the perspective of managed care plans, the next phase of the managed care revolution promis-es to be improved health care outcomes giving more value to the purchaser per expended dollar for health care. From the perspective of purchasers, the next phase may be even more mutation in the forms of the organiza-tions with which large employers do business. From the perspective of the individual customer, skill at understanding and navigating the "rules of the road" for one's own health plan will become increasingly important.

CASE STUDY

You are the newly appointed director of quality management at a medium-sized MCO that was originally a group model but now has about half of its members cared for by physicians in a network model arrangement. NCQA has recently adopted and promulgated a new set of measures for quality of care of diabetics and you know that the results will be publicized, with customers encouraged to use them to choose plans. Much of the information needed is available in your administrative data set, that includes frequency of visits, laboratory tests, etc. You note with both interest and concern that the performance of the network physicians is nowhere near as good as that of the large group practice that is the outgrowth of your old staff model arrangements. You are also very aware that patients must be active partners if your plan is going to do well on these measures, since so many of the events are ones in which patients must choose to receive care. What steps would you take to improve quality in this area? Should you use financial incentives or other means with the doctors? What will you do with respect to patients known to be diabetic? Is there any use you could make of the difference in baseline performance between the two sets of doctors?

DISCUSSION QUESTIONS

1. What are the essential differences between Medicare managed care plans and the commercial products offered by the same companies? Should it be possible for the federal government to achieve the same cost savings from managed care that large commercial insurers do?
2. What aspects of managed care are of the most concern to consumers, including your own friends and family? How do you think that states should regulate managed care plans to protect people from "worst case" results?
3. What kinds of information would you like to have to help you choose a plan? Should the government collect and distribute this information or should private vendors do it?
4. Many observers believe that the Internet will have a profound effect on medical practice that is only just beginning. Will the interest in Internet-based resources benefit MCOs? What kinds of steps ought MCOs take to make the best use of this new resource?

REFERENCES

Blendon, R., Brodie, M., Benson, J. M., Altman, D. E., Levitt, L., Hoff, T., & Hugick, X. (1998). Understanding the managed care backlash. *Health Affairs, 17,* 80–94.

Brewster, L. & Ginsburg, P. (2000, December). At the brink: How Harvard Pilgrim got in trouble. *Center for Studying Health System Change,* (Issue Brief 33).

Center for the Health Professions, University of California. (2001). *Managed care glossary of terms* (2nd ed.) [on-line]. Available: www.futurehealth.ucsf.edu/cnetwork.html

Diabetes Control and Complications Research Group. (1993). The effect of intensive treatment of diabetes on the development of long-term complications in insulin-dependent diabetes mellitus. *New England Journal of Medicine, 329,* 977–986.

Fox, P. (1997). An overview of managed care. In P. Kongstvedt (Ed.), *Essentials of managed health care* (pp. 3–16). Gaithersburg, MD: Aspen Publications.

Freudenheim, M. (2000, September 6). HMO costs spur employers to shift plans. *New York Times,* p. D1.

Group Health Cooperative. (2001). *Group health facts* [on-line]. Available: www.ghc.org

Grumbach, K., Osmond, D., Vlanizan, K., Jaffee, D., & Bindman, A. B. (1998). Primary care physicians' experience of financial incentives in managed-care systems. *New England Journal of Medicine, 339,* 1516–1521.

Health Care Financing Administration. (2001). *Centers for Medicare and Medicaid Services. 2000. Medicaid managed care enrollment* (on-line). Available: www.HCFA.gov

Himmelstein, D., Woolhandler, S., Hellander, I., & Wolfe, S. M. (1999). Quality of care in investor-owned vs. not-for-profit HMOs. *Journal of the American Medical Association, 282,* 159–163.

Iglehart, J. K. (1996). Managed care and mental health. *New England Journal of Medicine, 334,* 131–135.

Kaiser Permanente. (2001). *Newsroom: Fast facts* [on-line]. Available: www.kaiser-permanente.org

Kassirer, J. P. (1995). Managed care and the morality of the marketplace. *New England Journal of Medicine, 333,* 50–52.

Kovner, A. (1998). Health maintenance organizations and managed care. In A. Kovner & S. Jonas (Eds.), *Health care delivery in the United States* (6th ed., pp. 279–302). New York: Springer Publishing.

Lyles, A., & Palumbo, F. B. (1999). The effect of managed care on prescription drug costs and benefits. *Pharmacoeconomics, 15,* 129–140.

Mayer, T. R., & Mayer, G. G. (1985). HMOs: Origins and development. *New England Journal of Medicine, 312,* 590–594.

National Committee on Quality Assurance. (2001). *HEDIS: Health plan employer data and information and quality compass* [on-line]. Available: www.ncqa.org

National Health Policy Forum. (1999). *The ABCs of PBMs.* Washington, DC: George Washington University.

Plocher, D. (1997). Disease management. In P. Kongstvedt (Ed.). *Essentials of managed health care* (pp. 225–232). Gaithersburg, MD: Aspen Publications.

Reschovsky, J. D., & Hargraves, J. C. (2000, September). Health care perceptions and experiences: It's not whether you are in an HMO, it's whether you think you are. *Center for Studying Health Systems Change* (Issue Brief 30).

III

System Performance

P art III, "System Performance," provides a cross-sectional view of health care, focusing on functional characteristics, such as government regulation, governance and management, quality improvement, improving access, and cost containment.

In chapter 12, Sparer describes the different levels of government involved in health care and principal agencies of government and their activities. These include financing, purchasing, providing, and regulating health care. He explains the causes of change and variation in government roles, to include major changes in federal policy and sources of variations in state health policy. Sparer concludes by focusing on health policy issues: providing insurance coverage for the uninsured, providing insurance for prescription drugs and restructuring Medicare, and regulating the managed care industry.

In chapter 13, Kovner specifies how governance and management contribute to the performance of health care organizations. He identifies the pros and cons of for-profit, not-for-profit, and publicly owned organizations. Next he describes how performance is measured in health care organizations. He concludes by identifying ways to improve the governance and management of health care organizations.

In chapter 14, Horn describes the evolution of quality assurance, assessment, and improvement in health care, reviewing differing definitions and components of quality. She describes and gives examples of measures of quality related to structure, process, and outcomes, and describes and assesses various sources and methods for gathering information on quality of care. Horn critiques various mechanisms for assuring, promoting, and improving quality of care. She concludes by describing the new clinical practice improvement methodology, comparing it to the usual outcomes research, guideline development, and randomized clinical trials.

In chapter 15, Billings and Cantor frame the nature of the access problem to health care in the United States. They specify distinctions between economic and noneconomic barriers to health care. They present the characteristics of the uninsured and the policy implications of those characteristics. They describe how access barriers impinge on health and affect health care delivery. They conclude by presenting the range and limitations of options for increasing insurance coverage and reducing the barriers to health care.

In chapter 16, Thorpe discusses the factors that have contributed to the growth in health care expenditures in the United States. Next he describes the approaches employed by Medicare, Medicaid, and the private sector to control the growth in health care costs. He concludes by analyzing the historic and recent performance of these cost-containment strategies.

12

Government

Michael S. Sparer

LEARNING OBJECTIVES

- ☐ Review the evolution of government's role during the course of American history.
- ☐ Describe the roles of the federal, state, and local governments in the U.S. health care system.
- ☐ Examine the advantages and disadvantages of the trend toward devolving more authority to state and local levels.
- ☐ Examine the key issues and options on the current health policy agenda.

TOPICAL OUTLINE

Government as payer: The health insurance safety net
The government as regulator
Government as health care provider
Key issues on the health care agenda

KEY WORDS

government, regulation, federalism, Medicare, Medicaid, Child Health Insurance Program, Employee Retirement and Income Security Act (ERISA), public hospitals, the uninsured

Government is deeply entrenched in every aspect of the American health care system. The federal government provides tax incentives to encourage employers to offer health insurance to their employees, provides health insurance to the poor, the aged, and the disabled, and operates health care facilities for veterans. State governments administer and help pay for Medicaid, regulate private health insurance insurers and medical schools, license health care providers, and operate facilities for the mentally ill and developmentally disabled. Local governments own and operate public hospitals and public health clinics, and develop and enforce public health codes.

Even with this vast agenda, government officials seem certain to add new tasks and new programs. The nation is engaged in an ongoing debate over whether government should guarantee health insurance to the 43 million people that are currently uninsured. Federal and state officials are engaged in an equally controversial debate over the rise of managed care and the extent to which government should regulate the managed care industry. And the aging of the baby boom generation prompts many to suggest that the nation needs to do more to develop an adequate and affordable system of long-term care.

The goal of this chapter is to provide an overview of government's role in the health care system. The chapter is divided into three sections. First is a discussion of government as a payer for health care services. The theme is that government provides health insurance to many of those that are not covered by the employer-sponsored private health insurance system. The section describes the evolution of the private system, the gaps in that system, and the government efforts to aid those outside of the private system. Second is a summary of government as regulator of the health care system. The focus is on state and federal efforts to enact patient protection legislation. Third is a discussion of government as a provider of health care. The section reviews the health systems operated by the three levels of government: the Veteran's Administration facilities run by the federal government, the institutions for the mentally ill operated by the states, and the public hospitals and public health clinics owned and administered by local governments.

GOVERNMENT AS PAYER:
THE HEALTH INSURANCE SAFETY NET

For much of U.S. history, the national government and the states were minor players in the nation's health and welfare system. The nation's social welfare system was shaped instead by the principles that governed the English poor law system. Social welfare programs were a local responsibility, and assistance was to be provided only to those who were outside of the labor force through no fault of their own (the so-called deserving poor). National welfare programs were considered unwise and perhaps even unconstitutional. The main exception was the Civil War pension program, that provided federal funds to Union veterans, but even this initiative was administered and implemented at the local level.

Lacking federal or state leadership (and dollars), local governments tried to provide a social and medical safety net. The most common approach was to establish almshouses (or shelters) for the indigent aged and disabled. There was often also a medical clinic that provided health care to almshouse residents. These clinics eventually evolved into public hospitals, offering services without charge to the poor. Generally speaking, however, the clinics (and hospitals) provided poor quality care and were avoided by those that had any alternative. Similarly, the few private hospitals then in operation were charitable facilities that served only the poor and the disabled. These hospitals, like their public counterparts, represented only a small (and rather disreputable) portion of the American health care system.

Most 19th century Americans instead received health care in their homes, often from family members who relied on traditional healing techniques. At the same time, an assortment of health care providers (including physicians, midwives, medicine salesmen, herbalists, homeopaths, and faith healers) offered their services as well. Generally speaking, these providers charged low fees and people paid out-of-pocket, much as they would pay for other commodities.

As the 19th century drew to a close, however, two developments fundamentally changed the nation's health care marketplace. First, the physician community began to dominate the competition between the various individual providers. Americans increasingly believed that medicine was a science and that physicians were best able to deliver high quality health care. The status and prestige accorded to physicians grew and the role of alternative medicine providers declined.

The emergence of a physician dominated health care system was accompanied by dramatic growth in the size and the status of the hospital industry. Indeed, the nation's stock of hospitals grew from less than 200 in 1873 to 4,000 (with 35,500 beds) in 1900, to nearly 7,000 (with 922,000 beds) by 1930 (Rosenblatt et al., 1992). This growth was prompted by several factors. First, advances in medical technology (antiseptics, anesthesia, X rays) encouraged wealthier persons to use hospitals, thereby eliminating much of the prior social stigma. Second, the number of nurses expanded dramatically (as nurses evolved from domestics to professionals), and hospital-based nurses worked hard to improve hygienic conditions. Third, the growing urbanization and industrialization of American life produced an increasingly rootless society, that in turn lessened the ability of families to care for their sick at home. Fourth, the medical education system begin to require internships and residencies in hospitals as part of the training of the physician.

As the hospital industry grew, so too did the cost of care. By the mid-1920s, there was growing recognition that middle-income folks needed help in financing the rising costs of hospital-based and increasingly high-tech medicine. The onset of the Depression only made the situation more problematic. In response to the emerging crisis, various hospital associations formed health insurance companies to cover the high cost of hospital care (Blue Cross plans). At the same time, medical associations formed health insurance companies to cover the cost of physician care (Blue Shield plans). More and more Americans began to rely on private health insurance.

During the 1940s and 1950s, the federal government for the first time became a key player in the health care system, taking several actions that accelerated the trend toward a hospital dominated delivery system and an employer-sponsored health insurance system. The federal activity was spurred in large part by the era of American optimism that arrived with the end of World War II. Advances in medical technology had prompted confidence that the medical system would in time conquer nearly all forms of disease. This perception prompted the federal government (through the National Institutes of Health) to funnel billions of dollars to academic medical researchers. And with federal dollars so readily available, medical schools soon emphasized research and medical students increasingly chose research careers.

Around the same time, Congress enacted the Hill-Burton program, that provided federal funds to stimulate hospital construction and modernization. The policy assumption was that all Americans should have access to the increasingly sophisticated medical care rendered in state-of-the-art hospital facilities. The program was a success: a relatively small fiscal investment (approximately $4 billion) generated nearly 400,000 hospital beds (Thompson, 1981).

The congressional decision to exempt fringe benefits, such as health insurance, from the wage and price freeze enacted during the 1940s, also had a profound effect on the health care system, encouraging employers to provide health insurance in lieu of wage increases. The growth of employer-sponsored health insurance accelerated even more following the decision by the Internal Revenue Service that employers could take a tax deduction for the cost of health insurance provided to employees. Over the next several decades, the employer-based health insurance system became increasingly entrenched. By the end of 1999, private health insurance companies had enrolled more than 159 million Americans.

As the employer-sponsored health insurance system grew, so too did concern about those unable to access such coverage (such as the aged, the disabled, and the otherwise unemployed). For many years, liberal politicians had argued without success in favor of government-sponsored health insurance. In 1949, President Harry Truman had even proposed that health insurance was part of the "Fair Deal" that all Americans were entitled to. Neither Truman nor his liberal predecessors ever came close to overcoming the opposition to national health insurance (from doctors, businessmen, and others who viewed it as "un-American" and "socialistic").

With the growth of the employer-based insurance system, the likelihood of a government funded program became even more remote. As a result, by 1949 the mainstream democrats abandoned their visions of universal insurance and were proposing instead that the social security (retirement) system be expanded to provide hospital insurance to the aged. After all, the elderly were a sympathetic and deserving group, and hospital care was the most costly sector of the health care system.

Conservatives opposed the effort to provide hospital insurance to the aged, arguing that it unfairly (and unnecessarily) offered free coverage to many that were neither poor nor particularly needy. The conservatives argued instead that government's role is to be a safety net to those members of the deserving poor that are unable to access employer-sponsored coverage. The result was an amendment to the Social Security Act in 1950 that, for the first time, provided federal funds to those states willing to pay health care providers to care for welfare recipients. Interestingly, this "welfare medicine" approach passed with bipartisan support (Sparer, 1996; Stevens & Stevens, 1974). For liberals it was an acceptable, if inadequate, first step. At least some poor persons could now receive previously unavailable medical care. Conservatives also went along both because a medical safety net for the poor would undermine arguments for a more comprehensive health insurance program, and because responsibility for the program was delegated to state officials.

In 1960, newly elected President John F. Kennedy revived the effort to enact hospital insurance for the aged. Congress responded by expanding its "welfare medicine" model, enacting the Kerr-Mills program, which distributed federal funds to states willing to pay health care providers to care for the indigent aged. Congress later expanded the program to cover the indigent disabled. These initiatives again deflected support from the Kennedy social insurance proposal.

The political dynamic seemed to be quite different, however, in 1965. President Lyndon B. Johnson and the democrats now in control of Congress were enacting various laws designed to turn America into a "Great Society." This seemed to be an opportune time to renew the effort to enact national health insurance. Even longtime opponents of health insurance expansions expected Congress to enact legislation far more comprehensive than that embodied by the Kerr-Mills program. Perhaps surprisingly, however, Johnson followed the path set by Truman and Kennedy and proposed again hospital insurance for the aged. At the same time, various republican legislators, citing the nation's oversupply of hospitals, and proposing to return to a physician-centered delivery system, recommended that Congress enact physician insurance for the aged. And the American Medical Association (AMA), hoping to deflect yet again the social insurance model, urged Congress simply to expand the Kerr-Mills program.

As Congress debated the various proposals, congressman Wilbur Mills, the powerful chair of the House Ways and Means Committee, and an aspiring presidential candidate, convinced his colleagues to enact all three expansion initiatives. Johnson's proposal for hospital insurance for the aged became Medicare Part A. The republican proposal for physician insurance for the aged became Medicare Part B. The AMA's effort to expand Kerr-Mills became Medicaid. And the government for the first time became the health insurance safety net for those unable to access employer-sponsored coverage (Marmor, 2000).

Medicaid

Medicaid is not a single national program, but a collection of fifty state-administered programs, each providing health insurance to low-income state residents. Each state initiative is governed by various federal guidelines, and the federal government then contributes between 50% and 80% of the cost (the poorer the state, the larger the federal contribution). In 1998, the various Medicaid programs covered roughly 40 million persons at a cost of more than $176 billion (Kaiser Commission, 2001).

Given its decentralized structure, state officials have vast discretion to decide who in their state receives coverage, what benefits beneficiaries receive, and how much providers are paid. One not surprising result is that states like New York have more generous eligibility criteria than do Alabama or Mississippi. Interestingly, however, there is also stark interstate variation between states that can be classified as both large and liberal. In New York, for example, a nursing home receives roughly $140 per day for every Medicaid resident. In California, in contrast, a similarly situated facility receives approximately $75 per day (Sparer, 1996).

During the late 1980s, Congress (for the first time) imposed rules designed to reduce the level of interstate variation. In 1988, for example, Congress required states to cover pregnant women and infants with family income below 100% of poverty. State coverage for these populations had previously hovered around the 50% level. The next year, Congress required states to cover pregnant women and children under 7 years old with family income below 133% of poverty. Then, in 1990, Congress required states to phase in coverage for all children younger than 19 with family income below 100% of poverty. As a result of these mandates, the number of children on Medicaid nearly doubled between 1987 and 1995, growing from 10 million to 17.5 million. The overall number of beneficiaries increased from roughly 26 million to nearly 40 million.

During this era, the Medicaid expansions were the nation's main effort to reduce the ranks of the uninsured. At the same time, however, the Medicaid price tag grew from $57.5 billion in 1988 to $157.3 billion in 1995. State officials blamed the cost increases on these (and other) federal mandates. Federal regulators disputed the claim and suggested that the states themselves were largely responsible for the cost increases. There was significant intergovernmental tension (Holahan & Liska, 1997).

During the early 1990s, President Clinton, a former state governor (and critic of Medicaid mandates) stopped using Medicaid as the linchpin of an effort to reduce the number of uninsured. Clinton proposed instead to require employers to offer health insurance to their employees, thereby replacing public dollars with private in the effort to subsidize the cost of covering the uninsured. Clinton's proposal for national health insurance failed, but the shift away from Medicaid mandates remained. Instead of imposing Medicaid mandates, federal officials were approving state requests for waivers from federal Medicaid laws, thereby granting states additional flexibility and autonomy.

During most of the 1990s, there were two trends that dominated the Medicaid policy arena. First, states used their expanded discretion to encourage or require beneficiaries to enroll in managed care delivery systems. Between 1987 and 1998, the percentage of enrollees in managed care increased from less than 5% to more than 50%, from fewer than one million to more than 20 million. Second, the growth in the number of Medicaid beneficiaries ended, replaced instead by a slow decline in enrollees.

The most persuasive explanation for the enrollment decline was federal welfare reform, enacted in 1996. Before 1996, beneficiaries enrolled on Aid to Families with Dependent Children (AFDC) were automatically enrolled on Medicaid. Thereafter, however, those on welfare often need to apply separately for Medicaid, as must those no longer entitled to welfare (but still eligible for Medicaid). Millions do not know they are Medicaid eligible, the administrative hurdles deter others, whereas still others are dissuaded by the stigma that attaches to public benefits. For all of these reasons, the number of adult Medicaid beneficiaries declined by 5.5% between 1995 and 1997, while the number of child beneficiaries declined by 1.4% during the same period.

During the late 1990s, state and federal officials undertook a major effort to increase Medicaid enrollment. One strategy was to simplify the eligibility process (shortened application forms, mail-in applications, expanded eligibility sites). A second strategy was to simplify eligibility rules (eliminate asset tests and ensure 12-month continuous eligibility). A third strategy was to expand outreach and education (by increasing marketing activities and by encouraging community-based institutions to educate and enroll). The effort to increase enrollment achieved modest success. Beginning in mid-1998, Medicaid enrollment began to increase, a trend that has continued into 2001. The growth in enrollment, along with higher costs for prescription drugs and long-term care, may well lead to escalating Medicaid costs in the next few years.

Medicare

Like Medicaid, Medicare was enacted in 1965 to provide health insurance to segments of the population not generally covered by the mainstream employer-sponsored health insurance system. And like Medicaid, Medicare has become a major part of the nation's health care system, providing insurance coverage to nearly 34 million persons over the age of 65, and to roughly 5 million of the young disabled population, at a total cost of just over $216 billion (Kaiser Family Foundation, 1999).

In other respects, however, Medicare differs significantly from its sister program. Medicare is a social insurance program, providing benefits to the aged and the disabled regardless of income, whereas Medicaid is a welfare initiative, offering coverage only to those with limited income. Medicare is administered by federal officials (and the private insurers they hire to perform particular tasks), whereas Medicaid is administered by the states (pursuant to federal guidance). Medicare is funded primarily by the federal government (and by beneficiary co-payments and deductibles) while Medicaid is funded by the federal government and the states (without any beneficiary contribution). Medicare has a relatively limited benefit package (that excludes much preventive care, long-term care, and prescription drugs), while Medicaid offers a far more generous set of benefits.

Medicare also is comprised of two separate parts, with different funding sources and different eligibility requirements. Medicare Part A covers inpatient hospital care. It is financed by a 2.9% payroll tax (1.45% paid by the employer and 1.45% paid by the employee). All beneficiaries automatically receive Part A coverage. Medicare Part B, in contrast, is a voluntary program, providing coverage for outpatient care for those beneficiaries who choose to pay a $45 monthly premium (95% of beneficiaries choose to enroll). The balance of the Part B bill is paid by general federal revenues.

Prior to 1994, the revenue contributed to the Part A Trust Fund exceeded the program's expenses and the Trust Fund built up a significant surplus. Beginning in 1994, however, expenses began to exceed revenue, the surplus was used to pay bills, and the surplus began to decline. Medicare experts predicted that the surplus would be gone by early in the 2000s, that the Trust Fund would be unable to pay its bills, and that Medicare would therefore slide into bankruptcy.

In response to this crisis, Congress in 1997 enacted a broad effort to reduce Medicare costs, mainly by cutting provider reimbursement. The legislation also contained provisions designed to encourage beneficiaries to enroll in managed care. While the managed care initiative has had only mild success (roughly 15% of Medicare beneficiaries are enrolled in managed care), the effort to cut Medicare spending was remarkably successful. In 1999, for example, Medicare spending actually declined by roughly $1 billion, the first decline in the program's 25-year history.

The rapid shift in the economics of Medicare prompted an equally rapid change in the politics of Medicare. No longer were politicians claiming that the program was about to go bankrupt. No longer was there talk of greedy providers overcharging and generating excess profits. No longer was there an intense effort to enroll beneficiaries in managed care. There were instead three competing views about how to respond to the changed Medicare market. One camp emphasized the need to undo some of the cuts in provider reimbursement, others focused on the importance of expanding the Medicare benefit package, and still others argued against new spending measures (whether on behalf of providers or beneficiaries). This last group, the fiscal conservatives, proposed that any surplus remain in the Trust Fund to be used in years to come.

Faced with these options, Congress chose in 1999 to undo some of the cuts in provider reimbursement. Provider organizations argued that the prior cuts in reimbursement were unnecessarily endangering the financial health of thousands of health care providers. Even supporters of the cuts conceded that the extent of the reductions was far greater than expected. As a result, the Congress reduced the impact of the cuts by $16 billion (over the following 5 years) and $27 billion (over the following 10 years). The following year, Congress passed another giveback initiative, this time delivering to providers $35 billion (over 5 years) and $85 billion (over 10 years).

Following the provider giveback legislation, Congress turned its attention to prescription drug coverage. The issue became prominent in the 2000 presidential election, with both Al Gore and George Bush proposing drug coverage legislation. There were, however, significant differences in the two proposals. The democratic plan would enable all Medicare beneficiaries to purchase prescription drug coverage. The new Medicare coverage would cost $25 per month (rising to $50 over 5 years) and would cover 50% of all drug costs (up to a cap of $5,000). The democratic plan also would have paid for all prescription drug expenditures incurred after beneficiaries spent more than $4,000 out-of-pocket on drugs in a given year.

President Bush opposes the democratic approach and has countered with an initiative of his own. Bush points out that more than 70% of Medicare beneficiaries already have some prescription drug coverage (either from a private supplemental policy, a retiree health policy, a Medicare managed care policy, Medicaid, or a state pharmacy assistance program). Bush hopes therefore to focus his effort on those beneficiaries now without any coverage. He proposes that Congress provide states with $48 billion (over 4 years) to create or expand state programs that provide pharmacy assistance to low-income beneficiaries now without drug coverage. Beyond this short-term "helping hand," Bush hopes to encourage larger numbers of beneficiaries to enroll in managed care plans that offer drug coverage (with the federal government subsidizing the cost of the coverage for low-income seniors). Bush also proposes 100% Medicare coverage for all prescription drugs needed by those seniors who have spent more than $6,000 out-of-pocket on health care.

Bush's proposal on prescription drugs is designed, in part, to revive the effort to encourage beneficiaries to enroll in managed care. The managed care initiative was sagging, in part, because of declining health plan interest. In 1999, for example, 45 plans left the Medicare market while 54 others reduced their service areas. The exits affected 407,000 clients, 50,000 of whom had no other managed care option, and about half of whom chose to rejoin the traditional fee-for-service program. But while the health plans cite inadequate reimbursement as the main explanation for their exit, several studies also suggest that federal officials are actually losing money on the managed care initiative. The problem is that Medicare capitation rates are set based on the health care experience of the average client in a particular community, while the typical enrollee is healthier and less costly than average.

Recent Efforts to Help the Uninsured

Over the last decade, the number of persons without health insurance has grown from roughly 35 million to approximately 43 million (or more than 16% of the nation's population). There is much interstate variation in the percentage of uninsured residents. In Arizona, California, and Texas, for example, more than 25% of the population is uninsured, while in Hawaii, Oregon, and Wisconsin the number is less than 12%. Nonetheless, the growth in the number of uninsured occurred even in states with relatively few uninsured. In Oregon, for example, the uninsured population grew in 1998, reversing an 8-year trend of declining numbers. There was a similar pattern in Hawaii and Wisconsin.

Rather remarkably, the national increase in the number of uninsured has happened at a time of unprecedented economic growth, low unemployment, and relatively small rises in health care costs. Much of the increase also occurred during a time when the Medicaid rolls were expanding dramatically.

The best explanation for the rise in the number of uninsured is the decline in the number of Americans with employer-sponsored private health insurance. Between 1977 and 1996 the percentage of Americans under age 65 with employer-sponsored coverage dropped from 67% to 60%.

The decline in employer-sponsored coverage is due to several factors. Many employers have increased the share of the bill that the employee is required to cover, prompting some employees to abandon the coverage. Other employers are reducing dependent coverage (for spouses and children) or phasing out retiree health coverage. Still other employers are hiring more part-time workers and outside contractors, thereby avoiding the need to even offer health insurance. At the same time, much of the recent job growth is in the service sector of the economy. These jobs are relatively low paying and often do not provide health insurance.

In response to these trends, and to media and political attention to the problems of the uninsured, state and federal officials tried during the early 1990s to enact new programs for the uninsured (Brown & Sparer, 2001; Sparer, 1998). These proposals generally sought to require employers to provide health insurance to their employees (and to use public dollars as a safety net for those outside the labor market). The idea was to retain and reinvigorate the employer-sponsored health insurance system. By the mid-1990s, however, the various employer mandate proposals (including the plan proposed by Bill Clinton) had disappeared, defeated by vehement opposition from the business community. Business opponents argued that the mandate would be too costly and would force employers to eliminate jobs (rather than provide health coverage).

Following the collapse of the employer mandate strategy, policymakers (especially at the state level) enacted a host of efforts designed to make health insurance more available and more affordable in the small group and individual insurance markets. These reforms focused on three problems in the health care system. First, employers in the small business community often cannot afford to provide health insurance to their employees. These employers lack the market clout to negotiate a good deal, particularly given the high administrative costs associated with insuring a small group. Second, the self-employed and the employee in the small business community generally earn too little to purchase their own health insurance policy. Third, individuals with a high risk of catastrophic medical costs are often excluded from the individual insurance market regardless of their ability to pay.

The most common of the insurance reform initiatives seeks to ensure that health insurance is available to all. As of late 1997, for example, 47 states had enacted legislation that requires insurers in the small group market to provide insurance to all small group applicants (so-called "guarantee issue" provisions). The same number of states also limit insurer's ability to deny coverage for medical conditions that began prior to the insurance coverage. And 28 states subsidize special insurance products (known as high-risk pools) for individuals who have been denied health insurance because of their medical condition (Robert Wood Johnson Foundation, 2000).

Far more controversial, however, are state efforts that seek to make insurance more affordable. One strategy is to encourage small businesses to join state-run or state-regulated purchasing alliances. The goal is to supply increased market clout, decreased administrative costs, and therefore less expensive insurance premiums. Twelve states have launched such initiatives. In 1982, for example, California established the Health Insurance Purchasing Cooperative (the HIPC), that now purchases insurance on behalf of approximately 7,700 small business owners and 140,000 employees. In Colorado, in contrast, the state licenses and regulates privately administered small business purchasing cooperatives. In neither state, however, has the alliance model provided significant aid to the uninsured: In California, for example, nearly 80% of the businesses that participate in the HIPC had previously offered insurance to their employees (but because of the alliance can now do so at a lower cost).

A second strategy is to allow health insurers to sell no-frills insurance policies, presumably at a lower cost than the more comprehensive packages states often require. As of late 1997, for example, more than a dozen states had enacted this sort of "bare-bones" insurance program. By most accounts, bare-bones policies have also not sold well. Those that can afford health insurance prefer a more comprehensive policy, while those unable to afford the traditional policies are typically unable to afford even the scaled back insurance product.

There are also efforts in several states to prohibit insurers from relying on the health status of the insured when determining the individual or the small group premium. These initiatives challenge the underwriting that underpins the insurance industry: the practice known as experience rating, under which persons with a high risk of catastrophic medical care are charged higher premiums than are healthy young adults at low risk of incurring significant medical costs. The goal instead is to require a single rate (called a "community rate") for all insured, thereby requiring the healthy to subsidize the expected medical costs of the ill. By late 1997, several states had enacted some form of community rating, though most allowed some variation in rates based on age, gender, or location.

The various insurance reform initiatives have had a modest impact. According to one study, roughly 11% of the insured that work for small businesses owe their coverage to the various reforms. At the same time, however, the reform initiatives have themselves generated significant political controversy, especially from healthy younger workers who complain about paying higher rates to subsidize the older and the sicker, and from insurance companies threatening to exit reform-minded states rather than comply with the new rules.

By the late 1990s, state and federal policymakers had shifted their focus away from the (disappointing) insurance reforms and toward programs that expanded health insurance for children. There were several factors that explained the emerging consensus. Children are considered a deserving group: there is bipartisan agreement that youngsters should not go without health care services because their parents cannot afford to pay.[1] Children are also a relatively low-cost population. In 1993, for example, the average child on Medicaid cost just under $1,000; in contrast the typical aged beneficiary cost over $9,200, while the disabled population averaged just under $8,000. Child health initiatives are also consistent with the political agendas of both republicans and democrats. Republicans (along with many moderate democrats) support insurance expansions as a counterbalance to other social welfare cutbacks. Families that move from welfare to work will still have health insurance for their children. At the same time, liberal democrats, still reeling from the defeat of national health insurance proposals, see child insurance as an incremental step on the path to universal coverage.

Given this bipartisan support, Congress enacted the Child Health Insurance Program (CHIP) as part of the 1997 Balanced Budget Act. CHIP provides states with just over $40 billion (over a 10-year period) to expand insurance programs for youngsters. States are generally required to spend CHIP dollars on children that are not Medicaid eligible and that are in families with income below 200% of the federal poverty line. The main exception is for states that already provide Medicaid coverage to children in families with income more than 150% of poverty: these states can use CHIP dollars to raise their income levels by 50%.

States can use the CHIP funds to liberalize their Medicaid eligibility rules, or to develop a separate state program, or to do a combination of both. The main advantage to using the funds to expand Medicaid is administrative simplicity (for both the client and the state). This is especially so

---

[1] This is especially so for the very young. Older children are sometimes considered morally culpable when their behavior necessitates medical treatment. The best example is the teenager in need of substance abuse services.

for families in which some children are eligible for Medicaid and others for CHIP. At the same time, there are several advantages to creating a separate state program. Enrollment can be suspended when the dollars are spent (unlike Medicaid, which is an entitlement program). The state has more discretion when developing the benefit package. The state can impose co-payments and premiums (that are not allowed under Medicaid). Beneficiaries (and providers) may be more likely to enroll since the new program may lack the stigma associated with Medicaid. As of late 1999, 22 states were relying on a Medicaid expansion, 16 states had implemented a separate state program, and 13 states have a combination of both (Kaiser Commission, 1999).

By all accounts, the early efforts to enroll children into CHIP were disappointing. By the end of 1999, roughly 1.5 million youngsters were enrolled in the program, far fewer than predicted. The low enrollment was due to several factors. Large numbers of eligible families did not know they were eligible. Others were deterred by the administrative burden of the application process. Still others were dissuaded by the stigma associated with many government insurance programs. And the premiums and other cost-sharing requirements clearly discouraged others. As a result, by the end of 2000, 41 states had not spent their full allotment of federal CHIP dollars and may need to return some funds to the federal treasury.

Beginning in early 2000, however, the CHIP enrollment numbers began to significantly rise. By the end of the year, there were roughly 3.3 million enrollees, nearly double the number from the prior year. Policymakers attribute the turnaround to improved outreach and education initiatives and to simplified processes for eligibility and enrollment. Moreover, there is bipartisan support for expanding CHIP. In early 2001, for example, federal regulators authorized several states to use CHIP dollars to cover parents (as well as their children).

THE GOVERNMENT AS REGULATOR

One of the key issues in contemporary health politics is the extent to which the states and the federal government should regulate the managed care industry. Between 1997 and 2000, for example, 35 states enacted laws designed to protect patients that are enrolled in managed care. In 1999, both the United States Senate and the House of Representatives passed their own versions of a managed care bill of rights, and the effort to resolve the differences between the two bills has become a bitter partisan battle. During the 2000 presidential campaign, George Bush and Al Gore debated vigorously over the content of a good patient protection act, but both claimed to be fully in favor of the concept.

The focus on patient protection is prompted by the consumer backlash against managed care. Interestingly, however, the federal legislation, if enacted, would represent an important policy shift: there is little precedent for federal regulation of the health insurance industry. At the same time, state legislators, while more accustomed to regulating private insurers (as well as other sectors of the health care industry) complain that their efforts are undermined by a federal pension law that restricts state regulatory activity. These officials urge Congress to repeal or amend the pension law and thereby provide the states with far greater regulatory autonomy.

This tale of regulatory uncertainty begins with the general proposition that the states have traditionally played a dominant role in regulating all aspects of the nation's health care system. To be sure, the federal government also plays a role in regulating the health care system. Back in the late 19th century, for example, federal officials began regulating the nation's food supply, and ever since 1938 the Food and Drug Administration (FDA) has regulated the introduction and use of new drugs into the medical marketplace. Indeed, the speed (or lack thereof) of the FDA's approval of new drugs is an ongoing source of controversy. Moreover, federal officials also require providers that participate in federal health insurance programs (such as Medicare and Medicaid) to comply with a host of regulatory conditions.

Despite these federal efforts, however, there remains a long-standing bias in favor of state regulatory activity. The states supervise the nation's system of medical education, license health care professionals, and oversee the quality of care delivered by health care providers. States also administer the workers' compensation system (which provides benefits to workers injured on the job) and they govern consumer efforts to hold providers accountable (whether through medical malpractice litigation or otherwise). Beginning in the early 20th century, the states also began to regulate the nation's private health insurance system, establishing capitalization and reserve requirements, regulating marketing and enrollment activities, and (in some states) establishing the rates paid by insurers to various providers (especially hospitals).

Prior to the 1960s, however, state insurance departments rarely exercised their regulatory muscle, imposing few substantive requirements on insurance companies. Liberal critics complained that the relationship between providers, insurers, and regulators was far too cozy. Providers (especially hospitals) charged high rates, insurers paid the bill with few questions asked, and regulators did little to ensure that insurance companies were adequately capitalized (and even less to guarantee that clients were treated fairly).

In response to the critics, several states imposed new administrative requirements, most of which dealt with health plan finances, benefit packages, and marketing practices. In the mid-1960s, for example, New York regulated the rates that hospitals could charge insurers. Around the same time, states also imposed tougher capitalization and reserve requirements. Over the next 2 decades, states required insurers to cover certain medical services (from mental health to chiropractor visits) in every insurance package they issued. Indeed, there are now more than 1,000 of these benefit mandates. For example, 40 states require that insurers cover alcohol treatment services, 39 require coverage for mammography treatment, and 29 require mental health coverage.

The states' ability to regulate health insurers was limited, however, in 1974, when Congress enacted the Employee Retiree Income and Security Act (ERISA). Ironically, the issue Congress focused on when enacting ERISA was the unfair denial of pensions to employees. The law requires that pension plans be adequately funded, that vesting requirements be reasonable, and that companies provide employees with understandable information about their pension programs. But the law also contains a provision that prohibits states from regulating employee benefit programs unless the law is part of the traditional state regulation of insurance. This clause has in turn led to endless controversy and litigation.

Consider, for example, the convoluted legal reasoning that governs state efforts to require insurers to cover certain medical services. These laws clearly relate to employee benefit programs. The courts have ruled, however, that the validity of the laws depend on whether the coverage is provided by a traditional insurance company (like Blue Cross or Prudential) or by a company that self-insures.[2] The policies sold by the traditional insurers must include the mandated benefits, but the policies provided by the companies that self-insure need not. Indeed, following the same reasoning, the courts have held that companies that self-insure are exempt from state capitalization and reserve requirements, state taxes imposed on insurers, and all other state regulatory requirements (such as patient protection laws).

To be sure, companies that self-insure are required to implement any federal regulatory requirements: ERISA simply exempts them from state regulation. But federal officials have generally steered clear of imposing any such requirements. As a result, self-insured companies are generally unregulated: the states cannot regulate them and the federal government rarely does. Not surprisingly, this regulatory vacuum encourages firms to self-insure: by the mid-1990s, more than 70% of large firms offered self-insured plans to their employees (Dranove, 2000), and more than 45 million Americans were covered by self-insured health plans.

ERISA also makes it extremely difficult for subscribers to sue their health plan. Consider, for example, the situation in which an individual claims she was injured when her health plan wrongfully refused to authorize needed care. The woman seeks to sue the health plan for negligence. Prior to ERISA, she would have commenced such a lawsuit in state court

---

[2] Under the original insurance model, employers pay premiums to insurance companies, in exchange for which the insurer reviews health care utilization, processes claims, and pays the actual cost of covered health care. The insurer is at risk for the full cost of care. Over time, however, some companies chose to self-insure (to themselves pay the cost of all health care bills). These companies still hire insurers to do utilization review and to process claims, but the insurer is not at any financial risk.

and demanded damages to cover the cost of the denied services, as well as compensation for the injury and the unnecessary pain and suffering endured. She might also have won punitive damages (intended to punish the health plan for its wrongful behavior). Because of ERISA, however, our hypothetical victim cannot bring her case to state court (unless she is a government employee or is in a government funded health plan). She must instead proceed in federal court under a very different set of rules. For example, in her federal action, the most the woman could win would be the cost of the wrongfully denied care: she could not win compensation for pain and suffering, nor could she win punitive damages.

The impact of the ERISA barrier is illustrated by the case of Goodrich vs. Aetna. Mr. Goodrich was a government prosecutor in California, suffering from stomach cancer, whose request for surgical relief was wrongfully denied and delayed (even though Aetna's own doctors were in favor of the procedure). After Mr. Goodrich died, his estate brought a lawsuit in state court seeking damages for the wrongful denial of care. The jury awarded his estate $4.5 million in actual compensatory damages, and $116 million in punitive damages (Johnston, 1999). Rather remarkably, however, had Mr. Goodrich not worked for the government, his estate would have had to proceed in federal court, and could have collected a maximum of roughly $400,000 (the cost of the surgical procedure).

Until recently, ERISA was also viewed as a barrier to cases in which patients sue the health plan for the poor care delivered by an affiliated doctor. During the late 1990s, however, several states (led by Texas) enacted laws designed to overcome this barrier and to permit such cases to proceed in state court. While the Supreme Court has yet to rule on the validity of these laws, the lower courts have distinguished these "poor quality of care" cases from the "wrongful denial of care" cases described above, and have so far permitted the cases to proceed. Whether the health plan is then held liable for the malpractice of the provider depends on the relationship between provider and plan. Staff model HMOs, which exercise close oversight over their salaried doctors, are more likely to be liable than are independent practice associations, with their large and loosely controlled provider network.

ERISA has also emerged as a key component in the national debate over patient protection laws. As discussed earlier, more than 35 states have enacted such laws. Most of the laws require an appeal process when care is denied. Most also have rules governing access to the hospital emergency room. Some states require that subscribers have direct access to certain medical specialists. Others restrict the ability of health plans to censor what doctors say to their patients. Still others guarantee new mothers the right to spend at least 48 hours in the hospital following the birth of their child. Because of ERISA, however, none of these laws protect those persons enrolled in self-insured health plans.

The regulatory vacuum became especially controversial during the mid-1990s as there emerged a consumer backlash against much of the managed care industry. There was increased pressure on Congress either to amend ERISA (to allow state regulation of the self-insured) or to enact federal consumer protection legislation.

The effort to amend ERISA is unlikely to succeed. The sponsors of the self-insured plans (especially multistate employers and labor unions) are well-organized and influential. The lobbyists for the self-insured argue that the goal of the law is to avoid inconsistent state regulation that would undermine the effective administration of their organizations.

Congress has, however, begun to experiment with federal consumer protection legislation, and may move further in this direction. In 1996, for example, Congress enacted a law that guarantees new mothers the right to spend at least 48 hours in the hospital following the birth of their child. The next year, Congress enacted the Health Insurance Portability and Accountability Act (HIPAA), which seeks to make health insurance more available to the self-employed and to those that work in small companies.

More recently, in 1999, both the House of Representatives and the Senate enacted versions of a managed care bill of rights. There are two main differences between the House and Senate legislation. First is the scope of the bills. The House version would cover all Americans with private health insurance, while the Senate bill would cover only those persons that work for self-insured companies (and are thus beyond the scope of the state patient protection initiatives). The second difference is the right to sue: the House's bill enables consumers to sue their health plan; the Senate's bill does not.

GOVERNMENT AS HEALTH CARE PROVIDER

Each of the three levels of government owns and operates large numbers of health care institutions. The federal government provides care to veterans through the massive Veterans Affairs (VA) health care system. The states care for the developmentally disabled in both large institutional facilities as well as smaller group homes. And local governments own and operate acute care hospitals and public health clinics that provide a medical safety net for the poor and the uninsured.

The Veterans Affairs Health Care System

The Department of Veterans Affairs (VA) is required to offer health care to veterans and their dependents. There are approximately 70 million persons now eligible for these services (25 million veterans and 45 million dependents or survivors of deceased veterans).

In order to serve this population, the VA owns and operates 172 hospitals, 132 nursing homes, more than 600 outpatient clinics, and 73 home care programs. These facilities are divided into 22 integrated service networks. In 2000, more than 3.6 million people will receive care in one of these facilities, at a cost of more than $19 billion.

The VA health care system is also an integral part of the nation's system of medical education. There are 107 medical schools and 55 dental schools that use VA facilities to train students and residents. Indeed, more than 50% of the nation's physicians have received part of their education and training in the VA health care system.

In recent years, the VA system has engaged in a wide-ranging effort to improve the quality of care provided in its facilities. The focus is a system designed to reduce the number of medical errors. The VA created the National Center for Patient Safety (NCPS) to take the lead in the effort. The NCPS program is considered so innovative and important that it was recently nominated as a finalist in the Innovations in American Government Program, sponsored by the Ford Foundation and the Kennedy School of Government at Harvard University.

The issue of medical errors received national attention when the Institute of Medicine issued a report that estimated that between 44,000 and 98,000 persons die each year because of medical errors. Much of the effort to reduce medical error focuses on individual wrongdoing. If only Dr. Jones had operated on the right leg; if only Nurse Smith had given the right medication, if only Aide Wilson had held the patient and prevented the fall. As a result, hospitals and other providers respond to medical error (if at all) by trying to identify and punish the "culprit," while policymakers press for a practitioner data bank that will list those providers guilty of committing medical errors.

The NCPS focuses less on individual blame and more on finding the root cause of the error. For example, if the medication error is due to inadequate labeling of drugs, then with better labeling the likelihood of future error is reduced. In the NCPS system, health care staff are encouraged to report "close calls" as well as "adverse events." For example, if Patient Jones is given the wrong medication but suffers no adverse consequences, that is a close call. If the surgeon uses instruments that are not properly sterilized but the patient does not develop an infection, that is a close call. In the past, no one was likely to report or investigate the event. The nurse would be too embarrassed and the system too uninterested. The goal now is to encourage the nurse to report, promising that the report will be completely confidential; to create a 3–4 person team to investigate the root cause of the error; and to develop a plan of action to make it less likely that a similar error will occur in the future.

State Facilities for the Mentally Ill

Prior to the 1860s, caring for the mentally ill was considered a local responsibility, part of the safety net provided to the so-called "deserving poor."

Perhaps the most common strategy utilized by county governments was to house the indigent insane in almshouses (or shelters) for the poor. County officials also locked away many of the severely mentally ill in local jails. And, by the mid-19th century, several counties had also established hospitals for the mentally ill, though there was little effort at treatment in even the best of these facilities. The goal instead was to warehouse the mentally ill and keep them separate from the rest of society.

Dorothea Dix and other reformers slowly persuaded nearly every state legislature to assume responsibility for the mentally ill, and to construct state hospitals to provide for their care. The state hospitals generally were located in rural communities: reformers believed that the patients were more likely to improve in a quiet and serene environment (and of course most communities seemed perfectly content to ship their mentally ill off to distant facilities). State mental hospitals were also extraordinarily large, some with as many as 2,000 patients. In 1920, for example, the 521 state hospitals had an average bed capacity of 567. In contrast, the nation's 4,013 general hospitals then had an average bed capacity of only 78 (Starr, 1982).

By the turn of the 20th century, state governments had emerged as the primary providers of care for those with mental—and other behavioral—disorders. Behavioral health became the only health problem with a separately financed and managed treatment system, and state governments assumed responsibility for the entire system (Hogan, 1999). The system grew exponentially, as county governments transferred many of those still under their jurisdiction (such as the old and the senile) to the state facilities (thereby transferring the cost of their care as well). By 1959, there were roughly 559,000 patients housed in state mental hospitals across the country (Katz, 1989).

Beginning in the 1960s, however, a new generation of reformers challenged the conditions in many of the state institutions. Patients were generally warehoused rather than treated, were kept isolated from families and friends, and were often brutalized by staff or other patients. At the same time, medical researchers were developing a host of new drugs that enabled large numbers to cope (more or less) in the community, thereby avoiding the harsh and dismal conditions in the hospitals. Perhaps most importantly, the federal government provided funding (both directly and through Medicaid) for community-based mental health services, while restricting federal funding for services provided in the hospital. Medicaid, for example, prohibited coverage for inpatient care in psychiatric institutions for persons between ages 22 and 64, while providing coverage for a host of mental health services provided to those in community-based settings. Similarly, Congress provided direct funding to help establish a system of community mental health centers.

For all of these reasons, state governments began a massive effort to discharge patients from the state hospitals and to divert others from admission. As a result, by 1980, the number of persons in state mental hospitals had dropped to roughly 130,000 (from a previous high of nearly 560,000)

(Katz, 1989). In Ohio, for example, the number of patients in state hospitals dropped from 30,000 in the early 1960s to 1,200 today, while the number receiving publicly funded community care grew from 20,000 to around 250,000 (Hogan, 1999).

Despite the reallocation of resources, however, experts suggest that the new balance of responsibility for the mentally ill has replaced one set of problems (overcrowded and poor quality institutions) with another: large numbers of mentally ill are unable to find adequate housing (and often end up homeless), and many of those in need are unable to access adequate mental health services—despite the growth in community-based services. Interestingly, however, few advocate a return to large-scale institutionalization. The most popular alternative among state officials is to delegate the problems of the indigent mentally ill to managed care plans that mainly serve those with behavioral health problems. It remains to be seen whether the managed care revolution will provide solutions to the longstanding problems of the mentally ill. What is quite clear, however, is that state governments will continue to have the overall responsibility for the mentally ill population.

Local Government and the Safety Net for the Poor

Scattered throughout America are more than 1,500 publicly owned general hospitals, nearly all of which are owned and operated by local governments. More than two thirds are small (fewer than 200 beds), located in rural communities, and have low occupancy rates (generally well below 50%). Many of the urban institutions, in contrast, are quite large and have high occupancy rates. For example, the 100 largest average nearly 600 beds and have an occupancy rate of roughly 80%. Indeed, the average big city hospital is three times the size of the typical privately owned facility, has four times as many inpatient admissions, provides five times as many outpatient clinics visits, and delivers seven times as many babies.

The urban public hospital also treats a disproportionately high percentage of the poor and uninsured. In 1991, nearly 50% of their patient population was on Medicaid, 25% was uninsured, and only 12% had private insurance. These institutions also treat a sicker and more difficult population than do most of their commercial or nonprofit counterparts. These are the providers of last resort, treating the homeless mentally ill, the babies addicted to cocaine, and the victims of violence.

Local governments also fund and administer more than 3,000 public health departments. Each of these departments makes an effort, to at least some degree, to assess the public health needs of the community, to develop policies that address those needs, and to assure that primary and preventive health are provided to all.

For most of the last century, health department officials focused their efforts on assessment (such as collecting data on disease data epidemics) and general public health activities (regulating the quality of the water supply, enforcing local health codes, conducting health education campaigns). Indeed, the focus on populations and community-based services is what distinguished public health from the traditional medical system. Only rarely would health department doctors themselves deliver health care, and when they did it was usually to supplement a broader health campaign (immunizing children, for example, as part of an immunization campaign).

In recent years, however, local health departments have shifted resources away from infectious disease control (and other public health initiatives) and increased their efforts to become direct providers of primary and preventive care. Health departments have become an increasingly important part of the medical safety net. By the late 1980s, for example, 92% of local health departments were immunizing children, 84% provided other child health services, and nearly 60% offered prenatal care services. At the same time, many health departments provide large amounts of specialty care services, especially to populations underserved by the traditional medical community. For example, most county health departments provide mental health services. Others treat sexually transmitted diseases. Still others care for persons with AIDS (Wall, 1998).

The emphasis on direct-care services was prompted by the growing number of persons without health insurance and the by growing number of communities in which the local health department was the only (or the primary) source of care for the medically indigent. At the same time, however, the growing emphasis on direct-care services meant fewer resources for population-based activities. This shift prompts concern among many public health leaders. The public health department seemed to be retreating from its core mission (population-based activities) just as the nation seemed to be experiencing an epidemic of public health problems (from sexually transmitted diseases to tuberculosis to foodborne illnesses). Nonetheless, the local health department occupies such an important niche in the health care delivery system that it seems a flight of fancy to suppose its role might again quickly shift.

KEY ISSUES ON THE HEALTH CARE AGENDA

Health care policymakers are grappling with a host of difficult issues, ranging from the uninsured to the long-term care system to how best to serve those with special needs (such as mental illness or substance abuse). In this section, three such issues are identified, and the key options on the policy agenda are summarized.

The Uninsured

There are more than 42 million Americans without health insurance. Policymakers need to make a series of decisions about this population. Should government target its dollars on further expanding the various public insurance initiatives? How can government encourage those that are eligible but not enrolled in the public programs to sign up? Is it wiser to spend public dollars providing tax credits and other incentives to encourage persons to purchase their own private insurance policies? Are there other ways to help the uninsured (and if so are they politically and financially feasible)?

President Bush proposed (during the 2000 campaign) three strategies for helping the uninsured: (a) a tax credit ($2,000 per family) to enable the uninsured to buy health insurance in the individual market; (b) providing states with increased flexibility to implement CHIP; and (c) funding the creation of hundreds of new community health centers to provide health care to the poor and the uninsured. During that same campaign, Al Gore focused his proposals on expanding eligibility for the public insurance programs (Medicaid, CHIP, and Medicare), though he too suggested a small tax credit for the uninsured.

Medicare and Prescription Drugs

There is bipartisan support in favor of adding prescription drug coverage to the Medicare benefit package. There is even a large enough surplus in the Medicare trust funds to encourage supporters that there is a window of political opportunity. At the same time, however, there is no agreement on how extensive the drug benefit should be or on how it should be administered.

President Bush has proposed a prescription drug block grant, that would provide the states with $48 billion (over 4 years) to encourage states to expand (or establish) pharmacy assistance programs for those now without any drug coverage (those with income too high for Medicaid but too low to afford a Medi-Gap policy). Democrats oppose the Bush initiative, noting that it is contrary to the social insurance principles of the Medicare program (by targeting benefits based on income and by delegating responsibility to the states). Democrats also insist that relatively few of those eligible for the new benefit are likely to actually enroll and receive coverage. The democrats propose instead to offer some prescription drug coverage to all beneficiaries, for a premium of roughly $25 (different democratic plans cover anywhere from 50%–80% of drug costs, up to a cap of $5,000, with more expansive catastrophic coverage for those that incur over $4,000 in drug costs).

Regulating the Managed Care Industry

Just as in the debate over Medicare prescription drug coverage, there is bipartisan support for the concept of a nation patient protection act; but sharp differences exist between the parties as to the best way to achieve the goal. There are two key issues that dominate the debate. First, most liberals want the national law to apply to all those with private health insurance (roughly 158 million Americans). The republican leadership, in contrast, suggests that the bill cover only those 45 million or so that are in self-insured health plans and thus exempt from state patient protection laws.

Second, the more expansive proposal allows consumers to bring lawsuits to state court against HMOs for the denial (or delay) of needed health care treatment. In these state court proceedings, injured parties could receive compensation for pain and suffering, as well as punitive damages designed to punish especially malicious acts. The republican leadership opposes such a broad right to sue, preferring instead to allow lawsuits only in federal court (if at all), with limited rights to compensation for pain and suffering and without any right to punitive damages.

CASE STUDY

There are more than 10 million children without health insurance in the United States. In response to this crisis, Congress both expanded the Medicaid program and enacted the Child Health Insurance Program. Millions of uninsured children are eligible for these public programs but are not enrolled. Others are in families with income too high to qualify for eligibility. Why are so many youngsters eligible but not enrolled? What can government do to make it more likely that these youngsters will enroll? What should government do for those that are not eligible for these public programs? Respond from the viewpoint of a congressman, a state legislator, an insurance executive, a hospital manager, and a consumer advocate.

DISCUSSION QUESTIONS

1. What is and should be the role of the various levels of government in the health care system?
2. Should Congress enact a managed care bill of rights, and if so, what should be its content?
3. Should Medicare be amended to include a prescription drug benefit?
4. What should government do to aid the uninsured?
5. Is it good policy for the federal government to delegate authority over health care policy to the states?

REFERENCES

Brown, L. D., & Sparer, M. S. (2001, January/February). Window shopping: State health reform politics in the 1990s. *Health Affairs, 20,* 50–67.

Dranove, D. (2000). *The economic evolution of American health care.* Princeton, NJ: Princeton University Press.

Hogan, M. (1999, September/October). Public sector mental health care: New challenges. *Health Affairs, 18,* 106–111.

Johnston, D. (1999, January 21). $116 million punitive award against Aetna. *New York Times,* p. C1.

Kaiser Commission on Medicaid and the Uninsured. (1999, November). *Health coverage for low-income children.* Washington, DC: Author.

Kaiser Commission on Medicaid and the Uninsured. (2001, January). *The Medicaid program at a glance.* Washington, DC: Author.

Kaiser Family Foundation. (1999, September). *Medicare at a glance.*

Katz, M. (1989). *The undeserving poor.* New York: Pantheon Books.

Marmor, T. (2000). *The politics of Medicare* (2nd ed.). New York: Aldine de Gruyter Press.

Robert Wood Johnson Foundation. (2000, January). *The state of the states.* Princeton, NJ: Author.

Rosenblatt, R., Law, S., & Rosenbaum, S. (1997). *Law and the American health care system.* The Foundation Press.

Sparer, M. S. (1996). *Medicaid and the limits of state health reform.* Philadelphia: Temple University Press.

Sparer, M. S. (1998, May/June). Devolution of power: An interim report card. *Health Affairs,* 7–16.

Starr, P. (1982). *The social transformation of American medicine.* New York: Basic Books.

Stevens, R., & Stevens, R. (1974). *Welfare medicine in America: A case study of Medicaid.* New York: Free Press.

Thompson, F. (1981). *Health policy and the bureaucracy.* Cambridge: MIT Press.

Wall, S. (1998, May/June). Transformations in public health systems. *Health Affairs, 17,* 64–80.

13

Governance and Management

Anthony R. Kovner

LEARNING OBJECTIVES

- ☐ Specify how governance and management contribute to health care organization (HCO) performance.
- ☐ Identify the pros and cons of for-profit, not-for-profit, and public ownership.
- ☐ Describe how performance is measured in health care organizations.
- ☐ Identify ways to improve governance and management of health care organizations.

TOPICAL OUTLINE

Governance
Measuring organizational performance
Ownership of health care organizations
Current governance issues
Management
Managerial work in health care organizations
Educating health services managers
Current management issues

KEY WORDS

accountability, benchmarking, board composition, structure and function, chief executive officer, competencies, environmental scanning, governance, governing boards, integrated delivery system, mission, organizational autonomy and performance, managerial skills and performance, not-for-profit ownership, for-profit ownership, governmental ownership, political terrain, position description, product line management

Put simply, governance is the system for making important decisions, about matters such as mission, goals, budget, capital financing, and quality improvement. Management is responsible for implementing these decisions. Increasingly, in large organizations governance is differentiated from management. In smaller organizations, the owner-managers often govern as well as manage, and they may also arrange for patient care.

This chapter has two parts. The first, on governance, defines what governance is, describes the contribution of owners to measuring performance, reviews the advantages and disadvantages of different patterns of ownership, and discusses current governance issues. These include preferable ownership patterns; the extent of autonomy of health care organizations; and how these organizations are held accountable to payers and to users. The second part of this chapter, on management, describes what managers do and how managerial work is carried out in health care organizations, reviews how managers are educated, and discusses current management issues. These include who should control HCOs, reasonable management costs for an HCO, and the accountability of managers to those who govern HCOs.

GOVERNANCE

The governance system is the process for making important decisions such as what services the organization provides to whom at what price. Those who govern or own the organization exercise ultimate direction, control, and authority. They are accountable to payers and users for the use of resources by the organization to provide care. The governance process in any organization may be dominated by a few individuals or by many; it may be exercised in an authoritarian or participatory way.

Every organization has a set of stakeholders who have interests in organizational performance. For health care organizations the list of stakeholders includes payers, users, clinicians and other employees, accreditors, and regulators. Different stakeholders often want the organization to perform in very different ways—for example, in regard to what services are provided by whom, or how employees are to be paid. HCOs are dependent on the resources required to achieve their purposes and survive. Such resources include patients, clinicians, facilities, and legitimacy. Governance influences the supply of resources as well as their allocation. It also influences the futures of those who work in HCOs and those who are served by them.

Levels of Analysis

There are several levels at which governance can be analyzed. First, there are those decisions that affect governance made outside the HCO by government. For example, the Medicare and Medicaid legislation of 1965 provided its beneficiaries with better health benefits coverage than many of them had prior to enactment. This design was not made by individual HCOs but by the elected representatives of the American people, who decided to have government collect and reimburse more uniformly for services provided to the populations to be covered. Decisions are also made that affect HCO governance by frontline clinicians and by patients and consumers. For example, registered nurses may choose to work in a home care agency or a nursing home, rather than a hospital. Patients may choose to enroll in one or another competing health plans, such as United Health Care or Aeta/U.S. Healthcare.

In this chapter, governance will be examined at the level of the HCO, rather than that of government or customers. Within the HCO, the focus is on the level at which policy is determined rather than the level at which it is implemented.

Governance and Managers

Although those who govern are supposed to make policy and those who manage are supposed to implement policy, it is well known that there is no clear-cut boundary between governance and management. In practice, those who manage at the top are often key participants in governance, as they have the necessary time and information to define an issue or limit consideration among policy alternatives. In large part, this is what managers are paid to do. On the other hand, because they at least potentially have the power and will to do so, those who govern the organization may carry out policy or manage as well. A more useful distinction between governance and management therefore concerns the nature of the decisions and their relative importance. Decisions about who governs, mission of the organizations, and major capital investment decisions are governance—and not management—decisions. Hiring, scheduling, and coordinating frontline providers of care are typically day-to-day management decisions.

Griffith, Sahney, and Mohr (1995) specify four types of organizational decisions: what the mission/vision is, how resources are to be allocated, the design of the organization, and how its programs are to be implemented. They point out that these processes may be considered at a strategic (policy) or a programmatic (operations) level. For example, at the strategic level, mission/vision can be considered as assessing the environment and developing a strategic plan; at the programmatic level, as developing and carrying out a marketing plan or a joint venture with another organization. These decisions may involve governance, as they concern the scope of service and the generation of resources. Alternatively, they may involve management, in generating information and motivating workers to carry out policy decisions. Governance includes decisions about what services the organization provides to whom at what price. Management decisions concern implementing those governance decisions through specification of priority objectives and strategies, and reconsideration of objectives and strategies as circumstances change.

MEASURING ORGANIZATIONAL PERFORMANCE

One reason for attempting to specify effective or acceptable organizational performance is to focus attention on the question "whose organization is this?" If performance is acceptable to trustees, managers, and clinicians, does it matter what anyone else thinks? If it does matter, what are others going to do if they find performance unacceptable?

A second reason for developing measures of performance concerns the distribution of organizational resources. To adjudicate claims on resources, questions may have to be raised about what the organization's purposes are, if they are not clearly stated somewhere. (Or, if they are stated clearly but not being achieved, why that might be so. For example, "How is our HMO doing? How does what we do compare with what our physicians and nurses, accreditors and regulators, and customers and potential customers think we ought to be doing?")

Prior agreement about standards of performance helps to facilitate agreement on performance evaluation and pay. Statements such as, "The hospital made a $100,000 surplus this year, 1% of patients made formal complaints, and our turnover rate in nursing was 15%," are uncertain indicators of performance unless they can be related to agreed upon standards and purposes. The standards of performance for which the organization and its managers are to be held accountable must be made clear in measurable terms and in advance. Of course, as circumstances change, targets can be adjusted, with fully explained reasons backing up the adjustment.

Those individuals or institutions that own HCOs are typically concerned with organizational performance. This includes defining standards, specifying measures of acceptable and superior performance, and hiring, retaining, or firing the key managers who are responsible for achieving organizational objectives. Superior organizational performance is defined differently by different stakeholders. Employees want higher salaries, clinicians want the latest equipment, patients want more convenient and higher quality services, and payers want better cost containment. A most common way to evaluate HCO performance is in terms of market share or financial profitability. Those governing the organization must decide what is acceptable performance and how it is to be measured. If they do not formally decide this, the judgments on performance outcomes will be based on the behavior of individuals and groups at lower levels in the organization. Further, different parts of the same HCO obviously may operate at different levels of success relative to each other or to the organization as a whole.

Ownership of Health Care Organizations

As noted above, different sponsors or owners of HCOs govern in different ways and have different goals. HCO owners include physicians and nurses, cooperatives, government, churches, investors, employers, unions, and philanthropists. Different categories of owners establish an HCO for different reasons, although their motives are often mixed. A classification of the main reasons and goals by type of sponsor is shown in Table 13.1.

A word of explanation about Table 13.1. That a key goal of government is to gain votes, signifies, for example, that a politician running for election claims credit for building a local health facility and creating local jobs. Or an archdiocese may seek to gain members for a church by owning and operating a health care facility.

HCOs are commonly grouped as to whether they are for-profit, not-for-profit, or public. What kind of ownership makes the most sense varies according to circumstances (such as those served), and the interests of the sponsoring stakeholders. Ownership may change from one form to another. For example, a church may sell a nonprofit hospital to a for-profit corporation because church officials decide that the monies gained from the sale can be used elsewhere to better serve the poor, while the for-profit corporation can better attract the capital required to upgrade and expand hospital facilities.

Governing Boards

Most organizations have a governing body with legal responsibility for control of the organization. Corporations are required to designate membership of the governing body as a condition of incorporation by the state in which their home office is located.

Bylaws outline the purposes of the organization, the composition and duties of the governing board, the requirements for periodic meetings of the board and notice of meetings, the duties and nature of corporate officers and the method of their selection, the nature and purpose of board

TABLE 13.1   Governance by Group and by Key Goals

Group	Goals
Physicians and nurses	Autonomy
Cooperatives	Service to membership
Government	Votes
Church	Service to believers
Employer	Lower costs
Investors	Profit
Union	Jobs
Philanthropists	Prestige

committees, and how the bylaws can be amended. A physician partnership agreement, for example, may typically specify the responsibilities of the partners, how net income is shared and losses borne, disability provisions, termination of a partner's agreement, and the composition of the executive committee or board and its functions.

The legal powers of the governing board, as suggested in a model constitution and bylaws for nonprofit hospitals published by the American Hospital Association (1981), are the following:

> The general powers of the corporation shall be vested in the governing board which shall have charge, control, and management of the property, affairs, and funds of the corporation; shall fill vacancies among the officers for unexpired terms; and shall have the power and authority to do and perform all acts and functions not inconsistent with these bylaws or with any action taken by the corporation. (p. 11)

These bylaws can be used by any corporation.

Although in theory the governing board has the responsibility for making policy, in practice the power and function of governing boards vary widely, depending on population served, resource dependence, and local power structure. Policy for the HCO may be decided by different internal subgroups and by external organizations. For example, hospital capital funding allocation may be decided by the board of a multiunit health system of which it is a part, the scope of hospital services by the local governing board, the nature of clinical education program by professional staff and accrediting organizations, and initiatives in marketing and community relations by management.

Board members of nonprofits are often less clear than those of their for-profit counterparts as to their responsibilities and functions. In the nonprofit organization, board members may not even be aware that they are (technically) the HCO's owners. Board members serve for a variety of reasons: community service, contacts, pay, status, access for their own medical care, or belief that their skills and experience add value to HCO mission attainment.

Selection of Board Members

The functions and powers of a governing board are strongly influenced by its composition and its method of selecting members. At first, a governing board consists of the HCO's founders, who may be contributing the key resources to begin the enterprise. Officers are elected by members of the governing board. For investor-owned organizations, owners of shares elect the governing board. In nonprofits, board members usually elect themselves. Or board members may be chosen from superordinate nonprofit corporate bodies that, in effect, own the HCO. For example, an archdiocese may own several hospitals and appoint board members for each hospital. A hospital might also be owned by members in a community who pay a fee to join the hospital corporation.

Large HCOs typically have boards dominated by businessmen, bankers, and lawyers; white males between 50 and 70 years of age. Board composition varies widely by type of control. Unsurprisingly, government and religious hospitals have greater proportions of government officials and religious leaders on their respective boards. For-profit and osteopathic hospitals have a greater proportion of physicians on their boards.

Board members may be "insiders" (managers or clinicians) or "outsiders" chosen for some special expertise, status, or access to resources. The type of person selected often depends on the functions and role of the board. If the primary purpose of the board is to raise money or give advice and counsel to the chief executive officer (CEO), then outsiders will be selected. If the primary function is policy making, then the directors should have detailed knowledge of the business—in which case, insiders may be preferred. For example, nonprofit hospital boards have been dominated by outsider community influentials and for-profit group practices by insider physicians.

According to Bowen (1994), the principal functions of a board of directors or trustees are as follows:

- To select, encourage, advise, evaluate, and if need be, replace the CEO.
- To review and adopt long-term strategic directions and to approve specific objectives, financial and other.
- To ensure, to the extent possible, that the necessary resources, including human resources, will be available to pursue the strategies and achieve the objectives.
- To monitor the performance of management.
- To ensure that the organization operates responsibly as well as effectively.
- To nominate suitable candidates for election to the board and to establish and carry out an effective system of governance at the board level, including evaluation of board performance.

Most board members are not paid for their participation; the vast majority of nonprofits do not pay board members. Board service can require a great deal of time, though. Board members could be spending that time earning money. Payment to board members for their time might improve accountability or provide the realistic opportunity for lower income persons to serve.

Board Composition, Structure, and Function

Governing boards vary in their makeup, structure, and function. According to an Ernst and Young study (1997) the average hospital board membership number is 13, although some boards had fewer than 7 or more than

16 members. Boards usually meet on a monthly basis; some boards meet quarterly. Most boards have committees of two types: standing committees, and special committees, that are discharged on completion of a task. Typical standing committees include those focusing on long-range planning, finance, and nominating. Some boards will appoint nonboard members to serve on their committees.

Appropriate composition, structure, and function depend on organizational circumstances. The boards of a national for-profit nursing home corporation with facilities in 40 states and a nonprofit academic medical center with one site will in all likelihood not have the same composition, structure, or function. What makes the most sense for a health care organization depends on mission, strategy, resources, and expected board contribution to results.

The Changing Role of the Board

Views differ and are changing regarding the role of the board of directors. More than 40 years ago, Burling, Lentz, and Wilson (1956) argued that a not-for-profit hospital governing board has a responsibility to provide and maintain the hospital to serve a community need according the wishes of the donor(s). To Umbdenstock (1987) the board must be the "organization's conscience, constantly assessing proposed directions . . . in light of what these steps mean for the implementation of a mission to serve and care for all" (p. 12).

It is easy to say that the board should be concerned with policy and oversight functions and that the staff should be responsible for management and administration (Bowen, 1994). But how this is best worked out in any organization depends on, among other factors, the skills, experience, and trust of the board chair and the CEO; the particular challenges the organization is facing at any particular time; and the expectations of major stakeholders.

Board Relationship to Independent Medical Staff

According to Griffith (1995), in the nonprofit HCO, the governing board "owns" the organization, but obviously cannot practice medicine. The independently practicing physicians are appointed to the medical staff, given privileges in the hospital by the board, and practice medicine. The CEO is the board's designate on site. The privileges agreement between attending physicians and the HCO grants these physicians permission to practice medicine and collect private fees from patients in return for their commitment to the hospitals to abide by the requisite bylaws, rules, and regulations. Especially important are those pertaining to the quality of medical care. The board (and there may be some physicians on the board) participates in implementing and revising the medical staff bylaws. The medical staff organization develops and enforces the rules so long as the board agrees that these are beneficial—to the community, in nonprofits, and to the shareholders, in for-profits. Griffith specifies that the compact breaks down if the board does not act vigorously as trustees for community (or shareholder) interests.

CURRENT GOVERNANCE ISSUES

Some current governance issues include the following: What are preferable HCO ownership patterns? How can nonprofit governance be improved? To what extent should the autonomy of HCOs be limited? What should be the nature of HCO accountability to those served and potentially served?

Preferable Ownership Patterns

Does it make any difference whether HCOs are owned by government, by for-profit, or by nonprofit organizations? Does it make enough of a difference to justify tax exemption for nonprofits? Currently, government is the primary owner of facilities that provide long-term mental health care and those that serve veterans. For-profits dominate in the HMO, nursing home, and physician practice sectors. Nonprofits own most of the short-term community hospitals.

There is insufficient evidence to make scientific conclusions regarding the effect of the type of ownership per se on the cost and quality of medical care or as to whether the performance of nonprofit HCOs justifies continued preferential tax treatment. Tax exemption applies to income, state, and local taxes. Exempt status makes gifts to the organization tax deductible for donors and allows the organization access to tax-free bonds. A related issue concerns conversions from nonprofit to for-profit status and their valuations.

Those who argue against for-profit ownership say that for-profits concentrate on providing only those services that are profitable, leaving the nonprofit and public HCOs to provide services to those who lack adequate insurance. A corollary argument is that for-profits build facilities only in expanding, high-income communities, leaving nonprofits and governmental HCOs to provide services to the poor. Opponents argue that the monies allocated to the shareholders of for-profits can be better reinvested in the delivery of care to those lacking access and that care is of lower quality in for-profits than in other HCOs.

Those in favor of for-profit ownership counter that, even allowing for profit, these HCOs are more efficient, adding that for-profits pay taxes. Consumers should be charged for the costs of the services that they use, rather than overcharged (in most cases, have their third-party payers overcharged), as in the nonprofits, to subsidize the payment of costs for others who cannot pay. For-profits respond more quickly and more flexibly in meeting market demand, and the quality of care most of them provide is adequate and sometimes higher than that of competing nonprofits and public HCOs.

Proponents of public ownership argue that their total costs and unit costs are lower, signifying greater efficiency. Yet every user gets treated similarly, based on health needs and regardless of income or disease status. The quality of care is not lower than that provided by other HCOs. Those who disagree say that primary emphasis in public HCOs is on keeping costs low, especially in this area of continual tax cutting for the better-off, rather than on providing adequate health care. Moreover, government operations are bureaucratic and inflexible, and the quality of care is lower.

Those in favor of nonprofit ownership praise the high level of quality of care provided and their high level of community service; those opposed cite their high cost. Opponents add that, for certain nonprofits, the quality of care is low and the community services nonexistent.

In order to reach informed conclusions as to preferred auspices, further research relating ownership to performance must be carried out. To properly do this, conditions other than ownership, such as organizational size, must be held constant. Also, evaluators must agree as to what is adequate and effective HCO performance.

Nonprofit Governing Board Performance

What is the value added to organizations by the nonprofit governing board, and how can this added value be increased? Answering this question cogently assumes some agreement on the criteria for evaluating board performance. Boards represent an ownership interest that is different from management's. Different owners choose to maximize different values. Such values may include improving health care in a community at acceptable levels of cost and quality. In any case, nonprofit boards add value by holding management accountable for results and by helping plan the future to fulfill organizational mission and to meet certain objectives and expectations of stakeholders.

Are boards contributing enough to organizations, relative to the expectations in the community regarding their performance? Government HCOs are usually not run by boards but rather by executives, with oversight from the legislative branch. The goals of for-profits are usually clear-cut—to make more money now and in the future. Some of the critics of nonprofit boards point to the amount of time it takes for these boards to make policy decisions, the lack of relevance/utility of decisions when board members don't understand the business, and the time and effort it takes for management to educate boards and provide staff support.

The issue is what stakeholders should do when nonprofit boards do not perform well. Obviously where there is healthy competition, the market forces accountability, and how boards add value may be of less stakeholder concern. Although top management should assist the board in carrying out its responsibilities, obviously management should be accountable to the board, as owners, rather than the other way around. Government should at least set rules for governance and disclose the performance of health care organizations. Organizations that accredit HCOs have similar responsibilities. Setting the rules includes establishing personal liability for board members when they have committed a breach of fiduciary duty, as when they pursue self-interest for firms for whom they work that sell to the institution on whose board they sit. Disclosing performance includes that of measures related to board performance, such as limitation—if any—on terms of office, the presence or absence of measurable objectives for the board, and the numbers, types, and added value of board committees. Some have argued that government should set requirements for boards, such as who can serve, for how long, and whether meetings should be open to the public, as well as establish committees to review quality of care in HCOs.

The Extent of Organizational Autonomy

To what extent should an HCO determine what services to provide to whom at what price? The autonomy of HCO governing boards has been shrinking since 1960. Federal and state governments have passed legislation, for example, forbidding discrimination against patients who seek admission or persons seeking employment. As well, there has been legislation passed invalidating a requirement that staff physicians of a nonprofit hospital be graduates of a medical school approved by the Liaison Committee on Medical Education and be members of the county medical society. Government has removed the exemption of hospitals from state labor laws, specified standards to be met by HCOs in order to be licensed by a state or reimbursed by Medicare, and forbidden construction of hospitals, nursing homes, and related facilities in some states without prior approval by state planning authorities. Medicare and Medicaid limit payment for new technology; some states require community service for hospitals to retain nonprofit status; in West Virginia, community representation is required on hospital boards; some states cap hospital revenue; and, Medicare limits hospital reimbursement to average length of stay, regardless of cost. Some states require that all Medicaid beneficiaries enroll in managed care plans. Some states require managed care plans to pay for hospital stays of 48 hours following healthy baby births, and that physicians be allowed to discuss with patients treatments for which the HMO will not pay.

Different stakeholders in health care delivery have different responses to questions about the degree of HCO autonomy that is useful in deciding what services they offer, what prices they charge, and what populations they serve. The same stakeholders may answer questions differently depending on whether they are sick or well at the time. HCOs should have enough leeway to decide issues regarding when they have better information than government, so long as there are ways to change HCO behavior when it falls unaccountably short of stakeholder expectations.

Too little autonomy for HCOs will result in the withdrawal from leadership positions of highly qualified individuals who have helped HCOs adapt appropriately in their local communities. Excessive standardization and centralization of decision making in governmental bureaucracies will result in decreased HCO innovation and ultimately in lower productivity. On the other hand, too much HCO autonomy may have been responsible, at least in large part, for the present unevenness in age-adjusted mortality and morbidity rates by race and by income, for overutilization of acute care and underutilization of long-term care, uneven productivity across HCOs, uneven service to customers, and high cost.

Accountability to Those Served

How should HCOs be accountable and to whom? Some advocate more formal accountability mechanisms than presently exist, for example, insisting that HCO governing boards be controlled by consumer representatives. Opponents argue that such control will result in ineffective decision making by boards and eventual withdrawal of community resources formerly donated to the organization. They question what evidence there is that the newly chosen representatives will be any more accountable to users and payers.

At the same time, most stakeholders will agree that on major decisions directly affecting the interests of consumers and employees, appeal mechanisms in HCOs should be available to them. In some HCOs, consumers lack an organized voice to complain or make suggestions, for example regarding provider manner, time spent waiting for services, or the explanations they receive concerning diagnosis and treatment. Consequently, they may seek service elsewhere or sue for malpractice. Consumers who are poor or institutionalized often lack even these unsatisfactory alternatives. Formal accountability mechanisms include a special board committee, an externally appointed ombudsman, and the patient advocate.

Other ways to improve customer service involve quality improvement committees, consumer advisory councils, customer focus groups, market surveys, and manager hotlines. As with most solutions, there are difficulties in getting things right the first time and limitations to their usefulness. For example, to whom does the consumer appeal if dissatisfied with the response of a patient advocate, who reports, after all, to HCO management? Appeal mechanisms may be costly in relation to benefits obtained by the consumer from following through on them. And there are many aspects of care that consumers (and providers) find objectionable, but about which little can be done by the HCO, such as obtaining acceptable payment for services provided to the uninsured. Finally, appeal mechanisms may serve only as buffers that satisfy the occasional vocal complainant, but do little to change the system of care that may be a cause of much unreported dissatisfaction.

MANAGEMENT

Now we shall focus on managers in HCOs—what they do, how their work is organized, and how they are trained. We shall also consider certain management issues, such as what managers should do, how much money they should be paid, how they should be trained, and how management performance can be improved.

Managerial work can be viewed as occupying positions, carrying out functions, requiring competencies, and performing roles. Managers do, variably, what they are supposed to do, what they are asked to do, what they want to do, and what they can do. Managerial work is characterized by choice or discretion after constraints are obeyed and demands are complied with.

Positions and Functions

A job or position description is one way of looking at the work that managers do. (See Table 13.2 for the position description of an HCO operations coordinator.) Implicit in this job description are managerial functions, each of which comprises a group of activities. Longest (1980) views the basic managerial functions as

- Planning—involves the determination of goals and objectives.
- Organizing—the structuring of people and things to accomplish the work required to meet the objectives.
- Directing—the stimulation of members of the organization to meet the objectives.
- Coordinating—the conscious effort of assembling and synchronizing diverse activities and participants so that they work toward the attainment of objectives.
- Controlling—the manager compares actual results with objectives to provide a measure of success or failure.

Competencies

Boyatzis (1995) has developed a model that includes three groups of managerial competencies. These include, first, the primarily "people skills" of efficiency orientation: planning, initiative, attention to detail, self-control and flexibility (goals and action management), empathy, persuasiveness, networking, negotiating, self-confidence, group management, developing

TABLE 13.2   Position Description of Operations Coordinator

Reason position exists
   To assist in all operational aspects of the physician hospital organization (PHO).
   To provide analytical support, maintain PC systems and coordinate various
      implementation projects.

Reports to
   Executive director, PHO.

Duties and responsibilities
   Schedule, coordinate, and maintain minutes for all IPA and PHO board meetings and
      board committee meetings.
   Prepare written correspondence, including, but not limited to, position papers and
      research, education and information pieces, and memos and letters.
   Maintain PC files on database, spreadsheet, and word processing programs.
   Possible desktop publishing responsibilities.
   Maintain financial income and expense spreadsheets for preparation of financial
      statements; maintain bank accounts and perform banking functions; maintain files
      for budget preparation and presentation.
   Design and produce reports for distribution on IPA and PHO activity.
   Maintain and assist in the analysis of reports from utilization management, HMOs,
      hospital systems, and IDX to produce data, as needed to analyze PHO performance.
   Maintain, update, and assist in the preparation of reports on IPA membership
      demographics, finances, and utilization performance.
   Assist in other projects as needed.

Knowledge, skills, and abilities
   Knowledge of managed care reimbursement and operations, working knowledge of
      physician and hospital reimbursement.
   Proficiency in spreadsheet and database applications.
   Excellent writing, organization, and presentation skills.
   Motivation to initiate/recommend action or research options for problem solving or
      program enhancement. Ability to follow up appropriately and effectively to affect
      action.
   Superior interpersonal skills and judgment.
   Comfort level with financial issues and accuracy in financial work.

Education and experience
   Bachelor's degree in public administration, health care administration, or
      finance/accounting with health care course work or experience; master's degree
      preferred.
   Managed care experience in finance, analysis, utilization management, contracting,
      or a combination of the above; experience may be in a hospital, physician group,
      HMO, or regulatory setting.
   Proven organizational or project management experience.

others, and oral communication. The second set of skills include use of
concepts, systems thinking, pattern recognition, theory building, technology, quantitativeness analysis, and social objectivity. Thirdly, written communication (analytic reasoning) is an important competency.

Goleman (1998) has found that most effective leaders have a high degree of
what he calls emotional intelligence, it is twice as important as are technical

skills and IQ for managerial jobs at all levels. The five components of emotional intelligence in managerial work are self-awareness, self-regulation (e.g., the ability to think before acting), motivation, empathy (e.g., the ability to understand the emotional makeup of other people), and social skills.

Managerial Roles

Roles are aspects of behavior that can be isolated for analytical purposes, such as leading, or handling disturbances. Positions can be viewed as combinations of roles. Kovner (1984) has conceptualized managerial roles as four sets of activities: motivating others, scanning the environment, negotiating the political terrain, and generating and allocating resources.

Motivating Others

Managers spend a great deal of time recruiting and retaining their managerial and supervisory staff, and in making decisions about rewards and promotions, work procedures, and development and training. To carry out these activities, they use communications and analytical skills. Managers facilitate the work of subordinates in doing what is required and in doing what subordinates want to do, within organizational limits.

Managers motivate others through development, pay level, and training. And managers must be developed, appropriately rewarded, and trained themselves. Motivation is affected by a worker's self-image of her job performance in any particular job. Managers can help improve performance by starting from where the worker is and using what strategies the worker will buy into to attain organizational goals and objectives. Worker performance can be enhanced through improvement of systems and processes, rather than by workers working harder and smarter. Also important in improving quality and productivity is the organizational culture. For example, workers can be rewarded for treating patients as customers, with high expectations for quality and service, or paid as a necessary complement to the physician's work.

Scanning the Environment

Effective managers scan or search the environment for potential problems and targets of opportunity. Scanning activities include market and product research, long-range planning, and quality benchmarking. The development of management information systems may be essential for effective scanning. In large HCOs, scanning activities are usually performed by special units for marketing, quality improvement, fund-raising, and planning. In smaller HCOs, managers scan the environment themselves and are assisted by colleagues. Information about how similar organizations and managers perform is available from journals, books, the Internet, newsletters, and advertisements. Managers attend continuing education and trade association meetings, and are part of on-line networks where colleagues and experts communicate. Managers visit similar organizations to learn first-hand about ways to improve effectiveness and efficiency. Openness to such visits has been a hallmark of public and nonprofit HCOs.

Negotiating the Political Terrain

Effective managers maintain trust and build alliances with groups and individuals. A positive political climate contributes to effective decision making and implementation. New managers must find out "who is doing what to whom" across a wide variety of organizational issues and problems. Or put another way, "What is the ball park in which I am really playing, who are the players, and what are the rules?" Managers learn the informal power structure by looking and listening. The operative rules are not always easy to learn. Organizational cultures vary, and within organizations subcultures' impacts differ by issue. Stakeholders involved in overhauling a management information system are different from those establishing a new renal dialysis unit, for instance. Activities that managers carry out in negotiating the political terrain include public relations, lobbying, labor relations, negotiating with governing boards and medical staffs, arbitrating among units and departments, and making alliances with other organizations.

Generating and Allocating Resources

Effective managers spend a great deal of time looking for ways to increase revenues and decrease expenses. In this analysis, managers consider past performance, performance in best practice organizations, and industry standards. For example, managers streamline buying procedures, secure long-term and working capital at low rates of interest, maintain effectively buildings and equipment, set optimal prices, and sequence appropriately new construction and renovations. In managing stakeholder expectations, managers listen closely to what subordinates, clinicians, and customers say.

Effective managers make decisions about generating and using resources. This occurs as part of the budgetary process and in response to emergency or extraordinary requests. Less tangible resources, such as staff time, must also be allocated, as must resources that may be less amenable to negotiation, such as use of space.

MANAGERIAL WORK IN HEALTH CARE ORGANIZATIONS

Hilsendrath and others (1993) have reviewed Bureau of Labor Statistics data, estimating a total of 362,500 health care managers in 1990, with projections showing an increase to 517,800 in 2005. Organizations that employ health services managers include hospitals and health systems, nursing homes, health maintenance organizations and other insurance companies, group practices, neighborhood health centers, home care agencies, ambulatory surgery centers, medical day care programs, durable equipment companies, home infusion agencies, and hospices.

In simple organizations such as the physician's office, clinicians themselves may perform managerial functions such as billing patients or contracting with vendors to bill patients (see Figure 13.1). In a group practice, the hiring, paying, and firing of physicians is done either by the whole group, or generally in the larger groups, by a subset of physicians who also practice medicine, while the billing function is supervised by nonphysician managers. In the large hospital or health maintenance organization, specialized functional managers support clinician and nonclinician general managers. Such functions include human resources (personnel), finance, information services, and marketing, among others. In multiunit organizations (also called integrated delivery systems), which include hospitals, nursing homes, group practices, and HMOs, managers of these units report to divisional managers for a geographic area (e.g., the northeastern United States). Divisional managers, in turn, report to managers in corporate headquarters, which are accountable to the board of directors. In these large organizations certain management functions are allocated among headquarters, divisions, and local HCOs. Headquarter functions commonly include legal affairs, construction, capital financing, and corporate public relations. Other functions, such as quality improvement and production standards, may be divided among the three organizational levels.

A newer development in the organization of managerial work in HCOs is product-line management (see Figure 13.2). The health system, large hospital, or group practice is reorganized into several divisions, such as women's health services, emergency care, cancer care, and rehabilitation services, each product line with its own manager and budget (see Herzlinger, 1997). The logic behind such reorganization is that these services can be more effectively managed as separate "businesses" than as part of a large HCO. Whether or not this is so, is unproven.

Accountability of health care organizations is uncertain unless there are measurable objectives set in advance and negotiated with stakeholders. Managerial contribution to organizational performance in health care has been criticized, as managerial costs are high per dollar of expenditures, and managerial salaries are often high. It has been difficult to isolate managerial contribution to organizational performance. For example, despite substantial managerial contributions, an HCO may be floundering because of a hostile environment or poor decisions by previous managers. Or the reverse situation may be occurring; despite little or ineffective managerial contribution, an HCO may be growing rapidly and even improving the quality of service rendered, due to lack of competitors, excellent performance by previous managers, and because of the performance of dedicated clinicians.

A. Doctor's office

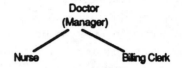

B. Group Practice

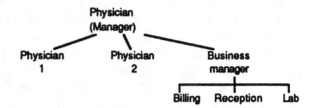

C. Hospital

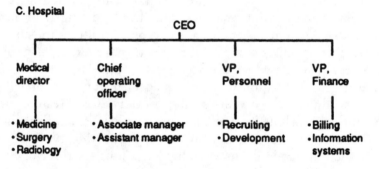

D. Multiunit hospital corporation

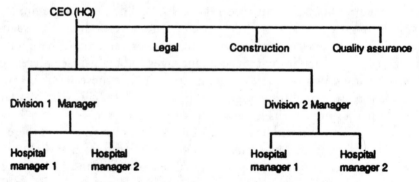

FIGURE 13.1   Organization of managerial work in HCOs.

EDUCATING HEALTH SERVICES MANAGERS

How do people learn to be health care managers? Can health care management be taught? Is it a science, an art, a craft, or something of all three? What can best be learned at school and on the job?

Learning health care management is done on the job, through continuing nondegree education, in undergraduate programs and in graduate

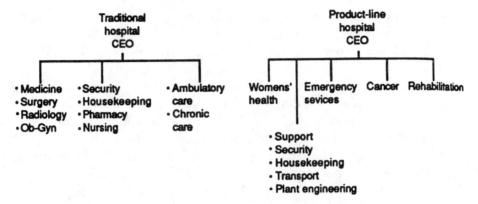

FIGURE 13.2 Traditional versus product-line organization.

programs leading to a degree. But despite the existence of large numbers of formal educational programs in management, much of what managers learn about what works in an organization and about how best they can work with clinicians and customers is taught on the job. Most large HCOs have formal orientation programs and offer special training courses on site as well. Managers can learn from others at work how to write what they mean, how not to always say what they are thinking, and how to more effectively influence others. Superiors, subordinates, and peers can assist managers in developing agendas and in forming and energizing networks through which goals and objectives may be accomplished.

Continuing nondegree educational programs are of various lengths and cover various subjects, such as developing an efficient and sustainable physician compensation system or developing an integrated information system for a HCO. These programs are offered by universities, by free-standing centers sometimes sponsored by professional associations or by vendors, and by large HCOs themselves.

Undergraduate programs train managers for intermediate level positions in large HCOs and for higher level positions in smaller organizations. The curriculum is often similar in subject matter to that of graduate programs. Courses that are generally required include introduction to the health care field, economics, law, management, human resources, financial management, and information and quantitative methods.

There are over 250 graduate programs in health care management in the United States today.[1] Programs are housed in various school such as business, public health, public administration, allied health, and medicine. Curricula commonly cover the following areas:

- Health status of populations: determinants of health and illness, and factors influencing the use of health services.

---

[1] For information about specific undergraduate and graduate programs, contact the Association of University Programs in Health Administration, 1110 Vermont Avenue, NW, Suite 220, Washington, DC, 20005.

- Organization, financing, and delivery of health services, drawing on the social science disciplines.
- Development of skills in economic, financial, polices and quantitative analysis.
- Values and ethical issues associated with the practice of health care management and the development of skills in ethical analysis.
- Positioning organizations favorably in the environment and managing these organizations for continued effectiveness.
- Development of leadership potential including stimulating creativity, and interpersonal and communication skill development.
- Management of human, capital, and information resources.
- Assessing organizational performance, and in particular, methods to assure continuous improvement in the quality of services provided.

(Accrediting Commission on Education for Health Services Administration [ACEHSA], 1994).

CURRENT MANAGEMENT ISSUES

Some current issues in HCO management are: Who should be in charge of HCOs: managers or clinicians? Are HCO managers overpaid? How can management performance be improved? How should managers be trained?

Who's in Charge: The Manager's Role in Health Care Delivery

Should health care organizations be run by managers or clinicians? Assuming they should be run by managers, should the managers have been clinicians, at one time in their careers, and have clinical degrees? What should be the role of nonclinician managers if they aren't in charge? Different stakeholders will respond differently to these questions.

Those in charge of HCOs should have the best set of skills, experience, and values to run them. HCOs in different situations require different types of leaders. Academic medical centers, neighborhood health centers, and large pharmaceutical companies do not require the same competencies in their leadership. One reason to have clinicians in charge of HCOs is that they tend to inspire more trust among other clinicians than do nonclinicians, whose high levels of performance are necessary for the organization to achieve its mission, goals, and objectives. So, in certain situations, chief executives of HCOs should be clinicians, with management training and experience. Not all managers of all types of HCOs need to have had clinical experience in order to function effectively, however. The bottom line is that any CEO, clinician or nonclinician, needs to have a deep understanding of the business of health care, and understanding of the process of health care delivery and organizational mission, in order to succeed in managing the HCO.

Given the increasing size and complexity of HCOs, the manager's job is becoming more important (and more highly paid) and less secure. New kinds of jobs are being created in large HCOs, such as the risk management specialist, medical service organization (MSO) director, and director of system development. The risk management specialist evaluates the actuarial health risk of a population in support of capitated contract negotiations. The MSO director solicits and negotiates contracts for hundreds of physicians and oversees administrative support across different physician groups. The director of system development leads joint venture discussions and continuously scans the market for merger and acquisition candidates (Advisory Board Company, 1996).

Managerial Compensation

The median total compensation in 1999 for hospital administrators and chief executive officers according to a survey by Hewitt Associates (Moore, 1999) was $210,000, and some health system CEOs make more than $800,000 per year. And of course, they get fringe benefits on top of that. Some CEOs have bonus arrangements keyed to organizational performance, which allows them to make more money in any particular year. Is that too much, or too little, relative to their contribution and relative to what other CEOs make outside of health care? Or relative to what physicians make? Once again, different stakeholders come up with different answers to these questions.

Part of the answer relates to what contribution top managers make to organizational performance, and part relates to determinations of what are acceptable profits in a just society. Proponents of paying managers more argue that health care is an increasingly competitive sector of the economy, as patients are choosing lower cost, higher quality, and better managed HCOs. They say the management function contributes to keeping costs down, and quality and revenues up, and that the best managers must be attracted to work in health care rather than in other sectors of the economy.

Opponents of higher managerial compensation argue that the money paid to high-salaried managers could be better spent on, for example, improving access of the uninsured to health care. Of course, this idea would not go very far as there are few highly paid managers and many uninsured. Opponents argue that since health care is a right not a privilege, HCOs should not be competing against each other for market share, but rather working cooperatively to improve population health. They also argue that health care managers should be paid like managers in other public service organizations such as education, welfare, and religion.

Improving Managerial Performance

To what extent does managerial performance in HCOs have to be improved? Why don't more HCOs have a greater capacity to change? Why do they invest so little in training? Why is quality so uneven and service to customers not sufficiently user-friendly?

In some HCOs, management has been transforming organizational performance. Costs per unit of service has been reduced, quality has been improved, and market share has grown, in part because service has improved. Disclosure to customers and stakeholders of HCO objectives and the degree of their attainment relative to best practice is an excellent way to hold managers' feet to the fire in terms of improving service, monitoring quality, cutting waste, and improving health status. It is the responsibility of stakeholders—government, owners, clinicians, and customers and payers, to expect improved performance and to act if expectations are not met. When the organization fails, the customers either try to change performance or they seek services elsewhere, and the managers are fired or forced to resign. This has been the American way. It has been highly regarded by other developed nations, even as we are criticized as a society for the high preference given to organizational performance relative to community solidarity.

CASE STUDY

What follows is the mission statement of the Henry Ford Health System of Detroit, Michigan:

> To enable a given population to maximize its present and future health and provide tangible benefit to its community the Health System will provide the highest quality service to prevent episodes of illness and provide coordinated episodes of care in a way that satisfies and delights both clients and system staff with efficient use of resources, appropriate facilities and labor capacity, and the financial performance to maintain and improve the above activities, while continuing to support research and education. (Henry Ford Health System, 1998)

Please answer the following questions about this statement of purpose:

1. How should organizational performance at Henry Ford be measured?
2. Why don't all HCOs have statements of purpose similar to Henry Ford's?
3. What contribution should the board of Henry Ford make to accomplish the statement of purpose?
4. What contribution should the management team of Henry Ford make to the attainment of the statement of purpose?

DISCUSSION QUESTIONS

1. What are the advantages and disadvantages of the different forms of ownership of HCOs?

2. What mechanisms of accountability are most effective for not-for-profit HCOs?
3. What are some of the ways to measure the performance of HCOs?
4. What are some of the ways to measure managerial performance in HCOs?
5. What skills and experience are required to own and manage HCOs?
6. Who should be in charge of HCOs and how should they be trained?

REFERENCES

Accrediting Commission on Education for Health Services Administration. (1997). *Criteria for accreditation* (2nd rev. ed.). Arlington, VA: Author.

Advisory Board Company. (1996). *The rising tide: Emergence of a new competitive standard in health care.* Washington, DC: Author.

American Hospital Association. (1981). *Guide for preparation of constitution and bylaws for general hospitals.* Chicago, IL: Author.

Bowen, W. G. (1994). *Inside the boardroom: Governance by directors and trustees.* New York: John Wiley.

Boyatzis, R. E. (1995). Cornerstones of change: Building the path to self-directed learning. In R. E. Boyatzis, S. S. Cowen, D. A. Kolb, & Associates (Eds.), *Innovation in professional education* (pp. 50–94). San Francisco: Jossey-Bass.

Burling, T., Lentz, E., & Wilson, R. (1956). *The give and take in hospitals.* New York: G. P. Putnam's Sons.

Ernst & Young. (1997). *Shining light on your board's passage to the future.* Cleveland, OH: Author.

Goleman, D. (1998). What makes a leader. *Harvard Business Review, 76*(6), 93–102.

Griffith, J. R. *(1995). The well managed health care organization* (3rd ed.). Ann Arbor, MI: Health Administration Press.

Griffith, J. R., Sahney, V. K., & Mohr, R. A. (1995). *Reengineering health care: Building on CQI.* Ann Arbor, MI: Health Administration Press.

Herzlinger, R. (1984). *Market-driven health care.* Reading, MA: Addison-Wesley.

Hilsenrath, P. E., Levey, S., Weil, T. P., & Ludke, R. (1993). Health services management manpower & education: Outlook for the future. *Journal of Health Administration Education, 11,* 407–419.

Kovner, A. R. (1984). *Really trying: A career guide for the health services manager.* Ann Arbor, MI: Health Administration Press.

Longest, B. B. (1980). *Management practices for the health professional.* Reston, VA: Reston Publishing.

Moore, J. D., Jr. (1999). Holding the line (for you down there). *Modern Healthcare, 29*(28), 43–46, 48.

Umbdenstock, R. J. (1987). Refinement of board's role required. *Health Progress, 68*(1), 47.

14

Improving Quality of Care[1]

Susan D. Horn

LEARNING OBJECTIVES

☐ Describe the evolution of quality assurance, assessment, and improvement in health care.
☐ Discuss differing definitions and components of quality.
☐ Describe and give examples of measures of quality related to structure, process, and outcomes.
☐ Describe and assess various sources and methods for gathering information on quality of care.
☐ Critique various mechanisms for assuring, promoting, and improving quality of care.
☐ Describe the new Clinical Practice Improvement (CPI) methodology and compare it to the usual outcomes research, guideline development, and randomized controlled trials.

TOPICAL OUTLINE

Historical perspectives
Definition of quality
Measuring quality
Promoting quality: Assurance and improvement
Quality assurance through the Continuous Quality Improvement (CQI) framework
Quality improvement through the Clinical Practice Improvement (CPI) framework
Organizational considerations in promoting quality
Current issues and questions

---

[1] Portions of this chapter have been adapted from chapter 13, Improving Quality of Care, by Beth Weitzman in the 6th edition of this book.

KEY WORDS

accreditation, certification, Clinical Practice Improvement (CPI), Joint Commission for the Accreditation of Healthcare Organizations (JCAHO), licensing, National Commission on Quality Assessment (NCQA), optimal care, outcomes, overutilization, peer review, process, peer review organizations (PROs), quality assurance, reliability (of criteria), structure, Total Quality Management (TQM), underutilization, utilization review, validity (of criteria)

The assessment and improvement of quality of care is a major challenge in health care today. Recent changes in health care delivery—especially the move to managed care—have intensified the focus on quality. Although it is agreed that high-quality health care is desirable, and despite substantial advances in the field, there continues to be much disagreement about its definition, its measurement, and methods for improving it.

Quality of care problems are diverse, and as new quality assessment tools have become available new problems have been identified. They include excessive or inappropriate surgery, variable outcomes of surgical procedures and pre- and post-surgical treatments, inappropriate diagnosis or treatment of common acute conditions, and excessive use, underuse, or inappropriate use of prescription drugs (Lohr, Yardy, & Thier, 1988).

Until early in the last century, there was little concern about the quality of care provided. "Do no harm," taken from the Hippocratic Oath, served as the guiding principle. In the latter half of the 20th century, however, quality has been pushed to the forefront of the health care debate, in part because of attempts to reduce health care costs and the worry that quality might be jeopardized by this (Blumenthal, 1996). New circumstances of health care practice, including declining hospitalization, industry consolidation through mergers, and growth of for-profit plans also raised concern about quality (Gabel, 1997). A recent report from the Institute of Medicine on quality of health care in the U.S. estimated that 98,000 people die each year from medical errors (Kohn, Corrigan, & Donaldson, 2000). Almost daily, both local and national newspapers describe detailed patient situations indicating significant quality of care problems. Thus, quality of care concerns are now widespread.

Our knowledge of methods to measure and improve the quality of care has been bolstered by new models for approaching questions of quality improvement in industries other than health care (Blumenthal, 1996). Using concepts taken from industry, a new methodology called Clinical Practice Improvement (CPI) has been used successfully to identify best medical practices in several areas where it has been applied (Horn, 1997). A detailed description of this new methodology is presented later in this chapter.

The chapter begins with a brief review of the history of quality assessment and assurance. Definitions and methods of measuring quality health care are explored, followed by discussions of strategies for promoting and improving the quality of health care services.

HISTORICAL PERSPECTIVES

Concern with quality has become a focal issue for the health care community only within recent decades. In the early 1860s, however, Florence Nightingale helped lay the groundwork for medical care evaluation by suggesting a uniform format for collecting and presenting hospital statistics (Christoffel, 1976). To her, statistics were more than a study, they were indeed her religion. Florence Nightingale believed—and in all the actions of her life acted upon the belief—that the administrator could only be successful if she were guided by statistical knowledge (Pearson, 1924). In the early 20th century Dr. Ernest Codman, a Boston surgeon, advocated the collection and evaluation of systematic information on the end results of patient care activities (Christoffel, 1976). Entitled "end result analysis," it was introduced at Massachusetts General Hospital in 1900 and featured a careful analysis of cases for which treatment was unsuccessful. End result analysis included data collection on large numbers of patient outcomes and a recognition that a poor outcome might result from a range of factors. Codman's ideas failed to gain widespread acceptance at that time, principally because application of his methodology found so many errors.

Despite the initial lack of enthusiasm for end result analysis, the Joint Commission on Accreditation of Healthcare Organizations (JCAHO) traces its inception back to certain elements of Codman's original proposal (Roberts, 1987). In 1917, the American College of Surgeons established and published the *Minimum Standard for Hospitals,* which contained the first formal requirements for the review and evaluation of the quality of patient care. Quality of care in hospitals that participated in the Hospital Standardization Program improved noticeably (Shanahan, 1983). In 1951 the American College of Surgeons joined with the American College of Physicians, the American Hospital Association, the American Medical Association, and the Canadian Medical Association to establish the Joint Commission on Accreditation of Hospitals (JCAH) to oversee the *Minimum Standards.* In recognition of the growing diversity of health care provider settings, the JCAH broadened its scope and in the mid-1980s became the Joint Commission for the Accreditation of Healthcare Organizations. By the early 1990s, the JCAHO moved toward a standard that stressed "optimal" care through continuous evaluation, assessment, and improvement (Joint Commission, 1991).

As the organization of health care has changed, other accrediting bodies have been created. For example, the National Commission on Quality Assessment (NCQA) accredits state-licensed managed care plans. Government has also played an active role in health care quality. With the funding of hospital facility construction through the Hill-Burton Act and the enactment of Medicare and Medicaid in the 1960s, the federal government became a major source of health care dollars, and quality standards for participation in these federal programs were established. By the 1970s, due to the large federal deficit and increasing federal health care expenditures, cost containment and its relationship to quality emerged as key issues in health care (Thurow, 1985). Using new initiatives such as utilization review, emphasis was placed on the elimination of the overuse of medical procedures (overuse occurs when the risks of the service outweigh the benefits) (Chassin, 1991).

In addition, the government began to take steps to ensure that needed care would not be sacrificed in the name of saving costs. As the mechanism for financing health care shifted from fee-for-service to per-case reimbursement and capitated payments, the insurance industry became another focus of the government's quality assurance activities. States, for example, began passing legislation to ensure reimbursement for minimum stays specified by law for routine childbirth and for procedures such as mastectomies, taking such determinations out of the hands of insurance companies.

Accompanying these changes in the financing and method of payment were dramatic changes in the organization and delivery of health care services. Traditionally, the focus of quality assurance programs has been on hospital care both because it is so expensive and because hospitals are more amenable to organizational constraint (Donabedian, 1985). Yet care outside the hospital setting has been growing rapidly since 1985. Thus, questions regarding the quality of care in ambulatory and long-term care settings started to be asked, and concerns about quality under various organizational arrangements, such as provider networks, also began to be addressed.

DEFINITION OF QUALITY

According to *Merriam Webster's Collegiate Dictionary* (7th edition), quality is defined as "degree of excellence" or "superiority in kind." This concept of quality is not unique to health care. As consumers we must assess the quality or degree of excellence of a broad range of products and services, whether we are selecting a restaurant, purchasing clothing, or making an airline reservation. Consumers use available information to try to identify the highest-quality product, relative to its cost. Given the complexity and diversity of health care services, however, there is not one quintessential definition of quality but rather several legitimate definitions.

The Components of Quality

Quality care aims to promote, preserve, and restore health; it is delivered in an appropriate setting in a manner that is satisfying to patients. Quality care is achieved when the improvements in health status that are possible are, in fact, realized. Quality has several components, including appropriateness (the right care is provided at the right time), technical excellence (care is provided in the correct manner), accessibility (care can be obtained when needed), and acceptability (patients are satisfied) (U.S. General Accounting Office, 1996).

In trying to define and measure precisely what can be called quality care, there is a dilemma or tension between focusing on that which is unacceptable or poor-quality care and that which is optimal or highest-quality care. For many purposes, *good-quality care* is a standard that focuses on minimal requirements for quality. Such definitions are often employed because they are easy to use and measure. In other cases, the definition aims to characterize an optimal or ideal standard of high quality. Often this sort of definition can be difficult to use in a meaningful way; the new Clinical Practice Improvement study methodology described below operationalizes the concept of optimal care by using data collected in actual practice to determine which treatments work best for specific patient types (Horn, 1997).

Various Definitions

How one defines quality varies by one's role in the health care delivery process. Traditionally, quality of care has been defined by clinicians, primarily in terms of the technical delivery of care: "the application of the science and technology of medicine, and of the other health sciences, to the management of a personal health problem" (Donabedian, 1980). From early in the development of medical practice in the United States, society delegated the establishment of quality standards to the medical profession (Caper, 1988). Peer review—a member of a profession being responsible for assessing the work of colleagues within that same profession—has traditionally been at the center of quality assessment and assurance efforts. These peer review efforts have emphasized the scientific aspects of quality, such as appropriate drug prescription, postoperative infection rates, and accuracy of diagnosis. Physicians' grip on the definition of quality has eroded in recent years, however, as both purchasers and patients have become more active in this arena.

In contrast to the physician's emphasis on the technical aspects of care, when assessing care patients tend to focus on interpersonal aspects of care and amenities of care. Lacking technical expertise and assuming technical competence on the part of providers, patients typically judge the quality of technical care indirectly, by evidence of the practitioner's interest in and concern for their health and welfare (Donabedian, 1985). Also, a significant body of research indicates that the quality of the patient-practitioner interaction may be a major contributor to treatment success, through greater patient compliance with treatment regimens and return for prescribed follow-up care (Cleary, Keroy, Karapanos, & McMullen, 1989; Danziger, 1986; Svarstad, 1986).

Thus, definitions of quality in health care are no longer left solely to physicians. Administrators, nurses, and other health care personnel emphasize different aspects of quality from those stressed by physicians and patients (Donabedian, 1980). Administrators, for example, tend to focus on the amenities of care, perhaps because this is the area over which they have greatest control. Nurses present a middle ground—looking both to indicators of technical competence and interpersonal relations. As health care becomes more of a team effort, and as more nonphysician professionals begin to practice independently, the definitions of quality of care will broaden (Lohr et al., 1988). For example, the recently organized Foundation for Accountability (FACCT) brings together the voices of payers, providers, purchasers, and consumers to define performance standards for the managed care industry. Further, there is growing recognition of the need to consider quality in terms of the consequences, or outcomes, of care rather than only its structure or process of delivery.

Quality of Care vs. Quantity of Care and Their Relationship to Reimbursement

More care does not necessarily equal better care. Sometimes, however, quality of care may be confused with quantity of care. Consumer ratings of quality do reflect, at least in part, how many services are received (Davies & Ware, 1988). Yet closer examination reveals that although there are times when more care does equal better care, there are also times when more is not only not better but actually worse. In the past the precise relationship between inputs and benefits has not been clear in all areas of health care. When the care received by any one patient is insufficient to bring about the potential benefits, the care is clearly poor in quality because of quantitative inadequacy (Donabedian, 1980). Underuse occurs when the benefits of an intervention outweigh the risks, but it is nevertheless not used (Chassin, 1991). An example is the failure to complete a vaccination series; more care is needed before the benefits of the intervention can be realized. Chassin (1997) argues that underuse is "ubiquitous in U.S. medicine." Where the existing quality of care is low because of inadequate quantity of care, improving quality may increase costs.

Eventually, however, care can become excessive and even harmful; such care is more costly but of equal or lower quality. Examples of care that may be unnecessary are annual Pap smears and routine use of fetal sonograms in low-risk pregnancies. Such care may be excessive but carries little risk; however, costs for unnecessary care are hard to justify and resources could be better spent elsewhere. Examples of care that may be excessive but also harmful are routine chest and annual dental X rays; they introduce a potential danger to the patient through excessive exposure to x-radiation. Overuse of procedures, including some that are highly invasive, has been documented also. A study of Medicare patients found that 17% of angiographic procedures and 32% of carotid endarterectomies were inappropriately performed (Brook, Park, Chassin, Solomon, Keesey, & Kosecoff, 1990); both procedures are associated with some risk. Eliminating the use of these unnecessary and potentially detrimental medical procedures and practices would clearly improve the quality of health care and lower cost.

In addition to unnecessary and excessive care, sometimes care is produced inefficiently. In such cases, reducing the costs of care can be achieved by producing it more efficiently, not by reducing the quantity or intensity of care. Substitution of a nurse-practitioner for a physician or the use of ambulatory rather than inpatient surgery are two examples of strategies aimed at maintaining good quality while reducing costs.

The relationship between the quantity and quality of care is of critical importance to policymakers as they decide on the relative merits of various health care reimbursement systems. The incentive structure built into traditional fee-for-service medicine may encourage overuse, because more money is made when more costly procedures are undertaken. Under capitated and managed care systems, the perceived risk is underuse. Fee-for-service medicine is expected to use resources inefficiently, while capitated systems are expected to be more efficient. Emerging evidence is that reality is not as clear as the theory might suggest. "There is little objective information that suggests that patients are greatly disadvantaged in one model of practice versus another" (Ogrod, 1997). Underuse, overuse, and inappropriate use all exist in both fee-for-service and managed care settings.

Supporters of managed care argue that "by focusing cost-containment efforts on reducing the inappropriate use of health services and avoiding preventable adverse effects, physicians can cut costs and improve quality at the same time" (Chassin, 1996). Although studies to date suggest that managed care results in lower costs with equal quality, these studies are limited because, for example, they have focused on short-term outcomes (Berwick, 1996). Very little is known about the effect of specific reimbursement or organizational arrangements on the quality of care (Enthoven & Vorhaus, 1997). Further, there is emerging evidence that the quality of care provided under capitated systems may differ across population groups. Whereas average patients fare well under managed care, chronically ill elderly and poor patients show poorer outcomes than those treated under fee-for-service arrangements (Ware, Bayliss, Rogers, Kosinsky, & Tarlov, 1996). This is discussed further under Economic Approaches.

MEASURING QUALITY

Structure, Process, and Outcome

Defining what is meant by the term *quality* is only the first step toward assessing it in the delivery of health care. Appropriate variables must be identified to determine the degree to which quality is present. Structure, process, and outcome are the three most commonly defined approaches to both establishing criteria and gathering information so that the presence or absence of the attributes that constitute or define quality may be determined. *Structure* has been defined as "the relatively stable characteristics of the providers of care, of the tools and resources they have at their disposal, and of the physical and organizational settings in which they work" (Donabedian, 1980). Structure includes those things that exist prior to and separate from interaction with patients, such as board certification for physicians, nurse/bed ratios for hospitals, availability and acceptability of facilities, and availability of laboratory services for HMOs. Structure, an indirect measure of quality, is useful to the degree that it can be expected to influence the direct provision of care.

Process concerns the set of activities that go on between practitioners and patient, and may be used to assess the quality of the technical management of care (e.g., was the appropriate laboratory test ordered?), as well as the interpersonal aspects of care (e.g., was the medical history taken in a sensitive and caring manner?). Process is what is done to patients; outcomes are what happens to patients as a result of the intervention(s) (Hogness, 1985). *Outcome* refers to a change or lack thereof in a patient's current and future health status that can be attributed to antecedent health care, such as mortality rates, postoperative infection rates, and rates of rehospitalization (Donabedian, 1980).

The Causal Model

The underlying causal model in most quality assessments is that structure influences the process of care, which in turn has an impact on the outcome of care. Most definitions of quality assume that the application of the appropriate process of care will maximize patient outcomes (Lohr et al., 1988). Justification of this inference must be established, however; there is considerable disagreement about cause and effect in health care. Also in this assessment, patient differences in severity of illness and preferences need to be taken into account.

Research methods are used to determine the links between particular structures and processes and desired outcomes, and to test whether changes in health status (outcome) are really the result of the care given, controlling for patient differences. Are board-certified physicians (structure) more likely to make appropriate use of laboratory tests (process)? And does the appropriate utilization of laboratory tests have a positive impact on patient recovery (outcome)? Do second surgical opinion programs (structure) influence the use of surgery (process)? And does this benefit patient health (outcome)? Structure is, at best, a crude predictor of the quality of care since it can only address general tendencies. Structural indicators are, however, generally easy and inexpensive to access, whereas information on the process and outcomes of care is often unavailable, incomplete, or expensive to obtain.

When the link between process and outcome has been validated, process indicators become an important tool for assessing and assuring quality in a direct and timely fashion. Another great virtue of process evaluation lies in the broad clinician involvement and education that is a consequence and may subsequently result in improved practices (Blum, 1974). Too often, however, what is described as high-quality care has not been demonstrated to have much impact on the health status of patients. The Congressional Office of Technology Assessment estimated that only 10%–20% of clinician practices were shown effective by randomized controlled trials (Eddy & Billings, 1988). In other words, many health care treatments lack scientific evidence of efficacy (better outcomes in controlled studies) and even fewer have evidence of effectiveness (better outcomes in actual practice settings).

Although the validity of elements of process depends on the contribution of process to outcome, outcome measures tend to be inherently valid, because change in health status and patient well-being is the ultimate goal of health care. When high-quality care is delivered, we expect improvement in such outcomes as mortality, morbidity, or social functioning. But before outcomes can be used to make inferences about the quality of care, it is necessary to establish that the observed outcomes can be attributed to that care, and vice versa. Intervening factors, such as differences in severity of illness, must be ruled out (Blum, 1974).

For example, the release of hospital-based mortality rates by the federal government's Health Care Financing Administration (HCFA) has been criticized on these grounds; many argue that there is insufficient evidence to attribute a particular mortality rate to poor hospital performance. Rather, preexisting health (severity of illness) differences among the patients served may instead be the cause for many of these differences. In 1993, when Bruce Vladeck was appointed administrator of HCFA, he decided to withhold the data because there was "something lacking in the methodology" (*Medicine and Health,* 1993). This debate reminds us that in the absence of good severity adjustment, the use of a health outcome such as mortality as an indicator of quality of care may be misleading.

On the other hand, some research on structure, process, and patient outcomes has demonstrated linkages. A recent study on the treatment of breast cancer illustrates this. Mastectomy was contrasted with a treatment protocol that included the less disfiguring lumpectomy combined with radiation. The researchers found that the use of lumpectomy resulted in similar clinical outcomes (Johantgen, Coffey, Harris, Levy, & Clinton, 1995). In another example, family physicians were found to be less likely than obstetricians to use epidural anesthesia, Cesarean sections, episiotomies, and other interventions with low-risk deliveries, and these differences in the process of care did not result in differences in the clinical outcomes of care (Hueston, Applegate, Mansfield, King, & McClafin, 1995). Evidence from either randomized trials or associations found in well-designed observational studies is needed to determine which treatments are associated with better outcomes, controlling for patient differences.

Measurement Issues: Reliability and Validity

Measurement is critical to the assessment and improvement of quality, for it is through measurement that we can make precise comparisons of benefits and risks. However, no single indicator can capture the entire concept of quality or even any major component of it. Therefore, it is better to use multiple operational definitions or measures that account for the broadest understanding of quality.

For example, in a study comparing costs and benefits of hospice and conventional care for terminally ill cancer patients, a broad range of criteria and measures had to be developed, including measures of pain, symptoms, and activities of daily living, as well as patient and family satisfaction (Kane, Wales, Bernstein, Leibowitz, & Kaplan, 1985). Any single measure would have provided an incomplete and misleading assessment of the quality of care provided. Furthermore, criteria and standards change over time; this is integral to the philosophy of quality improvement. The concept that there is some absolute level of quality was implicit in earlier work in the field of quality assurance. More recent work has stressed the concept of variable standards, depending upon situation and patient differences.

In assessing the quality of care, the criteria or measures used must be both valid and reliable. Reliable measures are those that do not fluctuate randomly from one episode of measurement to the next; this is called test-retest reliability. Reliable measures yield the same results regardless of who is making the rating; this is called interrater reliability. As examples, mortality data tend to be highly reliable, whereas psychiatric and social assessments may not be as reliable.

The validity of a measure concerns how well it really reflects the concept being assessed. The validity of a given measure may be evaluated by determining its correlation or convergence with other measures of the same concept; if several different measures of the same concept all lead to the same conclusions, we have greater confidence that the individual measures are valid. For example, if we are rating physician performance we might include a review of lab tests ordered, an assessment of the medical histories taken, and a judgment of the quality of the medical record; if all three measures lead to the same conclusion about the physician's performance, we would have greater confidence about the validity of any one measure. Validity of measures may also be examined by their ability to distinguish between cases that are known to differ and by their predictive ability of outcomes. For example, a valid severity of illness measure is expected to be a good predictor of mortality, cost, and length of stay.

The scientific validity of a measure is best based on a demonstrated causal relationship. In the absence of a scientifically demonstrated relationship, "normative validity" is often substituted. Normative validity comes from professional consensus (e.g., agreement among physicians) (Donabedian, 1980). In conducting an assessment of the quality of care, process elements are often used when there is general agreement that certain procedures are appropriate for certain situations, even though there is no "scientific proof' of appropriateness (Donabedian, 1980). The problem with relying on measures that have normative validity rather than scientific validity is that they can lead to the perpetuation of ineffective process.

Similarly, when there is a lack of information linking process to outcomes, there is also a tendency to apply the criterion of potential benefit. In this framework a practice is considered appropriate if it might have benefit (Eddy & Billings, 1988). The appeal of the criterion of potential benefit is that it is easy to apply and it deals with the uncertainty that surrounds many practices. As an example, rather than limit the use of fetal monitors to high-risk deliveries, in some hospitals all pregnancies are monitored because it may be difficult to assess risk and there may be rare cases where otherwise unidentified problems might be found. Unfortunately, the criterion of potential benefit translates easily into "when in doubt, do it."

Clinical Guidelines

Growing sophistication in the research on the relationship between the structure, processes, and outcomes of patient care, and federal support for this research through such agencies as AHCPR (Agency for Health Care Policy and Research, now called AHRQ, Agency for Healthcare Research and Quality), have made possible the development of what are called "clinical guidelines." It has been shown that their use can greatly enhance medical decision making. The efficacy of various methods and procedures as well as long established standards are being subject to scientific scrutiny—often for the first time and often with surprising results. CONQUEST 1.0 (Computerized Needs-Oriented Quality Measurement Evaluation SysTem) was released by AHCPR in 1996. It summarized information on approximately 1,200 clinical performance measures, developed by a variety of public, private, and not-for-profit organizations, and provided health care organizations the opportunity to use recent research to set standards and monitor the care provided. This increased availability of scientific information for health care decisions holds tremendous promise for improving quality of care.

Sources of Information

In trying to measure and promote good quality care, one can use computerized administrative records or data gathered through interviews, observations, or review of individual records. Data sources and collection methods differ in costs, acceptability, reliability, and validity (Gerbert, 1988). Generally, a method becomes more expensive and less feasible if it requires information that is not routinely collected. On the other hand, routinely gathered data may not have quality assessment as their primary focus and may be only an indirect and incomplete measure of quality.

Administrative Data and Computerized Systems

Administrative data on health care institutions and providers are regularly compiled by a range of public and not-for-profit agencies. These measures—number of beds, number of registered nurses, number of board-certified surgeons—have become a routine part of accreditation and certification procedures. Routinely collected data on insurance claims, drug prescriptions, and malpractice suits may provide information on the process of care. If properly organized, these data can permit relatively inexpensive, large-scale quality assessment activities. A centralized medical malpractice information system could help identify recurring problems, including problems with individual medical care providers, and focus attention on needed corrective and preventive actions (Baine, 1987). Similarly, health care organizations, state medical and dental boards, and professional societies are required to report adverse professional actions (such as actions against a practitioner's license). They are sources of data regarding some of the most egregious examples of "bad-quality" care.

The Medical Record

Medical records are the most commonly used source of information on the process of care. Record review or, "chart audit," is an integral part of many quality assurance and cost-containment programs such as utilization review. Ease of access is the most attractive characteristic of the medical record. The information is routinely gathered; using it for quality assessment involves limited additional expense or time.

Ideally, the medical record provides accurate and detailed information on patient symptoms, on the tests and procedures that were undertaken, and on patient progress. Unfortunately, in reality, medical records often do not reach the ideal standard. They may be incomplete and use practice-specific terminology; thus information on diagnosis, treatment, and outcome may not be linked across settings without developing standardized documentation (Lohr et al., 1988). Growing use of computerized systems for maintaining patient records and structured formats for such record keeping may enhance the quality of the patient record and therefore make it an improved tool for monitoring the quality of care.

Patient and Practitioner Interviews

In addition to record audit, information may be obtained by directly interviewing or surveying providers and patients. The provider is probably the most accurate source of reported information regarding the process of care (Gerbert, Stone, Stulborg, Gullian, & Greenfield, 1988). But physician interviews are an expensive source of information and may not be a good one on the nontechnical aspects of care. In contrast, getting information from consumers of care may be no more expensive than using traditional sources such as the medical record (Davies & Ware, 1988). There is good evidence that the information reported by patients is valid and reliable. Most crucially, the consumer is probably in the best position to rate the interpersonal aspects of care. It has become routine for managed care organizations to survey their members regarding their satisfaction and experience with network providers.

Perspectives of Assessment

Overall, methods may be characterized in terms of those that assess the quality of care relative to a positive standard (i.e., what should have been done), and those that assess it relative to a negative standard (i.e., what should not have been done). As an example of the latter, prescription patterns can be especially useful after drugs that are ineffective or hazardous have been identified. Assessments that focus on unnecessary or inappropriate care can be conducted prospectively (before care is provided) or retrospectively (after care is provided). For example, if we use unnecessary surgical procedures as an indicator of poor quality of care, second surgical opinions would provide a prospective quality measure (how often does the second opinion contradict the first physician's recommendation?). Tissue analysis provides a retrospective method of using the same indicator, unnecessary surgery (how often does the tissue analysis indicate that a healthy organ was removed?).

Utilization review is another example of quality assessment and assurance that identifies cases of poor quality or inappropriate care. Inappropriate hospital usage may arise from inappropriate admissions, delayed discharges, or extra days during which services are not fully provided (Donabedian, 1985). Rehospitalizations after hospital discharge may be used as an indicator of poor quality, that is, of the patient's being released too quickly.

PROMOTING QUALITY: ASSURANCE AND IMPROVEMENT

Measuring the quality of care does not result in immediate improvements in that care. Simply defining what is meant by high-quality care does not assure the measures to guarantee its implementation will be undertaken. Practice guidelines are established, yet little attention is paid to helping practitioners learn how to use and implement those guidelines (Laffell & Berwick, 1992). Quality-promotion activities—including assurance and improvement—are intended to translate the concepts and findings of quality assessment into programs that will improve the quality of care. The rest of this chapter is devoted to methods of controlling and improving the quality of care.

Quality Assurance Mechanisms

Regardless of the mechanism for assessment, there are different approaches to trying to ensure that care will be of high quality. Three such approaches of the structural type that have been used for quite some time are licensing, accreditation, and certification. They are similar in that they intend to assess an individual's or institution's ability to provide quality care on the basis of meeting established criteria at a particular time. These criteria include certain characteristics of the institution or individual such as education, experience, staffing patterns, and service availability. In contrast, other approaches promote quality by reviewing specific instances of provider-patient interaction. These approaches, used for example by peer review organizations and the malpractice litigation system, tend to focus on the processes and outcomes of care.

Licensing

Licensing is backed by the force of law. Under the U.S. Constitution, states have been empowered to license both individuals and institutions, and to restrict the performance of certain activities (e.g., surgery or a dental exam) to those individuals and institutions that it has determined meet defined standards. Occupations that are licensed by all states include medicine, dentistry, pharmacy, nursing, nursing home administration, and podiatry. In some states, occupations such as laboratory technicians, midwives, and psychologists are also licensed. Generally, each profession establishes standards for educational attainment, experience, and performance on a written exam that each applicant must meet.

Individual licensure as a method of ensuring quality is a source of great controversy. Rather than protecting the public, licensure may protect the professional group and its members from competition and public scrutiny, and make it difficult to change occupations within the health care sector, or to move from one state to another. There is little evidence to indicate that application of the criteria used in licensing can actually predict the quality of care delivered.

Licensing of facilities is usually accomplished by a state agency, for example, the state health department. All states license hospitals (short- and long-stay, general, and/or psychiatric), nursing homes, and pharmacies; many also license facilities for the mentally ill or developmentally disabled (Wilson & Neuhauser, 1987). Certain services, such as ambulance and home health care, are also licensed in some states. The criteria for licensing typically emphasize structural elements like nurse/bed ratios and the presence of appropriate equipment.

Accreditation and Certification

Although licensing is critical to understanding the role of government in the assurance of quality, voluntary self-regulation has long provided a primary approach to quality assurance in health care (Luke & Modrow, 1983). This approach is reflected both in accrediting bodies for institutions, such as the JCAHO, and in professional certification boards. Accreditation is limited to institutions, whereas certification applies to individuals.

The basic principles of accreditation are similar to those of licensure; it is assumed that if the institution meets certain standards of physical and organizational structure, then good-quality care will be delivered at that time and will continue into the future. Although accreditation is not a legal procedure, there are strong legal and financial incentives for undergoing accreditation. For example, state education departments will not recognize diplomas from medical schools that are not accredited.

The JCAHO is perhaps the oldest and best known of the accrediting bodies in health care. As already noted, recent changes in the Joint Commission's accrediting standards are reflective of shifts in the approach to quality taken throughout the field. Traditionally reliant on minimal structural standards, JCAHO rewrote its standards to raise them from the "minimal essential" to the "optimal achievable" level.

The NCQA is the accrediting organization for HMOs, as well as the developer of the Health Plan Employer Data and Information Set (HEDIS). Started in the late 1970s as a creation of the managed care industry, NCQA became an independent body in the early 1990s. Just as the JCAHO came to define what is good quality of care for hospitals, the NCQA has increasingly become the arbiter of good quality for HMOs. As of 1996, 57% of all HMOs operating in the country had asked for accreditation. Compared to the JCAHO process, denials and provisional accreditation were common ("NCQA," 1996). The NCQA accreditation process gives enormous weight to quality improvement indicators (evidence that improvements are being made) and the ongoing monitoring of performance. Accreditation also plays a critical role in medical education. Medical schools are accredited by the Liaison Committee on Medical Education, made up of representatives from the American Medical Association and the Association of American Medical Colleges. Training for other health care occupations also takes place in accredited programs or schools.

Certification, like accreditation, represents a form of voluntary self-regulation, and although certification is not backed by law, there are incentives that encourage individual practitioners to seek certification. For example, most hospitals limit privileges to board-certified specialties. Certification uses standards of education, experience, and achievement on examinations to determine qualification.

PSROs and PROS

Professional Standard Review Organizations (PSROs) were established by the 1972 amendments to the Social Security Act. The purpose of the law was to involve local practicing physicians in the ongoing review and evaluation of health services covered by the Medicare, Medicaid, and Maternal and Child Health Programs of the U.S. Department of Health and Human Services. Although PSROs were charged with the dual role of quality assurance and utilization review, most PSRO activity focused on utilization review and cost containment rather than on overall quality assurance.

In 1984, peer review organizations (PROs) became the successor to the PSROs. Unlike PSROs, PROs reviewed only Medicare; Medicaid review was left to the states. Physician-based organizations were given a prominent role in the control of the PROs, which were awarded fixed-price contracts that specified, in numerical terms, the results to be achieved. For example, some PROs focused on reducing inappropriate admissions; others focused on reducing admissions overall. Because of the specific nature of the objectives, PROs were given an increased incentive to actually try to change physician behavior. The results, however, have been disappointing. For example, an independent review of medical records for hospitalized Medicare patients found that approximately 18% of them had received below standard care; yet the PRO had found only 6.3% (Rubin, Rogers, Kahn, Rubinstein, & Brook, 1992).

Malpractice Litigation

Malpractice litigation may also be seen as an approach to quality assurance by focusing on extreme instances of poor-quality care. Using it as a tool for quality assurance shifts the focus away from frequent but low-cost errors toward infrequent and high-cost ones.

Several studies have suggested that malpractice litigation may not be an effective tool for identifying problems in the quality of health care. The Harvard Medical Practice Study found that in a random sample of more than 30,000 cases, approximately 1% had evidence of an adverse event that was caused by negligence (Localio, Lawthers, Brennan, Laird, Herbert, Peterson, et al., 1991). Yet malpractice claims were filed in only about 1.5% of these latter cases. Given the relative rarity of malpractice claims, only very incompetent physicians could be identified in this way (Rolph, Kravitz, & McGuigan, 1991). In a more recent study in Colorado and Utah, using data from 1992, medical malpractice claims data were linked with clinical data from a review of 14,700 medical records (Studdert et al., 2000). The study found poor correlation between actual medical negligence and the filing of malpractice claims; the incidence of negligent adverse events exceeded the incidence of resulting malpractice claims by 40:1. The study also found that when a physician was sued, there was a high probability that it would be for rendering nonnegligent care. The authors concluded that the malpractice system demonstrated an inability to deter injury-causing medical practice and did not compensate most patients injured by substandard care. In addition, they stated that subjecting physicians to meritless malpractice claims is costly, wasteful, burdensome, and unjust, while at the same time most victims of medical negligence are never compensated for their injuries.

Economic Approaches and the Managed Care Context

"The problem with using incentives to shape physicians' behavior is the bluntness of the method" (Berwick, 1996). Although such activities are often primarily concerned with cost containment, they serve a quality assurance function to the degree that they reduce unnecessary or excessive use of care. Second surgical opinion programs, preadmission review, and diagnosis-related groups (DRGs) all aim to reduce costs by eliminating unnecessary or excessive care. Most broadly, capitated payments—wherein the provider is paid for the ongoing care of the patient rather than for individual instances of care—may be seen as the strongest economic incentive to eliminate duplication, waste, and unnecessary services.

Unfortunately, economic solutions seem to have as much impact on appropriate care as they do on inappropriate care (Brook, 1988). Evidence from the RAND Health Insurance Experiment suggests that cost sharing for inpatient and outpatient care reduces the use of effective and presumably needed services about as much as it lowers the use of ineffective or unnecessary services (Lohr et al., 1988). Before cost-containment efforts can be expected to have a positive impact on quality, *economic solutions must be coupled with medical solutions.* Some have argued that medicine must be codified (Brook [1988] called for a "gourmet cookbook" of practice guidelines) and physicians must be rewarded for appropriate medical practice.

An example of an economic approach that led to poor outcomes was limiting the number of prescriptions to three per patient per month for New Hampshire Medicaid recipients. The outcome was more institutionalization and increased Medicaid costs. There was a 220% increase in nursing home admissions, greatly exceeding the 35% decrease in drug costs. In fact, the increased health care costs were 17 times higher than the drug cost savings. The program was cancelled after 9 months (Soumerai, 1991, 1994).

Another example of a failed economic approach to improving quality/ containing costs comes from a study called the Managed Care Outcomes Project. This study followed 15,000 HMO patients with at least one of five specified diseases for a year. It found that several common HMO cost-containment practices were associated with lower quality of care, such as higher numbers of emergency department visits and hospitalizations. For example, limiting access to medications through stricter drug formularies was associated with higher health service utilization, including more office visits, more emergency department visits, more hospitalizations, and even more drug use and cost (Horn et al., 1996; Horn, Sharkey, & Gassaway, 1996). Also, in some instances drug use limitation affected elderly more than nonelderly (Horn, Sharkey, & Phillips-Harris, 1998).

A recent study of almost 23,000 Medicare patients enrolled in three settings within one managed care organization found that, after controlling for age, gender, and severity of illness, pharmaceutical capitation patients had 14% higher total health costs than noncapitated patients (an additional $376 per patient per year) and 29% higher pharmaceutical costs (an additional $110 per patient per year) (Popovian et al., 1999). Thus, using capitation reimbursement mechanisms to influence quality may not work either. One economic approach that may result in better quality is called "pay-for-performance." Pay-for-performance basically involves a return to fee-for-service but with added performance incentives focused on *paying for the value received.* An example is when a payer indexes payments to the provider on something like a Resource-Based Relative Value Scale (RBRVS) and gives the provider 80% of RBRVS. However, the payer may also give providers the opportunity to earn up to 125% of RBRVS by clearly demonstrating a series of measurable behaviors and results related to high-quality care and outcomes (*Medical Network Strategy Report,* 1997). Also, some employers, such as Merrill Lynch, are finding that expanding health care benefits and using clinical guidelines (see below) to deliver care, but not restricting access to services, including not requiring use of generic drugs, has lowered total health care costs *Wall Street Journal,* 2000).

Technological Approaches

The growth in sophisticated computer technologies offers new promise to those concerned with quality assurance. New information systems can greatly modify provider practice, improve information dissemination, and prevent individual instances of error. In a study examining the impact of "computer alerts" on individual patient care, Safran, Rind, and Davis (1996) found that the computer generated prompts to practitioners based on clinical practice guidelines programmed into the computer significantly improved the care of HIV-infected patients and promoted the adoption of practice guidelines. Another study examining the effects of implementation of an antibiotic practice guideline through computer-assisted decision-making support found that patient-level computer-assisted guidelines can improve quality of care. Although about twice the number of patients received antibiotics in the treatment year compared to the control study year; the costs of antibiotics decreased about $350,000; the antibiotic-associated adverse drug events decreased by 30%; and the mortality rate decreased about 1% (Pestotnik, Chassen, Evans, & Burke, 1996). Technology holds much promise for quality improvement.

QUALITY ASSURANCE THROUGH THE CONTINUOUS QUALITY IMPROVEMENT (CQI) FRAMEWORK

Dramatic shifts in the activities surrounding quality promotion have resulted from the widespread adoption of the Continuous Quality Improvement (CQI) paradigm. The thrust of CQI, based on the industrial concepts of Total Quality Management (TQM), is to integrate methods of measurement and assessment with those of change and improvement on an ongoing basis in the operation of the enterprise. The Deming Cycle—plan, do, check, act, and analyze—was invented by and named for the creator of TQM (the American industrial engineer, Edwards Deming) (Gabor, 1990). CQI uses statistical methods to raise the norm of performance, rather than to weed out "bad apples" (Joint Commission, 1991). The goal is to obtain more uniform, or predictable, results through the analysis of process (Gabor, 1990).

Whereas the quality assurance methods discussed above, such as licensure and certification, have traditionally relied on fixed minimal standards, CQI encourages change and growth. While PROs have relied on punitive actions to enforce their recommendations, CQI requires collaboration, cooperation, and compromise. Quality improvement "does not seek to identify errors in order to assign blame, but instead assumes that faulty systems of care are very often responsible for errors" (Chassin, 1996). The use of sophisticated methods of measurement and statistical analyses are, slowly, becoming the everyday tool of managers, who can feed information back to practitioners in order to help them enhance their manner of care. If CQI is to fulfill its promise, the delivery of high-quality care must be the central goal of all players in the health care field. The promise made by CQI is noble. It remains to be seen whether it has the ability to transform the health care delivery system.

QUALITY IMPROVEMENT THROUGH THE CLINICAL PRACTICE IMPROVEMENT FRAMEWORK

One challenge presented by the usual CQI studies is the limited range of data they often use. Clinical Practice Improvement (CPI) is a new multidimensional outcomes methodology that has direct application to the clinical management of individual patients. It is designed to overcome the barriers presented by the limited availability of patient, process, and outcomes data in CQI studies. Clinicians in actual practice help create a large database of detailed patient and treatment/process variables that are important elements of the particular problem under study, reflecting the complexity of clinical practice and the multiple variables that affect patient outcomes. Multivariate statistical techniques identify clinically relevant relationships that explain complex clinical phenomena. The multidisciplinary nature of the CPI inquiry involves many different types of clinicians who participate in posing clinically relevant questions, determining what variables will be measured, and implementing decisions about the treatment and care process based on the data. Clinicians who treat patients develop the definitions of all the study variables so that they understand exactly how to change their practices based on the findings of the study.

CPI methodology encompasses a comprehensive view of the complex care process. By collecting and analyzing measures of patient differences (e.g., physiologic severity of illness and psychosocial derangements presented at each visit or at each admission), care process steps (i.e., all treatments that are part of the care process for that condition and patient), and outcome variables, clinicians can evaluate objectively the effects of the treatments they give to similarly ill patients. Without all three types of data from the care process (e.g., if one has only process and outcome data, but not detailed patient data), clinicians cannot tell if the outcomes achieved are due to the process steps or to differences in patient severity levels (see Figure 14.1).

Dimensions in a Clinical Practice Improvement Study Design

Patient Variables

Patient variables are key characteristics of the study population: demographics, specific indications for treatment, severity of illness, psychosocial factors, etc. Within a well-defined group of similarly ill patients, one would expect that care processes of equal effectiveness would result in similar outcomes. In order to have enough detail describing patients and their needs so that clinicians will agree to stabilize their processes of care, one usually requires disease-specific physiologic data, such as those contained in the inpatient and outpatient components of the Comprehensive Severity Index (CSI®) (Horn, Buckle, & Carver, 1988; Horn, Sharkey, Buckle, Backsten, Averill, & Horn, 1991; Horn, 1995; Horn, Sharkey, & Levy, 1995; Horn, Sharkey, & Gassaway, 1996; Horn, Sharkey, Stacy, et al., 1996; Horn, 1997; Iezzoni, 1998). Detailed physiologic severity data are needed to create decidable and executable treatment protocols that are based on signs and symptoms found in patients.

Medical Care Process Variables

A process of care is a sequence of linked steps designed to produce a set of desired medical outcomes. For CPI, the goal is to find a measurable factor that describes each major process step. Examples include which drugs are dispensed, what dose, what route of administration, and what duration; how often prescriptions are filled; etc. Timing data are collected for all process steps.

Outcome Variables

Processes of care should be designed to achieve specific patient outcomes. Among the outcomes commonly assessed are diagnosis-specific complications, adverse events, diagnosis-specific long-term medical outcomes (that may be assessed by both clinicians and patients), patient functional status, patient satisfaction, and cost. Outcomes may be thought of as analogs of the assessment endpoints in a randomized controlled trial.

Analytic Methods Used in Clinical Practice Improvement

A CPI study database typically includes a great many variables that describe patient characteristics, processes of care, and patient outcomes. When more

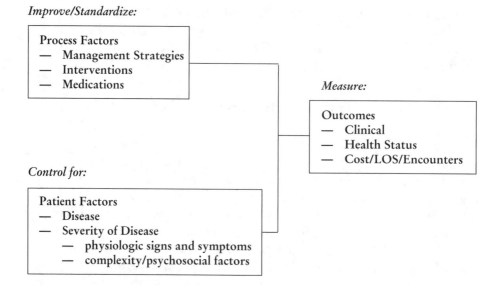

Improve/Standardize:

Process Factors
— Management Strategies
— Interventions
— Medications

Measure:

Outcomes
— Clinical
— Health Status
— Cost/LOS/Encounters

Control for:

Patient Factors
— Disease
— Severity of Disease
— physiologic signs and symptoms
— complexity/psychosocial factors

FIGURE 14.1   Three essential components for a Clinical Practice Improvement study.

than three or four patient and process (independent) variables must be taken into account, multiple regression analysis is used to model the effects of these factors on the outcome (dependent) variables. Multivariate statistical methods allow comparisons of alternative treatments while controlling for other variables that may be driving observed differences between the outcomes of the treatments. These statistical methods allow the researcher to examine relationships far more complex than those defined using only one or two explanatory variables at a time. The coefficients of the independent variables in the regression equations identify key process steps that, when controlling for patient factors, are associated with better outcomes. Interactions of certain process steps with other process steps or patient variables can be modeled explicitly.

Clinical Practice Improvement Goes Beyond Outcomes Research

Outcomes research typically uses large, existing insurance claims databases to find better or worse outcomes and to flag outcome failures (poor outcomes beyond some statistical threshold) such as high mortality rates. But most outcomes research does not scientifically relate the outcomes to detailed process steps and does not control for differences in severity of illness of patients having the same diagnosis code(s), so it is unclear what is driving the outcomes.

In addition, concerns about the completeness, accuracy, and relevance of large claims databases raise questions about their appropriateness as a basis for health services research, performance monitoring (such as identification and reduction of medical errors), or inspiring changes in clinical practice (Fisher et al., 1992; Hannan, Kilburn, Lindsey, & Lewis, 1992; Iezzoni, Burnside, Sickles, Moskowitz, Sawitz, & Levine, 1988; Jollis, Ancukiewicz, DeLong, Pryor, Muhlbaier, & Menk, 1993; Kennedy, Stern, & Crawford, 1984). A fundamental problem exists with outcomes data: data collected for one purpose (e.g., claims administration) may not be useful for other purposes (e.g., outcomes research) if they lack reliable detailed information about patient differences and medical care processes.

Clinical Practice Improvement Goes Beyond Guidelines

Because most clinical practices have no firm basis in published scientific research, developers of clinical guidelines often resort to expert consensus. But expert consensus is an inexact tool even when generated using formal methods. Different consensus groups often develop different, even conflicting, guidelines on the same topic (Audet, Greenfield, & Field, 1990; Kellie & Kelly, 1991; Leape, Park, Kahan, & Brook, 1992). And within a single consensus panel, the experts often disagree, and their assessments change when guidelines developed in a theoretical setting are applied to real patients (Park et al., 1989). Perhaps most troubling, physician experts show wide disagreement when they assess underlying probabilities essential to consensus judgments (Eddy, 1984; 1992; O'Connor, Plume, Beck, et al., 1988).

Most of the effort to develop guidelines is characterized by two weaknesses that hamper their relevance to local practice reform:

- Guidelines are developed nationally or centrally, based on expert consensus and literature review/synthesis.
- Guidelines are often too general or inconclusive to be useful to clinicians and do not address subgroups within a sample.

Thus, clinicians are unwilling to follow many current guidelines.

At present, "evidence-based" methods of guideline development are favored over consensus-based methods. However, the patient populations the "evidence" comes from (usually as a result of randomized controlled trials) are often different from those in which local translations of the guideline will be used. Since evidence-based guidelines must be all things to all people, they are often encyclopedic and equivocal. They are not decidable (they give a vague description of the patient) and are not executable (they give a menu of process steps to follow) and thus frequently do not have credibility with local clinicians. CPI provides the necessary data from everyday practice to develop decidable and executable guidelines, that is, guidelines that give specific process steps to follow based on deviations of a patient's signs and symptoms from normal values.

Clinical Practice Improvement Differs
from Randomized Controlled Trials (RCTs)

The randomized controlled trial (RCT) has a long history as the gold standard for establishing causality in scientific research. Randomization of study patients to the intervention/nonintervention groups being studied, in order to diminish potential selection bias and strict control of the intervention(s) of interest, are important tools for scientists of all types. However, the use of RCTs has been limited in some domains of inquiry because of problems such as

- ethical or practical inability to randomize patients to intervention/nonintervention groups or to control the specificity of the intervention to be studied;
- prohibitive cost when sizes of study groups are extremely large; and
- exclusion of large numbers of individuals who do not meet strict inclusion criteria. Therefore, patients in the initial study population with either secondary problems or more severe disease are often rejected from the trial, resulting that only a small percentage of patients—usually 10%–15%—are eligible for most trials. The idea is to eliminate all patients whose characteristics might adversely affect or bias the outcome of the comparison between the treatment and the control arm.

The alternative study designs used in Clinical Practice Improvement provide a pragmatic balance of study cost, clinician participation, rapid patient accrual, and the need for timely information vs. potential bias. Achieving this balance is especially important when examining operational process-of-care factors (in contrast to testing new treatments) and when data collection systems routinely track patient and process factors, so that invalid inferences are likely to be found and corrected over time.

RCTs use a protocol document to create an artificial practice environment that allows for valid statistical inference. While that structure eliminates practice variation, it usually covers a very limited subset of patients and practices. CPI addresses the same issues—practice variation and valid statistical inference—from another point of view. In a CPI study, valid statistical inference is possible because in large populations, groups of similar patients receive the same treatment. RCTs also tend to be limited in time; in most circumstances, they explicitly modify clinician behavior only for the duration of a study and only for the individuals directly involved in the trial. In contrast, CPI establishes a feedback loop aimed at all clinicians in an institution. It integrates research into daily practice, giving individual clinicians the information necessary to understand and modify their own activities at a detailed, operational level. CPI analyses help providers evaluate current practices and use the results to develop fact-based quality improvements. Changes to the process of care rest on clinical data rather than on clinical opinion.

The design of a CPI study allows for the inclusion of large numbers of patients likely to have been excluded from an RCT, thus improving generalizability and external validity. The ability to measure patient severity and control for confounding variables across multiple domains permits identification of associations rather than causality; however, the results of sensitivity analyses and the concurrence of findings with other research can help to determine whether the identified associations are real and are relevant to existing practices (Magi, Douglas, & Schwartz, 1996; Pestotnik et al., 1996).

Advantages of Clinical Practice Improvement Methodology

A key advantage of CPI methodology is the naturalistic view of medical treatment that is provided by retrospective data recorded routinely by medical providers. This view is critical to determine the implications and outcomes of treatment alternatives. In everyday practice, patients are assigned to different treatments based on the provider's medical judgment; patient compliance is not artificially influenced; and monitoring of results is based on the provider's need for information about how a patient is doing. All these factors can impact the effectiveness of medical treatment. This retrospective view is in direct contrast to that of traditional randomized controlled trials. Because their participants are screened, selected, and subjected to scrutiny and intervention beyond that occurring in everyday treatment, RCTs sometimes report results that are not broadly applicable in everyday medical treatment.

A second key advantage of CPI study methodology is cost. Using existing data from medical records and computerized databases is generally much less costly than implementing a prospective RCT. Other advantages of retrospective data include the large number of observations that can be available for analysis and the usefulness of the data for hypothesis generation and refinement.

There are numerous examples of areas where CPI studies have discovered process steps associated with the same or better clinical outcomes while reducing cost. For example, implementation of process changes based on a CPI study of adult patients (>18 years) undergoing abdominal surgery, resulted in fewer wound infections, less increase in severity of illness during hospitalization, a decrease in length of stay by more than 1.5 days for bowel surgery patients and by more than 2.0 days for appendectomy patients, and a calculated decrease in cost of $4,000/patient (Horn, 1997). One of the process steps that was associated with better outcomes related to nutrition. Even though they were sicker (had higher severity of illness scores), those patients fed early (within 48 hours after surgery) and sufficiently (greater than 60% of their protein and calorie needs) had between 1.4 and 2.9 days shorter average length of stay and between $1,940 and $5,281 lower average cost per case than patients fed either not early and/or not sufficiently. In another study, CPI-developed process changes resulted in pressure ulcer prevention at a rate of 302/year for a $1,268,400 cost savings/year in one hospital setting (Horn, 1997). Similar improved outcomes occurred when CPI methodology was used to create protocols for the use of heparin in adult patients with deep vein thrombosis (Horn, 1997). In a study of 762 asthma patients, extensive variation in practice was found across 10 pediatric hospitals regardless of severity of illness. If the best practices discovered in the CPI study were used in each study institution, we would expect less increase in severity during the stay, along with, on average, a 0.5 day decrease in length of stay and a $1,679 decrease in cost per case. In a study of 804 bronchiolitis patients, extensive variation in practice was again found across the same 10 pediatric hospitals, regardless of severity of illness. If the best practices discovered in this CPI study were used in each study institution, we would expect less increase in severity during the stay along with, on average, a 2.0 day decrease in length of stay and a $4,982 decrease in cost per case (Willson, Horn, Smout, Gassaway, & Torres, 2000; Willson, Horn, Hendley, Smout, & Gassaway, in press).

Recent literature has supported the use of well-designed observational studies such as CPI to discover what works best in medicine. Two separate studies found that treatment effects from observational studies and randomized controlled trials were remarkably similar (Benson & Hartz, 2000; Concato, Shah, & Horwitz, 2000). Both studies concluded that they found little evidence that estimates of treatment effects in well-designed observational studies were either consistently larger than or qualitatively different from those obtained in randomized, controlled trials. These findings should encourage greater use of the CPI methodology in future studies.

Today, data needed to conduct a Clinical Practice Improvement study are typically abstracted by hand from existing paper medical records. In the future, most hospitals will use computerized clinical information systems (CIS). Then, rather than relying on labor-intensive manual data abstraction, the needed patient, process, and outcome data will be found electronically in the hospitals' CISs. The efficiency and logistics of this new data acquisition modality will make it easier and less costly to conduct iterative Clinical Practice Improvement studies to determine best practices. Also, the resulting empirical evidence-based dynamic protocols can be programmed into hospitals' clinical information systems to flag for clinicians the appropriate protocol steps for a specific combination of patient signs and symptoms. This should result in more consistent implementation of protocol steps than without these flags. Although the up-front costs of clinical information systems may be high, they have the potential to decrease the cost of health care by 30%–50%, as demonstrated in various CPI studies.

Summary of CPI

Clinical Practice Improvement studies involve a rigorous form of quasi-experimental research. Quasi-experimental designs cover a variety of strategies that need not include a control group or random assignment. Although they are weaker than RCTs on internal validity, Clinical Practice Improvement studies better represent actual conditions of practice, and they cost less and take less time. Because they do not require homogeneous patient populations, they can include patients with comorbidities or complications. To avoid confounding the link between the interventions and patient outcomes, they measure relevant patient characteristics using severity assessment tools and statistically adjust for treatment variations by carefully monitoring and measuring actual treatments; they then use these data in the statistical analyses. Because this approach does not disqualify large numbers of patients, it facilitates generation of the number of cases needed for comparisons. Using multiple regression and other statistical techniques, researchers test which process steps are associated with desirable quality and cost outcomes for different kinds of patients. Clinical Practice Improvement studies are designed to be replicated easily so they can be undertaken at multiple sites.

Methodology alternatives such as CPI do not replace the RCT, but rather provide additional sources of systematic outcomes information that improve on the anecdotal and informal knowledge base that underlies much of clinical practice. Clinical Practice Improvement studies used by clinical teams have enormous power to enable health care providers, managed care organizations, and individuals to evaluate current practice and improve clinical decision making. The CPI methodology can be used in all health care settings. To date, CPI has been used to study various medical and surgical conditions in inpatient settings, including congestive heart failure, asthma and bronchiolitis (in children), coronary artery bypass graft surgery, abdominal surgery, bone marrow transplant, and colon cancer. In ambulatory settings CPI has been used to study asthma, congestive heart failure, hypertension, ulcers, arthritis, and ear infections. In long-term care, CPI has been used to study prevention and treatment of pressure ulcers and optimal treatment for residents with dementia. In rehabilitation, CPI is being used to study post-stroke rehabilitation. And in hospice, CPI is being used to study pain control, dyspnea control, and self-determined life closure. For more information see web site: www.isisicor.com.

ORGANIZATIONAL CONSIDERATIONS IN PROMOTING QUALITY

In order to assure good-quality care, we also need to know something about changing or modifying the behaviors of providers and the organizations in which they practice. Organizational change creates strain and tension; it raises conflict between the norms of professional freedom and bureaucratic autonomy (Hetherington, 1982).

Professional autonomy has been one of the most important impediments to health institutions becoming more fully accountable for the care they provide. Physicians have traditionally operated as free agents within the hospital structure. As quality assurance activities have grown, however, new restrictions and requirements have been imposed on physicians. Accountability obligations of health institutions have been formalized and the economic imperatives have become explicit. Thus, the potential for conflict has grown between institutional goals of self-regulation and survival and the autonomy requirements of clinicians.

Even within the context of a change-resistant environment, we know a great deal about the ways in which health care delivery can be modified. For example, we know that quality-promotion activities are more likely to succeed when professionals play an active role in developing the study questions, creating the study variables, assisting in data analyses, and administering the empirical evidence-based protocols. Evidence suggests that to change physician behavior, information must come from a credible source (Ball, 1988).

Within the continuous quality improvement (CQI) framework, organizational change must begin with commitment at the very top of the organization (Berwick, 1988). Quality improvement requires resources, and that the methods of quality measurement be taught and learned. Traditional quality assurance methods that attempt to identify and discipline an unruly few are antithetical to true improvement, which emphasizes change in the overall system and its processes. In this model, fear must be replaced by shared commitment and trust. CPI offers a methodology to accomplish this.

CURRENT ISSUES AND QUESTIONS

Who Should Define Quality?

Who shall define quality of care? Is it, ultimately, the consumers who decide the critical elements of what constitutes good quality? Or, will health care professionals continue to play the leading role? How will differing perspectives—of government, insurers, providers, and consumers of care—be reconciled? Will a negotiated definition of quality care satisfy any of the key constituents?

Who Should Assure Quality?

Who is, ultimately, responsible for assuring that high-quality care is provided? What role should government play? Is this to be a federal or state responsibility? How will individual institutions and organizations balance their responsibility for ensuring the quality of care against the responsibility of individual health care providers? In a rapidly changing environment, who will make sure that consumers are receiving the best possible health care?

Why Is There Poor Quality?

What are the organizational structures and systems that are associated with more quality problems? How much of poor quality is due to staffing factors, such as lack of sufficient training or too few qualified staff to handle the level of patient care needs? How much of poor quality is due to lack of a scientific basis for care delivered?

What Should Be Done About Poor Quality?

Today, the tools exist to discover what treatments work best for specific patient types. Computers can evaluate many variables simultaneously to help make these complicated assessments. A paradigm shift that encourages health care providers to spend 90% of their time treating patients and 10% of their time involved in studies to discover how to improve quality of care, would greatly benefit health care in particular, and society in general.

CASE STUDY

You are the medical director of a cardiology clinic and find that there is large variation in the number of hospitalizations for your congestive heart failure patients. You wonder how much of the variation in hospitalization rates is due to differences in patient severity of illness and how much of the variation is due to differences in patient treatments, patient psychosocial factors, organizational structure factors, etc.

You decide to do a study to determine why the hospitalization rates vary so much and what areas to target to reduce that variation if appropriate. Who would you include on a team to study this question? What patient, treatment, organization, and provider variables would you measure to determine the strongest predictors of higher hospitalization rates?

DISCUSSION QUESTIONS

1. Provide at least two indicators of quality based on structure, on process, and on outcomes. What are their strengths and weaknesses?
2. Can a physician be the "best" if patients are dissatisfied with the care that they receive?
3. In what ways does the CPI study methodology represent a real shift in the approach to quality assurance?
4. What barriers are overcome using the CPI methodology?
5. How are quality assurance activities affected by the move away from solo practice medicine?
6. What are the most critical factors to consider in designing a program for quality improvement?

REFERENCES

Audet, A. M., Greenfield, S., & Field, M. (1990). Medical practice guidelines: Current activities and future directions. *Annals of Internal Medicine, 113*(9), 709–714.

Averill, R. F., McGuire, T. E., Manning, B. E., Fowler, D. A., Horn, S. D., Dickson, P. S., Coye, M. J., Knowlton, D. L., & Bender, J. A. (1992). A study of the relationship between severity of illness and hospital cost in New Jersey hospitals. *Health Services Research, 27*(5), 587–617.

Baine, D. P. (1987, July 21). *Department of Defense health care.* Statement given by the General Accounting Office before the U.S. House of Representatives Subcommittee on Military Personnel and Compensation, Washington, DC.

Ball, J. R. (1988, June). *Physician payment: Why money doesn't buy quality.* Paper presented at the Association for Health Services Research, San Francisco, CA.

Benson, K., & Hartz, A. J. (2000). A comparison of observational studies and randomized, controlled trials. *New England Journal of Medicine, 342*(25), 1878–1886.

Berwick, D. M. (1988). Quality assurance and measurement principles: The perspective of one health maintenance organization. In E. F. X. Hughes (Ed.), *Perspectives of quality in American health care* (pp. 203–210). Washington, DC: McGraw-Hill's Healthcare Information Center.

Berwick, D. M. (1996). Quality of health care, part 5: Payment by capitation and the quality of care. *New England Journal of Medicine, 335,* 1227–1231.

Blum, H. L. (1974). Evaluating health care. *Medical Care, 12,* 999–1011.

Blumenthal, D. (1996). Quality of health care, part 4: The origins of the quality-of-care debate. *New England Journal of Medicine, 335,* 1146–1149.

Brook, R. H., Park, R. E., Chassin, M. R., Solomon, D. H., Keesey, J., & Kosecoff, J. (1990). Predicting the appropriate use of carotid endarterectomy, upper gastrointestinal endoscopy and coronary angiography. *New England Journal of Medicine, 323,* 1173–1177.

Brook, R. H. (1988, June). *Physician payment: Why money doesn't buy quality.* Paper presented at the Association for Health Services Research, San Francisco, CA.

Caper, P. (1988). Defining quality in medical care. *Health Affairs, 7,* 49–61.

Chassin, M. R. (1991). Quality of care: Time to act. *Journal of the American Medical Association, 266,* 3472–3473.

Chassin, M. R. (1996). Quality of health care, part 3: Improving the quality of care. *New England Journal of Medicine, 335,* 1060–1063.

Chassin, M. R. (1997). Assessing strategies for quality improvement. *Health Affairs, 16,* 151–161.

Christoffel, T. (1976). Medical care evaluation: An old idea. *Journal of Medical Education, 51*(2), 83–88.

Cleary, P. D., Keroy, L., Karapanos, G., & McMullen, W. (1989). Patient assessments of hospital care. *Quality Review Bulletin, 15*(6), 172–179.

Concato, J., Shah, N., & Horwitz, R. I. (2000). Randomized, controlled trials, observational studies, and the hierarchy of research designs. *New England Journal of Medicine, 342*(25), 1887–1892.

Danziger, S.K. (1986). The use of expertise in doctor-patient encounters during pregnancy. In P. Conrad & R. Kern (Eds.), *The sociology of health and illness.* New York: St. Martin's Press.

Davies, A. R., & Ware, J. E., Jr. (1988). Involving consumers in quality of care assessment. *Health Affairs, 7*(1), 33–48.

Donabedian, A. (1980). *Explorations in quality assessment and monitoring (volume I): The definition of quality and approaches to its assessment.* Ann Arbor, MI: Health Administration Press.

Donabedian, A. (1985). *Explorations in quality assessment and monitoring (volume II): The methods and findings of quality assessment and monitoring.* Ann Arbor, MI: Health Administration Press.

Eddy, D. M. (1984). Variations in physician practice: The role of uncertainty. *Health Affairs, 3,* 74.

Eddy, D. M. (1992). *A manual for assessing health practices and designing practice policies.* Philadelphia: The American College of Physicians.

Eddy, D. M., & Billings, J. (1988). The quality of medical evidence: Implication for quality of care. *Health Affairs, 7*(1), 19–32.

Enthoven, A. C., & Vorhaus, C. B. (1997). A vision of quality in health care delivery. *Health Affairs, 16*(3), 44–57.

Expansion of pay-for-performance will change the way payers compensate health systems. (1997). *Medical Network Strategy Report, 6*(7), 1–8.

Fisher, E. S., Whaley, F. S., Krushat, W. M., Malenka, D. J., Fleming, C., Baron, J. A., & Hsia, D. C. (1992). The accuracy of Medicare's hospital claims data: Progress has been made, but problems remain. *American Journal of Public Health, 82*(2), 243–248.

Gabel, J. (1997). Marketwatch: Ten ways HMOs have changed during the 1990s. *Health Affairs, 16,* 134–145.

Gabor, A. (1990). *The man who discovered quality.* New York: Penguin Books.

Gerbert, B. (1988, June 28). *Validity of patient report: A comparison with other methods of physician quality assessment.* Paper presented at the Association for Health Services Research conference, San Francisco, CA.

Gerbert, B., Stone, G., Stulborg, M., Gullian, D. S., & Greenfield, S. (1988). Agreement among physician assessment methods: Searching for the truth among fallible methods. *Medical Care, 26,* 519–535.

Hannan, E. L., Kilburn, H., Jr., Lindsey, M. L., & Lewis, R. (1992). Clinical versus administrative data bases for CABG surgery. Does it matter? *Medical Care, 30*(10), 892–907.

Hetherington, R. W. (1982). Quality assurance and organizational effectiveness in hospitals. *Health Services Research, 17,* 185–201.

Hogness, J. R. (1985). What about the patient? *New England Journal of Medicine, 313,* 689–690.

Horn, S. D. (1995). Clinical practice improvement: Improving quality and decreasing cost in managed care. *Medical Interface, 8*(7), 60–70.

Horn, S. D. (1997). *Clinical practice improvement methodology: Implementation and evaluation.* New York: Faulkner & Gray.

Horn, S. D., Buckle, J. M., & Carver, C. M. (1988). The ambulatory severity index: Development of an ambulatory case mix system. *Journal of Ambulatory Care Management, 11,* 53–62.

Horn, S. D., Sharkey, P. D., Buckle, J. M., Backofen, J. E., Averill, R. F., & Horn, R. A. (1991). The relationship between severity of illness and hospital length of stay and mortality. *Medical Care, 29,* 305–317.

Horn, S. D., Sharkey, P. D., & Gassaway, J. (1996). Managed care outcomes project: Study design, baseline patient characteristics, and outcome measures. *American Journal of Managed Care, 2*(3), 237–247.

Horn, S. D., Sharkey, P. D., & Levy, R. (1995). A managed care pharmacoeconomic research model based on the managed care outcomes project. *Journal of Pharmacy Practice, 8*(4), 172–177.

Horn, S. D., Sharkey, P. D., & Phillips-Harris, C. (1998). Formulary limitations in the elderly: Results from the Managed Care Outcomes Project. *American Journal of Managed Care, 4,* 1105–1113.

Horn, S. D., Sharkey, P. D., Tracy, D. M., Horn, C. E., James, B., & Goodwin, F. (1996). Intended and unintended consequences of HMO cost containment strategies: Results from the managed care outcomes project. *American Journal of Managed Care, 2*(3), 253–264.

Hueston, W. J., Applegate, J. A., Mansfield, C. J., King, D. E., & McClafin, R. R. (1995). Practice variations between family physicians and obstetricians in the management of low-risk pregnancies. *Journal of Family Practice, 40,* 345–351.

Iezzoni, L. I., Burnside, S., Sickles, L., Moskowitz, M. A., Sawitz, E., & Levine, P. A. (1988). Coding of acute myocardial infarction. Clinical and policy implications. *Annals of Internal Medicine, 109*(9), 745–751.

Iezzoni, L. I. (1998). *Risk adjustment for measuring health care outcomes.* Ann Arbor, MI: Health Administration Press.

Johantgen, M. E., Coffey, R. M., Harris, D. R., Levy, H., & Clinton, J. J. (1995). Treating early-stage breast cancer: Hospital characteristics associated with breast-conserving surgery. *American Journal of Public Health, 85,* 1432–1434.

Joint Commission on Accreditation of Healthcare Organizations. (1991). *An Introduction to quality improvement in health care.* Chicago: Author.

Jollis, J. G., Ancukiewicz, M., DeLong, E. R., Pryor, D. B., Muhlbaier, L. H., & Mark, D. B. (1993). Discordance of databases designed for claims payment versus clinical information systems. Implications for outcomes research. *Annals of Internal Medicine, 119*(8), 844–850.

Kane, R. L., Wales, J., Bernstein, L., Leibowitz, A., & Kaplan, S. (1985). A randomized controlled trial of hospice care. In L. Aiken & B. Kehrer (Eds.), *Evaluation studies review annual* (vol. 10, pp. 159–169). Beverly Hills, CA: Sage.

Kellie, S. E., & Kelly, J. Y. (1991). Medicare peer review organization preprocedure review criteria. *Journal of the American Medical Association, 265*(10), 1265–1270.

Kennedy, G. T., Stern, M. P., & Crawford, M. H. (1984). Miscoding of hospital discharges as acute myocardial infarction: Implication surveillance programs aimed at elucidating trends in coronary artery disease. *American Journal of Cardiology, 53*(8), 1000–1002.

Kent, C., & Jee, M. (1993). Perspectives. Feds, States look for flexible health reform. *Faulkner & Gray's Medicine and Health, 47*(25), Suppl. 4.

Kohn, L. T., Corrigan, J. M., & Donaldson, M. S. (Eds.). (2000). To err is human: Building a safer health system. Washington, DC: National Academy Press.

Laffell, G., & Berwick, D. M. (1992). Quality in health care. *Journal of the American Medical Association, 268,* 407–408.

Leape, L. L., Park, R. E., Kahan, J. P., & Brook, R. N. (1992). Group judgments of appropriateness: The effect of panel composition. *Quality Assurance in Health Care, 4*(2), 151–159.

Localio, A. R., Lawthers, A. G., Brennan, T. A., Laird, N. M. T., Herbert, L. E., Peterson, L. M., Newhorse, J. P., Weiler, P. C., & Hiatt, H. H. (1991). Relation between malpractice claims and adverse events due to negligence: Results of the Harvard Medical Practice Study III. *New England Journal of Medicine, 325,* 245–251.

Lohr, K. N., Yardy, K. D., & Thier, S. (1988). Current issues in quality of care. *Health Affairs, 7*(1), 15–18.

Luke, R. D., & Modrow, R. E. (1983). Professionalism, accountability, and peer review. In R. D. Luke, J. C. Krueger, & R. E. Modrow (Eds.), *Organization and change in health care quality assurance.* Rockville, MD: Aspen Publications.

Magi, D., Douglas, J. M., Jr., & Schwartz, J. S. (1996). Doxycycline compared with Azithromycin for treating women with genital Chlamydia trachomatis infections: An incremental cost-effectiveness analysis. *Annals of Internal Medicine, 124*(4), 389–399.

Medicine and Health, 47(25), 4, June 21, 1993.

Merriam-Websters 7th New Collegiate Dictionary. (1963). Springfield, MA: Merriam-Webster.

Moskowitz, D. (1996). Perspectives. NCQA: Setting the standard in setting the standard. *Faulkner & Gray's Medicine and Health, 50*(35), Suppl. 1–4.

NCQA: Setting the standard in setting standards. (1996). *Medicine and Health: Perspectives.*

O'Connor, G. T., Plume, S. K., Beck, J. T. (1988). What are my chances? It depends on whom you ask. The choice of a prosthetic heart valve. *Journal of Medical Decision Making, 8*(4), 341.

Ogrod, E. S. (1997). Compensation and quality: A physician's view. *Health Affairs, 16*(3), 82–86.

Park, R. E. (1989). Physician ratings of appropriate indications for three procedures: Theoretical indications vs. indications used in practice. *American Journal of Public Health, 79*(4), 445–447.

Pearson, K. (1924). *The life, letter, and labours for Francis Galton* (vol 2.).

Pestotnik, S. L., Classen, D. C., Evans, R. S., & Burke, J. P. (1996). Implementing antibiotic practice guidelines through computer-assisted decision support: Clinical and financial outcomes. *Annals of Internal Medicine, 124*(10), 884–890.

Popovian, R., Johnson, K. A., Nichol, M. B., & Liu, G. (1999). The impact of pharmaceutical capitation to primary medical groups on the health care expenditures of Medicare HMO enrollees. *Journal of Managed Care Research, 5*, 414–419.

Roberts, J. S., Coate, J. E., & Redmen, R. R. (1987). A history of the joint commission on accreditation of hospitals. *Journal of the American Medical Association, 258.*

Rolph, J. F., Kravitz, R. L., & McGuigan, K. (1991). Malpractice claims data as a quality improvement tool; II. Is targeting effective? *Journal of the American Medical Association, 266*, 2093–2097.

Rubin, H. R., Rogers, W. H., Kahn, K. L., Rubinstein, & Brook, R H. (1992). Watching the doctor-watchers: How well do peer review organization methods detect hospital care quality problems? *Journal of the American Medical Association, 267*, 2349–3354.

Safran, C., Rind, D. M., & Davis, R. B. (1996). Effects of a knowledge-based electronic patient record on adherence to practice guidelines. *M.D. Computing, 13*, 55–63.

Shanahan, M. (1983). The quality assurance standard of the JCAH: A rational approach to patient care evaluation. In R. D. Luke, J. L. Krueger, & R. E. Modrow (Eds.), *Organization and change in health care quality assurance.* Rockville, MD: Aspen Publications.

Soumerai, S. B., McLaughlin, T. J., Ross-Degnan, D., Casteris, C. S., & Bollini, P. (1994). Effects of a limit on Medicaid drug-reimbursement benefits on the use of psychotropic agents and acute mental health services by patients with schizophrenia. *New England Journal of Medicine, 331,* 650–655.

Soumerai, S. B., Ross-Degnan, D., Avorn, J., McLaughlin, T. J., & Choodnovskiy, I. (1991). Effects of Medicaid drug-payment limits on admission to hospitals and nursing homes. *New England Journal of Medicine, 325,* 1072–1077.

Studdert, D. M., Thomas, E. J., Burstin, H. R., Zbar, B. I. W., Orav, J., & Brennan, T. A. (2000). Negligent care and malpractice claiming behavior in Utah and Colorado. *Medical Care, 38,* 250–260.

Svarstad, B. L. (1986). Patient-practitioner relationships and compliance with prescribed medical regimens. In L. H. Aiken & D. Mechanic (Eds.), *Applications of social science to clinical medicine and health policy* (pp. 438–459). New Brunswick, NJ: Rutgers University Press.

Thurow, L. C. (1985). Medicine versus economics. *New England Journal of Medicine, 313,* 611–614.

U.S. General Accounting Office. (1996). *Medicare: Federal efforts to enhance quality of care* (GAO: HEHS-96-20). Washington, DC: U.S. GAO Health, Education, and Human Services Division.

The Wall Street Journal, May 23, 2000.

Ware, J. E., Bayliss, M. S., Rogers, W. H., Kosinski, M., & Tarlov, A. R. (1996). Differences in 4-year health outcomes for elderly and poor chronically ill patients treated in HMO and fee-for-service systems. *Journal of the American Medical Association, 276,* 1039–1047.

Willson, D. F., Horn, S. D., Smout, R. J., Gassaway, J., & Torres, A. (2000). Severity assessment in children hospitalized with bronchiolitis using the pediatric component of the Comprehensive Severity Index (CSI®). *Pediatric Critical Care Medicine, 1*(2), 127–132.

Willson, D. F., Horn, S. D., Hendley, J. O., Smout, R., & Gassaway, J. (in press). The effect of practice variation on resource utilization in infants hospitalized for viral lower respiratory illness (VLRI). *Pediatrics.*

Wilson, F. A., & Neuhauser, D. (1987). *Health services in the United States: Second edition with 1987 revisions.* Cambridge, MA: L. Ballinger.

15

Access

John Billings and Joel C. Cantor

LEARNING OBJECTIVES

- ☐ Understand the nature of the access problem.
- ☐ Understand the distinction between economic and noneconomic barriers to care.
- ☐ Understand the characteristics of the uninsured and the policy implications of those characteristics.
- ☐ Understand how access barriers impinge on health.
- ☐ Understand how access barriers affect the health care delivery system.
- ☐ Understand the range and limitations of options for reform—increasing coverage and reducing barriers to care.

TOPICAL OUTLINE

Economic barriers to care
Noneconomic or quasi-economic barriers to care
Health care reform: Improving access

KEY WORDS

access barrier, noneconomic barriers, quasi-economic barriers, underinsurance, cost-shifting, resource availability/performance, ambulatory care sensitive conditions, safety net, ERISA, pay or play, SCHIP, Clinton Health Plan

For most of the 20th century, the U.S. health care system has struggled in efforts to assure access to health care services for all Americans. There have been major steps forward. The growth of private, employer-based health insurance following World War II, the passage of the Medicare and Medicaid programs in 1965, and the growth of federal programs in the 1970s to expand direct service programs (such as community health centers) for low-income patients helped improve access for many. But the debate surrounding the proposed Clinton health reform plan of 1993 and its subsequent failure illustrate the difficulties that are entailed in making further progress.

Access is often viewed as a one-dimensional problem: too many Americans lack health insurance coverage. By this measure, approximately 42 million persons were estimated to be uninsured in 1999—more than 15% of the U.S. population (U.S. Census Bureau, 2000). Moreover, the situation has actually deteriorated over the past 20 years, with the rates of uninsurance growing.

The potential impact of lack of insurance on patients is obvious—delaying or forgoing needed care can lead to adverse health outcomes, and the costs of obtaining necessary care can be financially ruinous. The impact large numbers of uninsured patients have on the health care delivery system is also serious, as providers of uncompensated care struggle to subsidize to other payers the expense incurred by patients without coverage. These efforts by providers can create structural distortions in the health care delivery system, steering uninsured patients toward "safety-net" providers, further increasing the costs of care for these patients, undermining the financial integrity of many institutions, and reinforcing the development of a two-tiered health care delivery system in many communities. With the expansion of managed care and emergence of stronger market forces, the situation is expected to get worse.

The problem of access itself, however, is enormously more complex than insurance coverage. An insurance card alone does not eliminate barriers to access. First, there are issues of the extent and adequacy of coverage. Are outpatient services covered as well as inpatient care? Are prescription drugs included? Mental health and substance abuse services? What about long-term care? And what about the levels of co-payments and deductibles? As many as 29 million Americans are estimated to be "underinsured," with levels of coverage inadequate to assure financial access to care (Short & Banthin, 1995). Another important factor is the adequacy of payments to providers made by third-party payers. For example, low payment levels to physicians have historically plagued the Medicaid program, discouraging participation of many private physicians and limiting where Medicaid patients can receive care.

In addition, patients with an insurance card can also face serious noneconomic barriers to care that can have a dramatic effect on access, utilization patterns, and health outcomes. The delivery of care remains largely disconnected, creating substantial barriers for many users. Moreover, to the extent that the health care delivery system fails to respond to differences in language, culture, health care beliefs, care-seeking behavior, or educational levels, additional impediments to access can be created. These nonfinancial barriers are often aggravated for low-income patients by quasi-economic barriers. Obtaining timely care for a child may require that a parent get off work, forgo wages, arrange child care for siblings, or get transportation—all of which may be difficult for families with limited resources or who are socially isolated.

In this chapter, the nature and extent of all of these barriers to care are examined. In the next section, economic barriers to care are explored, including an overview of the characteristics of the uninsured, a discussion of problems associated with extent and adequacy of coverage, and an examination of the consequences that lack of adequate insurance has on patients and providers. In the following section, barriers other than economic are described, and their impact documented. In the final section, reforms are examined, their potential impact and limitations are discussed, and future issues related to access are explored.

ECONOMIC BARRIERS TO CARE

Who Are the Uninsured?

It is important to note that the level of uninsurance among the elderly is very low (1.3%), reflecting the impact of the Medicare program that provides almost universal coverage for Americans age 65 and over (see Table 15.1). Although there are important limitations in coverage for the elderly and some noneconomic barriers for this population, the Medicare program has done much to reduce barriers to access for the elderly.

Among the nonelderly, the highest rates of uninsurance are among the young adult population (ages 18–34). The higher rates among these age groups reflect two important factors: a dependence on employer-based coverage for private insurance, and the impact of the federal/state Medicaid program. When employers in the U.S. fail to provide or offer insurance to their workers or when an individual becomes unemployed, the risk of becoming uninsured increases enormously. The cost of individual coverage is prohibitive for most persons without coverage, especially low-income workers or the unemployed. Young adults have higher rates of unemployment, are often recent entrants to the workforce (often with lower wage/part-time jobs).

Young adults also often have difficulty establishing eligibility for Medicaid coverage, which varies among states. Medicaid eligibility is limited to low-income persons who fall into one of the following eligibility categories: child, elderly, blind/disabled, pregnant woman, single parent, or unemployed parent (in some states). Employed parents or childless adults simply cannot become eligible for Medicaid, regardless of income (unless they become blind, disabled, or pregnant), although some states provide coverage through state-financed programs (home relief, medically indigent, etc.) for some of these noncategorically eligible individuals. The

TABLE 15.1 Persons Without Insurance Coverage by Demographic Characteristics—1999 Current Population Survey

Characteristics	Percentage of total uninsured	Percentage who are uninsured
Total	100.0	15.5
Male	51.9	16.5
Female	48.1	14.6
< 18	23.6	13.9
18–24	18.1	29.0
25–34	20.6	23.2
35–44	17.3	16.5
45–64	19.5	13.8
< 65 total	99.0	17.4
65+	1.0	1.3
White (Non-Hispanic)	50.7	11.0
Black (Non-Hispanic)	17.9	21.2
Asian	5.4	20.8
Hispanic	26.0	33.4
Native U.S.	77.8	13.5
Foreign Born	22.2	33.4
Citizen	4.5	17.9
Noncitizen	17.8	42.6
< 100% Poverty	36.5	38.7
100–149%	15.7	30.7
159–199%	13.1	26.8
200–299%	15.1	16.2
300%+	19.7	6.9
Northeast	15.6	12.8
Midwest	16.6	11.1
South	39.7	17.6
West	28.1	19.1
< High School	28.0	26.7
High School	35.7	17.6
Some College (No Degree)	18.6	15.2
Associate Degree	5.8	12.9
Bachelor's or Higher	11.8	8.2

Source: U.S. Census Bureau. (2000). *Health Insurance Coverage: 1999.*

targeted nature of the Medicaid program is also reflected in the lower rates of uninsurance for children (categorically eligible) and women (more likely to be single parents or to become eligible through pregnancy).

Most uninsured persons work at least part-time. About 85% of the uninsured live in households where the family head has been employed during the past year. Accordingly, the problem of uninsurance is typically due to the failure of an employer to offer insurance or to the refusal of coverage by an employee. The highest rates of uninsurance are in the retail, service, construction, and agricultural sectors, with much higher rates of uninsurance among small employers (and the self-employed). Low-wage earners (incomes less than 200% of the federal poverty level) represent more than half of the working uninsured and have rates of uninsurance (40.9% uninsured) more than 6 times greater than higher income workers (6.9%) (see Table 15.2).

Rates of uninsurance also differ significantly among states. For example, less than 10% of the nonelderly are uninsured in Connecticut, Rhode Island, and Minnesota, while rates of uninsurance are above 22% in Louisiana, Texas, and New Mexico (U.S. Census Bureau, 2000). In addition to the categorical requirements noted above for Medicaid coverage (children, aged, blind/disabled, etc.), there are also minimum income standards for eligibility. These standards are set by the states and have been historically tied to welfare payment levels,[1] again with vast differences among states (e.g., eligibility limited to incomes below $2,280 for a family of 3 in Louisiana compared with $6,972 in Connecticut).

The profile of the typical uninsured person might be a young adult in a low-wage job working for a small employer in the retail/services sector. Accordingly, any realistic solution to the problem of uninsurance cannot be dependent on the uninsured themselves—more than half of the uninsured earn less than 200% of the federal poverty level (U.S. Census Bureau, 2000). The uninsured tend to be in the weakest sectors of the economy, among smaller employers, with very low wage levels. Adding insurance coverage would represent a large percentage increase in labor expense for these employers, and resistance to "reform" among these groups. The situation is likely to worsen—small employers in the services and retail sectors are where much of recent job growth has occurred.

Underinsurance and Other Limitations of Coverage

An insurance card does not always assure financial access to care, as private insurance often excludes mental health services, preventive care, and long-term care. Most plans have exclusions or waiting periods for preexisting conditions that were present at the time of enrollment. These limits affect those most in need of coverage and subject them to substantial financial risk if workers change jobs. Many plans also lack adequate coverage for catastrophic illnesses, with maximum lifetime benefit limits too low to cover the costs of serious illness or accident. Moreover, virtually all private insurance plans, even most managed care plans, have some form of co-payment

---

[1] Recent federal reforms have broken this link and give states more flexibility in setting eligibility standards.

TABLE 15.2   Nonelderly Workers Age 18–64 Without Insurance Coverage Employment Characteristics—1999 Current Population Survey

Characteristics	Percentage of total uninsured	Percentage who are uninsured
Total	100.0	17.5
Full-time/Full-year	55.4	14.1
Full-time/Part-year	23.1	27.8
Part-time/Full-year	10.5	21.9
Part-time/Part-year	11.0	22.9
Agriculture	5.0	35.8
Cleaning/Laborers	23.7	25.4
Craft/Repair	14.4	23.3
Food Service	10.2	37.6
Health Service	2.5	21.7
Managerial/Professional	14.2	8.4
Personal Service/Household	6.2	22.9
Tech/Sales/Administration	23.7	14.0
< 25 Workers	45.7	28.4
25–99	14.5	19.6
100–499	11.3	14.2
500–999	3.6	11.5
1000+	24.9	11.0
< 100% Poverty	24.7	49.1
100–149%	17.0	39.9
159–199%	15.4	32.9
200–299%	18.3	19.6
300%+	24.7	7.3

Sources: Kaiser Commission on Medicaid and the Uninsured. (2000). *Health Insurance Coverage in America—1999 Data Update.*

U.S. Census Bureau. (2000). *Health insurance Coverage: 1999.*

or deductible, which can have the effect of discouraging patients from seeking needed preventive care, especially lower income patients most sensitive to out-of-pocket costs.

While almost 97% of Americans over age 65 have Medicare coverage, the program has substantial patient cost-sharing provisions and serious gaps in coverage. The deductible is more than $700 for hospital care and $100 for outpatient care, with substantial co-payments (20%) also required in many cases. Moreover, Medicare provides no coverage for prescription drugs and has substantial restrictions on long-term care (only 2% of nursing home costs of the elderly are paid by Medicare). As a result of these limitations in coverage, Medicare is estimated to pay less than 50% of the total costs of health care for the elderly. Many elderly have supplemental coverage for some of these expenses (Medi-Gap plans), either through their employer/retirement plan or by purchasing such coverage directly. More than 20% of the elderly (35% of low-income elderly) have no supplemental coverage, however, exposing them to serious financial risks and potentially creating substantial barriers to access.

Low-income elderly qualify for coverage by Medicaid. Medicaid coverage is generally very comprehensive, covering most services (including drugs and long-term care) and having few restrictions or co-payments. However, Medicaid suffers from serious problems of provider nonparticipation. While hospitals historically have been guaranteed payment levels that were reasonably related to costs, physician payments are set by state administrative agencies facing staggering increases in program costs. Not surprisingly, payment levels for physicians and other noninstitutional providers have often been set below market rates. For example, in New York, the office-based physician payment rate for an "intermediate office visit" was set at $11, a level unchanged since 1985.

The Impact of Economic Barriers to Care

For patients, the impact of a lack of insurance can be profound. Uninsured patients are less likely than those who are privately insured to have a usual source of care (24% vs. 8%). Among patients with health problems, uninsured patients are more likely to have had no physician visits during a 12-month period than those with private insurance (22% vs. 9%) and have had fewer average number of physician contacts (9.1 vs. 14.8)—and these differences persist, even after adjusting for socioeconomic status among the insured and uninsured (Millman, 1993).

The impact of coinsurance on utilization is also significant, especially among lower income patients. While one goal of coinsurance is to discourage frivolous utilization, lower rates for preventive services (such as immunizations for children or screening tests for cervical cancer for adult women), suggest these barriers to care affect other utilization as well.

The lack of insurance can also affect hospital utilization. Uninsured patients are more likely to be admitted for preventable/avoidable conditions, such as asthma, diabetes, cellulitis, or other infections (Billings & Teicholz, 1990). In one study, hospitalized uninsured patients were found to have substantially lower rates for common diagnostic tests (colonoscopy, endoscopy, coronary arteriography, etc.) and for costly surgical procedures (bypass surgery, joint replacement, eye surgery, etc.), even after controlling for socio-demographic and diagnostic case-mix factors (Hadley, Steinberg, & Feder, 1991).

While it is difficult to document the effect of insurance status on health status and health outcomes, since the lack of insurance tends to be somewhat episodic (with individuals going on and off of insurance periodically), substantial differences for the uninsured have been observed. Uninsured mothers have been found to begin prenatal care later and to have fewer total visits than privately insured mothers (Braveman, Egerter, Bennett, &

Showstack, 1991), and uninsured newborns have been shown to have more adverse outcomes than babies with insurance (Braveman, Oliva, & Miller, 1989). Uninsured women have also been found to present with later stage breast cancer than privately insured patients and have lower survival rates (a 49% higher risk of death among uninsured patients; Ayanian, Kohlker, & Toshi, 1993).

Most dramatically, overall mortality rates for uninsured patients have also been shown to be higher than for those with insurance. In a study of a national cohort of patients between 1971 and 1987, uninsured patients were found to have a 25% increased risk of dying during the study period, even after adjusting for differences in socio-demographic characteristics, general health status, and health habits (Franks, Clancy, & Gold, 1993).

Although the cost of uninsurance and underinsurance is high in human terms, there is also a serious impact on the health care delivery system that can affect all patients. First, distortions in utilization patterns can increase total costs. While uninsurance promotes underutilization, it also has the effect of steering uninsured patients to providers who are willing to provide care regardless of ability to pay. These providers tend to be institution-based providers, such as hospital outpatient departments, emergency rooms, and community-based clinics. Costs in these institution-based settings are often higher, therefore increasing total costs for the health care delivery system.

Potentially worse are the financial disequilibriums these utilization patterns can create for providers. Providers serving large numbers of uninsured patients must cover the costs of unreimbursed care. These same providers usually serve substantial numbers of Medicaid patients for whom costs of care often exceed reimbursement rates, which may subject them to arbitrary payment limits and restrictions. These expenses can either be "cost-shifted" to other payers (by raising charge levels for these payers sufficiently above actual costs to raise enough revenue to cover unreimbursed expenses), or providers can seek government or private subsidies. Although some states have established elaborate pooling systems to offset some of these costs and many publicly operated providers receive direct subsidies, in most jurisdictions providers are dependent on the cost-shift.

Today, market forces make cost-shifting less viable. Managed care plans steer their patients to facilities with lower charges, making cost-shifting even more difficult, as the base of paying patients shrinks and even larger increases in charges are required to shift costs. The wholesale movement of Medicaid patients into managed care plans that has begun in most states will further worsen this situation for many providers.

The impact of hospital closures and provider failures on access to care for low-income patients may be serious. The providers most at risk are those with the highest levels of care to vulnerable populations. With the loss of these traditional safety-net providers, it is not clear that these patients will be assured access to needed care from the remaining providers, who may be located further away and who have previously avoided provision of care to these patients.

NONECONOMIC OR QUASI-ECONOMIC BARRIERS TO CARE

Is an Insurance Card Enough?

The impact of uninsurance on health outcomes and utilization was documented previously—however, in many of these studies it was possible to analyze Medicaid patients separately. Rates of preventable hospitalizations for Medicaid patients were below those of uninsured patients, but were still found to be almost 75% higher than the rate for insured patients (Billings & Teicholz, 1990). Incidence of late detection of breast cancer and survival rates for the cancer among the uninsured and Medicaid patients were found to be comparable (Ayanian et al., 1993), and pregnant women on Medicaid had rates of late initiation of prenatal care and average total prenatal care visit rates similar to those of uninsured mothers (Braveman, Egerter, Bennett, & Showstack, 1991).

For these patients, Medicaid coverage failed to eliminate all barriers to needed care. Vulnerable populations face special problems in dealing with the complexities of our fragmented health care delivery system, creating impediments to timely and effective care for many.

Race/Ethnicity

Large and persistent differences in health status, utilization, and outcomes among racial and ethnic groups are well documented. Black and Hispanic/Latino populations have been shown to be less likely to have a usual source of primary care, to have fewer physician visits, higher rates of no/late prenatal care, lower rates of immunizations and screening tests, and worse self-reported health status. Large racial differences have also been documented in rates for infant mortality, low-birthweight infants, late-stage diagnosis of cancer, and mortality from all causes (Council on Ethical and Judicial Affairs, 1990; Fiscella, Franks, Gold, & Clancy, 2000; Millman, 1993).

In American society, socioeconomic status and race/ethnicity are intertwined, and research has attributed a part, but not all, of racial/ethnic disparities in health to socioeconomic conditions. A growing body of research that attempts to control for socioeconomic and other factors, suggests that minority status itself is an important determinant of utilization and health outcomes. For example, after adjusting for differences in insurance coverage, minority adolescents were found to be less likely to have a usual source of primary care, to have fewer annual physician contacts, and lower levels of continuity of care (Lieu, Newacheck, & McManus, 1993). Among children enrolled in managed care plans, minority status was linked to lower rates of utilization, even after controlling for differences in health status (Riley, Finney, & Mellits, 1993).

In other research that could adjust for insurance coverage differences, African Americans with end-stage renal disease have been found to be 50% less likely to receive kidney transplants, and those ultimately receiving surgery had been on waiting lists significantly longer than nonminority patients (Gaston, Ayres, Dooley, & Diethelm, 1993). Similarly, among patients with coronary artery disease, black patients have been found to receive fewer angiographies and to have lower rates of coronary artery bypass surgery controlling for insurance status and disease severity (Johnson, Lee, & Cook, 1993).

Similar differences in rates for invasive cardiac procedures have also been observed for Hispanic/Latino populations (Carlisle, Leake, Brook, & Shapiro, 1996). A study of patients visiting a trauma center emergency room with bone fractures found that nonHispanic whites were more than twice as likely to receive pain medication as Hispanic patients, even after accounting for patient differences in injury severity, pain assessment, insurance status, gender, and language (Todd, Lee, & Hoffman, 1994; Todd, Samaroo, & Hoffman, 1993). Other studies have documented additional differences among Hispanic/Latino subgroups, with Mexican American, Puerto Rican, and Cuban American populations experiencing different rates of no usual source of care, no preventive care, and no physician visits (Council on Scientific Affairs, 1991).

Large racial/ethnic disparities in utilization have also been observed within the Medicare program. African American beneficiaries have fewer physician visits and lower rates of preventive care, such as influenza immunizations. African Americans with Medicare coverage also have lower rates for many diagnostic procedures (such as CT scans, barium enema X rays, mammography, etc.), surgical procedures (coronary bypass, prostatectomy, hysterectomy, orthopedic surgery, etc.), and other services (Friedman, 1994; Gornick et al., 1996). Even within the Veterans Administration hospital system, white veterans have been shown to be significantly more likely to receive coronary surgery than black veterans (Whittle, Conigliaro, & Good, 1993).

Of course, there are many potential explanations for these differences in utilization, outcomes, and health status associated with race/ethnicity. In research, controlling for factors such as socioeconomic status, education, disease incidence/prevalence, illness severity, resource availability, and even insurance coverage can be extraordinarily difficult, and interpretation of these research findings must be tempered by recognition of these methodologic limits. However, these differences by race/ethnicity are substantial and persistent across numerous studies that use a variety of research designs. But even isolating race as the determining factor in these differences leaves many unknowns. The impact of overt or latent racial/cultural bias at all levels of the health care delivery system cannot be discounted. A landmark study in which a large sample of physicians were presented with computerized patient scenarios in which actors were interviewed about their hypothetical chest pain showed that race and sex were important independent determinants of physicians' decisions to refer patients for advanced diagnostic procedures. That study showed that referral rates for cardiac catheterization were lower for women and blacks (84.7% of each group) compared to white men (90.6%) (Schulman et al., 1999). However, further research is required to understand more about the factors that contribute to or mediate any bias, and to identify how patient preferences (e.g., in weighing risks and benefits of medical intervention), care-seeking behavior, and attitudes toward the health care delivery system affect utilization and outcomes.

Managed care offers the hope of establishing a "medical home" for all enrollees, but it may erect other barriers to appropriate care. In one national survey, African American, Asian, and Hispanic respondents with private coverage were 25%–100% *more* likely than their white counterparts to lack a usual source of care, but these differences were much smaller between minority and white members of managed care plans. In contrast, minority managed care members were much more likely to report dissatisfaction with their usual source of care compared to minority members of traditional (nonmanaged care) health plans, while dissatisfaction among whites was low whether they were in managed care or not (Phillips, Mayer, & Aday, 2000).

Culture/Acculturation/Language

The effect of culture and acculturation on health care use and outcomes is not well understood. It is often hypothesized that cultural barriers may contribute to lower or less optimal utilization patterns by Hispanic/Latino and Asian immigrant populations in the U.S. These barriers can involve a broad range of potential problems, including social isolation, distrust of Western medicine, unfamiliarity with U.S. delivery system, differences in concepts of disease/illness, alternative care-seeking behaviors, perceptions of provider disrespect, fears about immigration status, or language difficulties.

Several studies have attempted to evaluate how increased acculturation tends to ameliorate these impediments to access. This research is limited by the difficulty of assessing levels of acculturation. One of the better designed studies suggests that language proficiency may be either the best indicator of acculturation or the most important component of these cultural factors in facilitating access. In that study, better language skills resulted in more use of preventive services such as physical exams, cancer screening, and dental checkups (Solis, Marks, Garcia, & Shelton, 1990).

Of course, acculturation itself may create new problems and new barriers. For example, many immigrant families have stable family structures, including strong intergenerational ties. To the extent that these relationships become more attenuated in urban America, the ability to cope with the requirements of managing a health condition or chronic disease may be impaired.

Gender

Less research has been conducted on gender-related barriers to health care. Similar differences in rates of procedures have been documented, however, with female end-stage renal disease patients less likely to receive a kidney transplant than male patients (Held, Pauly, & Bovberg, 1988; Kjellstrand, 1988). Women have also been shown to have lower rates of cardiac surgery than men (Udvarhelyi, Gatsonis, & Epstein, 1992), although these differences were not associated with higher mortality rates for women (raising an important issue about whether access to more surgical care is always beneficial).

Again, the impact of patient preferences and attitudes toward risk/benefit when considering surgical and diagnostic procedures requires further study to understand their influence on utilization rates. However, there are three emerging lines of research that underscore the potential seriousness of gender-related impediments to health care for women. First, it is well established that women have historically been systematically excluded from clinical trials for new drugs and procedures (Cotton, 1990a, b). The impact of bias in medical research is not yet fully established, but the potential is obvious. To the extent that medical practice is based on findings of medical research, many practitioners may be reluctant to prescribe medications or recommend surgical/diagnostic procedures that have not been fully tested for women. Accordingly, access to newly emerging drugs and technologies may be delayed for women, and resource utilization patterns significantly altered. But the corollary also raises serious concerns: when care provided to women is based on research that has been generalized from gender-biased studies, it may be inappropriate, creating impediments to optimal medical care for women.

A second body of research has begun to document how physician gender can affect practice patterns and utilization rates of care for women. For example, in one study of preventive care it was documented that patients of female physicians were more than twice as likely to receive cervical cancer screening tests (Pap smears) and 40% more likely to receive mammograms than women whose physicians were male (Lurie, Slater, & McGovern, 1993). Again, the full impact of how differences in physician gender can influence the care provided to female patients has not yet been determined. While the number of female physicians is growing, the potential for serious barriers to needed health care services for female patients is large.

Finally, many women do not have access to family planning, abortion counseling, or abortion services. There are explicit restrictions on use of Medicaid funds for these services, and many religiously affiliated providers simply do not offer such services. Moreover, the aggressive tactics of many antiabortion groups has deterred many providers from offering these services and discouraged many women from seeking care. Medicaid and provider restrictions tend to affect low-income patients disproportionately since they are likely to have fewer alternatives, but the chilling effect of politicization of abortion-related care affects access for all women (Henshaw, 1995; Mathews, Ribar, & Wilhelm, 1997; Rosenblatt, Mattis, & Hart, 1995).

Education

As with other indirect barriers to health care, it is difficult to isolate and quantify the effect of education on health care utilization and outcomes. Parental education deficits, however, have been shown to be associated with lower levels of well-baby and other preventive services (Short & Lefkowitz, 1992), and lower overall use by their children (Newacheck, 1992). Differences in education have also been linked to lower rates of breast cancer screening, even after adjusting for a broad range of economic and socio-demographic factors (Lantz, Weigers, & House, 1997). In another study, Medicaid patients with limited education were found to be less likely to use preventive services, have greater difficulties following medical regimens, miss more appointments, and seek care later in the course of an illness (Weiss, 1994).

A growing body of research has begun to document the impact of "functional health literacy," or the ability to use reading, writing, and computational skills in typical, everyday patient situations, such as reading prescription labels, following diagnostic test instructions, or understanding treatment directions. Because 40 million Americans are estimated to be illiterate and another 50 million marginally literate (Kirsch, Jungeblut, Jenkins, & Kolstad, 1993), the potential impediments to timely and effective care are serious. In a study conducted in two public hospitals, 42% of patients could not understand directions for taking medication on an empty stomach, 26% could not comprehend information on an appointment slip describing the scheduled follow-up visit, and more than 25% could not follow instructions for preparing for a gastrointestinal radiological exam. Overall, almost 30% of patients using the facilities were determined to have inadequate functional health literacy, and another 14% to have only marginal levels (Williams, Parker, & Baker, 1995).

Resource Availability/Performance

The supply of health care resources has obvious implications for access. In remote rural areas, the absence of a primary care practitioner, an obstetrician/gynecologist, or even a hospital can have a serious impact on the ability of area residents to obtain timely care (Kindig & Ricketts, 1991; Nesbitt, Connell, & Hart, 1990). In urban areas, supply issues are often more complex. There are huge differences in physician supply across and within communities that have been well documented (Cooper, 1995; Grumbach, 1995; Politzer, Harris, & Gaston, 1991), with some central city areas having serious shortages of practitioners.

The issue for access is availability of providers, however, not supply. Many large urban hospitals (and their associated medical office buildings) are located in or nearby lower income neighborhoods—but this proximity does not assure access. While many hospital outpatient departments accept patients without restrictions on ability to pay (or charge on a sliding-fee schedule), this is certainly not necessarily the case for the privately practicing physicians clustered nearby. Moreover, the low Medicaid reimbursement rates for physician visits noted previously discourage many of these physicians from participating in the Medicaid program, creating potential barriers even for Medicaid cardholders. Therefore, while a simple physician-to-population ratio for the areas surrounding these hospitals would suggest a sufficient supply, a substantial portion of the supply is simply not available to low-income residents.

There is little known about the performance of the primary care delivery system and access to care. Clearly a more efficient provider that can serve more patients has the potential to reduce barriers in its service area. But more important, providers can create care delivery approaches that reduce many of the indirect barriers to care discussed previously (e.g., eliminating language barriers, reducing wait times, developing a culturally sensitive environment, using telephone consultations more effectively, and developing more effective compliance techniques for chronic disease patients with literacy problems).

Recently, for middle-class medicine, patient satisfaction has become the focus of many health care delivery systems as they struggle to attract and maintain their patient base. These developments have spawned a mini-industry of researchers and consultants attempting to assist providers in becoming more responsive to this new world. A parallel effort needs to be targeted at understanding the indirect barriers to care for low-income patients and helping safety-net providers better adapt their care delivery approach to these needs. This is not yet on the horizon.

One Example of the Impact of Noneconomic and Quasi-Economic Barriers: Preventable Hospitalizations

As illustrated in many of the studies described previously, the impact of noneconomic and quasi-economic barriers on utilization patterns and health status can be substantial. A growing body of analysis has also begun to explore how barriers to primary care services can result in increased utilization of other health care services, such as more costly hospital care (Billings, Anderson, & Newman, 1996; Billings, Zeitel, & Lukomnik, 1993; Bindman et al., 1995; Weissman, Gatsonis, & Epstein, 1992).

This research is based on the simple premise that timely and effective primary care can often (a) prevent the onset of an illness (e.g., congenital syphilis, pertussis, tetanus, etc.), (b) control a condition before it becomes more acute (e.g., ear infections in children, urinary tract infections, dehydration, etc.), or (c) manage a chronic disease or condition to help reduce the chances of a serious flare-up (e.g., asthma, diabetes, congestive heart disease, hypertension etc.). To the extent that barriers exist for ambulatory care services, and that a patient may delay or be unable to obtain care, an

illness or condition may deteriorate beyond control in an outpatient setting, resulting in the need for hospitalization for effective management.

By analyzing hospital admission rates for diagnoses related to these
conditions, referred to as ambulatory care sensitive (ACS) conditions,
researchers have documented huge differences in rates among areas (see
Table 15.3). Areas with high ACS rates have been found to have higher
levels of self-reported barriers to access than low ACS rate areas (Bindman
et al., 1995). Moreover, these differences have been found to be strongly
associated with area income, with more than 80% of the variation in admission rates among zip codes in some communities being explained by the
percentage of low-income persons living in an area. Admission rates for
ACS conditions in low-income areas have been found on average to be
2.5–3.5 times higher than more affluent areas, with individual zip code rates
in some low-income neighborhoods as much as 20 times higher than rates
in high-income zip codes in the same community. (See Figures 15.1 and
15.2 illustrating these differences.)

Of course, not all admissions for these ACS conditions are preventable.
However, the extraordinarily high rates among low-income areas and the

**TABLE 15.3 Preventable/Avoidable Hospitalizations, Ambulatory Care
Sensitive (ACS) Admissions/1,000, Age < 65, 1990**

	All Zip/FSA areas		
MSA	ACS adms per 1,000	Association with income (Rsq)	Ratio low-income/ high-income
Boston	11.84	0.581	2.58
Buffalo	8.90	0.840	2.92
Jersey City/Bergen/Passaic, NJ	13.20	0.675	3.21
Los Angeles	10.34	0.518	2.09
Miami	10.90	0.371	1.58
New York City	15.16	0.663	3.13
Newark	14.48	0.827	3.51
Oakland	8.90	0.674	2.55
Orlando	10.29	0.557	2.36
Portland	6.85	0.586	2.59
Rochester, NJ	8.21	0.734	2.95
San Diego	7.15	0.756	2.64
San Francisco	8.55	0.633	3.70
Seattle	6.92	0.606	2.32
Tampa/St. Petersburg	9.63	0.513	2.05
Hamilton	7.25	0.409	1.58
Ottawa	7.43	0.672	1.79
Toronto	7.38	0.103	1.39

* More than 40% households with income < $15,000
** $20,000 Canadian $

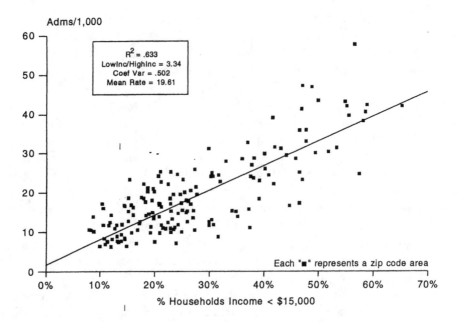

FIGURE 15.1   New York City: Ambulatory-care-sensitivity (ACS) admission, ages 0–64 (1995).

Source: SPARCS, UHF, NYU Health Research Program.

strong association between area rates and the level of poverty suggest that significant barriers to primary care exist in most low-income areas. Insurance coverage is undoubtedly an important factor—differences in rates among Canadian urban areas (with universal insurance coverage) have been found to be significantly lower than U.S. urban areas (Billings et al., 1996; see Table 15.3). Nevertheless, lack of insurance coverage is unlikely to be the sole or even predominant cause for the disparities documented in most U.S. urban areas, since the overwhelming majority of low-income patients admitted had Medicaid coverage. The impact of the noneconomic and quasi-economic barriers discussed above is undoubtedly substantial. A low-income patient who has no regular source of care, who is dissatisfied with available providers (because of long wait times, language difficulties, or lack of cultural sensitivity), or who has difficulties arranging child care, getting off work, or simply coping with problems associated with illness, is clearly at significant risk of delaying or not getting needed care.

The potential relationship between these noneconomic factors and access is illustrated by the findings for ACS admission rates in Miami, Florida. Although like most U.S. urban areas, Miami has significant concentrations of poverty and minority populations, the difference in ACS admissions rates between low- and high-income areas is much smaller (only about 1.6 times higher in low-income areas) and the association between area rates and income is also lower. This lack of a large difference

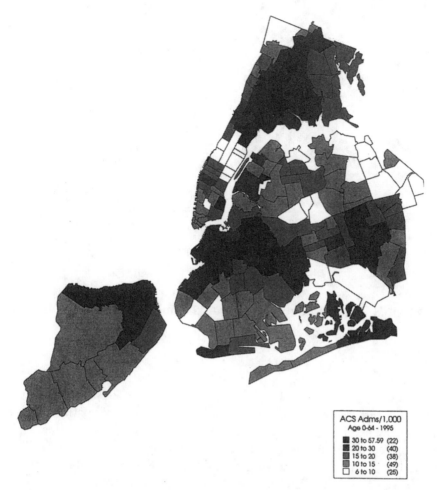

FIGURE 15.2   New York City: ACS admissions/1,000, ages 0–64 (1995).
Source: SPARCS, UHF, NYU Health Research Program.

between low- and high-income areas is particularly evident among Cuban American zip codes (see Figure 15.3), where admission rates were virtually identical, regardless of area income. In fact, in the other non-Latino zip code areas, the association was comparable to other U.S. metropolitan areas (Billings et al., 1996). These data offer some promise that the noneconomic and quasi-economic barriers to care for other low-income persons are not insurmountable. Further research is needed, however, to help sort out the impact of various factors, such as family/social structure of the Cuban-American immigrant population, their health status and care-seeking behavior, and the organization/performance of the primary care delivery system servicing this population (including a substantial cadre of Cuban American physicians who also left Cuba).

The extent and nature of some of these indirect barriers to care are illustrated in a study of patients hospitalized for ACS conditions in New York

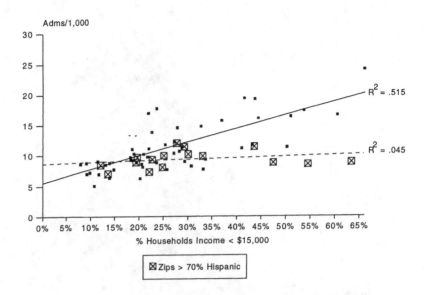

FIGURE 15.3   Dade County (Miami): ACS admissions age 0–64 (1990).

City (Billings, Mijanovich, & Blank, 1997). In interviews after hospital admission and medical stabilization, 60.9% of low-income patients reported that they had received no care prior to the admission and another 17.4% had received care only in the emergency room (compared with 31.4% of higher income patients receiving no care and 5.8% with only emergency room care). More than half of low-income patients reported that they had delayed or not obtained needed care (compared with about one fourth of higher income patients). The leading explanations for delay or the failure to obtain care among low-income patients were not directly related to the costs of care (the overwhelming majority had Medicaid coverage) but rather a range of social and quasi-economic problems reflecting the difficulties encountered by low-income patients and their families in their daily lives and in negotiating the complexities of the health care delivery system. Over 25% of adult patients indicated they were "too nervous or afraid," "too busy with other things," or simply "not up to going," reflecting serious ambivalence about the health care delivery system. Substantial numbers also reported difficulties arranging child care, problems with transportation, concern about having to wait too long, uncertainty about where to go, or apprehensions that providers wouldn't understand their needs (see Table 15.4).

These nonfinancial barriers to timely and effective care are substantial and serious. It is clear that successful interventions go beyond simply providing an insurance card to the uninsured. Part of the solution will require development of a care delivery system that recognizes that low-income

TABLE 15.4   Type of "Access" Problems Reported by Low-Income Patients Hospitalized for Preventable/Avoidable Conditions

Reason for problem	% of low-income patients with "access" problem who reported type of reason[1]		
	Age 6-mos–17 yrs.	Age 18–64 yrs.	All ages
Not up to going	5.1	36.1	29.2
Too nervous or afraid	10.2	33.8	28.6
Unable to get free time to get care	8.1	27.2	22.9
Had to wait too long to get appointment	20.3	20.4	20.4
Problems with child care	32.8	14.3	18.2
Costs too much	13.8	18.1	17.2
Unable to keep medical appointment	7.4	20.2	17.1
Couldn't fill prescription	16.4	16.9	16.8
Transportation difficulties	19.3	15.8	16.5
Didn't know where to go to get care	8.6	13.8	12.7
Not sure provider would understand needs	22.4	9.1	12.2
Care not available when needed it	11.3	12.1	12.0
Denied care	13.4	9.7	10.6
Didn't like usual place to get care	17.2	7.9	9.9
Lose pay/trouble getting off work	12.1	6.0	7.3
Language problem	1.8	4.7	4.3

[1] *Note:* Percentages total more than 100% because some patients indicated multiple reasons.

Source: Hospitalized Patient Interview Study, United Hospital Fund.

patients are struggling with many other aspects of their lives (as well as their health care problems)—these patients are "busy with other things" and do have difficulty getting off work or arranging child care. Longer clinic hours, home visits, and special outreach may be required to better serve them. Many of these problems necessarily will require that social service, education, and other programs become more responsive to the needs of these populations.

HEALTH CARE REFORM: IMPROVING ACCESS

At the Federal Level: Failure of the Clinton Health Plan and Beyond

In 1992 public support for some form of national health insurance reached a 40-year high of 66%. During the presidential election of that year, voters ranked health care as the third most important issue facing the nation after the economy and the federal budget deficit. By the time President Clinton took office in 1993, the issue had risen to second place, with 90% of Americans indicating they believed there was a crisis in health care (Blendon, Brodie, & Benson, 1995).

Clinton responded by appointing a task force that developed a proposal for a "Health Security Act" in the fall of 1993. The plan assured coverage for a comprehensive benefits package for almost all Americans. The elderly would continue to be covered by Medicare (although the coverage was to be expanded to include prescription drugs and expanded long-term care benefits for the severely disabled). The plan excluded undocumented immigrants and prisoners. However, coverage for everyone else would be provided through competing plans that would administer enrollment, collect premiums, and pay participating health plans. Large employers (5,000+ employees) could opt out, but would be required to offer comparable coverage from an array of competing plans and would be assessed a 1% payroll tax to support medical education and care for low-income/high-cost individuals insured in regional health alliances.

Almost all employers were to be required to offer coverage to all of their employees and dependents and pay 80% of the average premium costs. Premium subsidies were to be provided for small employers and for low-income workers. Medicaid coverage would be provided through the health alliances (state/federal funding for these patients would be maintained at prior levels) and unemployed workers would also obtain coverage through the alliances (with premium subsidy support based on income). Employer and individual premiums would be community rated (i.e., cost the same regardless of health status of those being insured), although payment levels to plans would be risk adjusted to account for differences in health status of plan enrollees. The restructuring of the health care marketplace by inducing competition among competing health plans was expected to help control health costs, but there was also a mechanism to impose caps on premiums if costs began to rise more than expected.

The proposal also included other provisions to help reduce barriers to access. Expanded funding was to be provided for public health services and for programs to support "essential" community providers. This latter group included so-called safety-net providers, which have traditionally provided care to uninsured and Medicaid patients. The support for these entities was intended to assure continuation of patient outreach programs, and to ease the transition to a more competitive health care environment.

The Clinton health plan avoided any new broad-based taxes to support the coverage expansions and premium subsidies, but rather relied on a combination of funding sources such as mandated employer contributions, Medicaid/Medicare savings (lower provider payments), assessments of large employers who opted out of alliances, and an increase in the tobacco tax. The expected costs of the program ($300+ billion by 2002) would be offset by these program savings and new revenues, making the proposed plan budget-neutral.

Of course, the plan failed. Large employers never supported the proposal, even though they were exempted from many of its requirements and the approach had promise of eliminating their financing of the cost-shift for uninsured patients embedded in their current premiums. Small employers were strongly opposed to the mandate coverage, although many would have been insulated from some of its effects by premium subsidies. Insurance companies strongly resisted the proposal, perhaps concerned that not all would survive in the competitive managed care environment contemplated by the approach of the alliances. Conservatives saw further encroachment of government into health care, with the complex system of quasi-governmental alliances and premium caps. Many liberals were concerned that the plan did not go far enough, or had discomfort with the concept of managed competition. Virtually everyone had reservations about the numbers: Was it really possible to create such a huge expansion of coverage and restructuring of the system without large amounts of new revenue?

The net effect of the failure of the Clinton plan has been to virtually extinguish comprehensive health reform from the national public policy debates. Only 5% of voters in the 1996 elections indicated that reforming health care was a top issue for the new administration (Blendon, Benson, & Brodie, 1997). Since the 1996 elections, the percentage of Americans who rank health care (including Medicare) as one of the two most important issues for the government to address has fluctuated between about 10% and 20% (Blendon, Benson, Brodie, Altman, & James, 2000). Not surprisingly, the focus at the federal level has largely returned to consideration of incremental reforms and cost control. In 1996, the Kennedy-Kassebaum proposal was enacted to assure greater portability of insurance coverage when an employee changes jobs (an important issue for many middle-class workers, but having only a small effect on the 40 million uninsured). The 1995–1997 budget battles focused primarily on how much savings can be extracted from Medicare and Medicaid. In fact, the Balanced Budget Act of 1997 included Medicare/Medicaid reductions of almost $140 billion (mostly from reduced payments to providers), an amount comparable to the $190 billion savings contemplated by the Clinton Health Plan. Of course, these savings were targeted for budget deficit reduction, whereas in 1993 the monies were intended to expand coverage for the uninsured and to broaden Medicare benefits.

However, two important features of the Balanced Budget Act of 1997 address access issues more directly and also provide a strong indication about the probable locus of near- and medium-term health reform activity. First, states obtained greater flexibility in the administration of Medicaid programs. Many states have begun to examine strategies to use managed care more effectively for Medicaid patients and/or to expand coverage to populations who are ineligible for Medicaid (because of the "categorical" requirements noted previously). These initiatives have historically required a discretionary federal "waiver," an uncertain process that usually caused substantial delay and inevitably entailed limitations on state initiatives. Under the new law, states are not required to obtain waivers for many of these reforms. While there are concerns that states may abuse this new flexibility, it will also undoubtedly encourage even greater state-level activity and innovation.

The Balanced Budget Act also included $24 billion to provide coverage for some of the estimated 10 million uninsured children in the U.S. through the State Children's Health Insurance Program (SCHIP). Again the action is at the state level, with funding distributed to states based on the number of low-income, uninsured children in the state, adjusting for differences in wages and the cost of health care. States can use the funding, which must be matched with local support (up to 35% depending on current Medicaid match rates), to expand Medicaid coverage for children up to 200% of the poverty level or to create new programs targeted at providing coverage for low-income, uninsured children. Up to 15% of the funding can be used for direct service programs and outreach services. After a slow start, the SCHIP program has become a major new source of coverage in many states, extending coverage to over 3.3 million previously uninsured child (http://www.hcfa.gov/init/fy2000.pdf; March 12, 2001).

State Initiatives to Improve Access: Innovations and Limitations

Most state activities or proposed approaches fit into one of the following major categories: (a) initiatives to stimulate/facilitate voluntary action by employers or individuals to purchase insurance, (b) efforts to coerce employers to provide coverage ("pay or play" approaches), (c) support of direct services for uninsured (e.g., community-based clinics), and (d) purchase of coverage for targeted uninsured populations (with or without federal assistance).

Many of the initial efforts in the 1980s focused on coping with the apparent failure of the insurance market for small employers where rates of uninsurance were observed to be high (see Table 15.2). Because of the inherently high marketing costs for small employers and the difficulties of spreading risks for small groups, it was believed that new products needed to be developed that could lower premiums for small employers. Attempts were made to stimulate development of larger groups or cooperative purchasing pools that could centralize marketing and spread risks, giving small employers some of the advantages of larger employers and reducing premiums by 10%–20%. While some of these initiatives have had some successes (Jacobson, Merritt, & Bartlett, 1994), most faced the difficult problem that for many small employers any premium was perceived as too much, and a relatively small number of small employers previously not providing coverage opted to purchase care from the pools.

Many states also established pools for high-risk individuals who could not get coverage in the private market because of their health status or history of high utilization. These programs have historically tended to reach only a small number of individuals. Without significant subsidies, the premiums for individuals using these pools is typically very high and beyond the means of many who are most in need. Second, the overwhelming majority of uninsured individuals lack coverage not because it has been denied for health reasons, but because their employer simply does not offer coverage and the individual insurance market is beyond their means.

While these voluntary efforts have met with only limited success, more coercive approaches have not fared well either. The approach considered by many states has been a "pay or play" strategy, where employers who do not offer coverage to their employees ("play") are assessed a tax ("pay") sufficient to support state-sponsored plans for uninsured workers. The goal is either to induce employers to offer insurance plans to their employees or to raise enough revenue to finance state-subsidized plans for employees of firms not offering coverage.

These approaches have faced two major obstacles: legal challenge and political feasibility. The legal challenge relates to the federal Employee Retirement Income Security Act of 1974 (ERISA), which has been interpreted to preempt state law in regulation of state employee benefit plans. To the extent that the "pay or play" requirement is interpreted as a mandate to provide coverage, it may be subject to legal challenge. The political obstacle is obvious—small employers strongly oppose the approach, even when subsidies or exemptions for new and very small employers are included. Of the several states that have considered or even initially legislated some variant of "pay or play," none has actually fully implemented the approach.

Initiatives to support direct services for the uninsured, such as community-based clinics, have generally fared better. The financial support typically goes to publicly operated facilities or, in some cases, to not-for-profit entities. Financing can come from general tax revenue, earmarked taxes (e.g., sales tax add-ons, tobacco/alcohol taxes, etc.) or from assessments on providers (usually hospitals). The smaller scale of these initiatives makes them more politically feasible, but also limits their reach. The federal government shares the cost of direct service support programs, particularly for hospitals, through Medicare and Medicaid disproportionate share (DSH) funding. Federal policy decisions in the late 1990s (most significantly thorugh the Balanced Budget Act of 1997), however, have limited the availability of DSH payments, further limiting the reach of state direct provider subsidy programs.

The area that has generated the most interest at the state level is the last category, efforts to purchase coverage for targeted groups of the uninsured. In the 1990s, several states have used the Section 1115 waiver process to expand Medicaid coverage to those groups that would otherwise not be "categorically" eligible or who are above income eligibility thresholds. These Section 1115 waiver coverage expansion initiatives attempt to avoid increasing total costs of the Medicaid program (a requirement of the waiver) by use of managed care/provider payment limits (e.g., Tennessee) or by cutting the services covered by the program (e.g., Oregon). Through the late 1990s, state initiatives in health coverage reform held significant promise, but also had serious limitations. First, most were narrow in scope, typically reaching a relatively small portion of the uninsured. Of the 14 states with the most developed initiatives in 1995, only 5% of the total uninsured had been reached. Because of the targeted nature of these initiatives (children, pregnant women, etc.), even if they reached their enrollment goals, only about 20% of the uninsured would receive coverage, assuming current levels of uninsurance and no dropping of coverage to take advantage of the new programs (Lipson & Schrodel, 1996). Moreover, the focus on children and pregnant women, although important and politically understandable, tends to overlook the more serious problems of uninsurance among the adult population, which often experiences the most serious barriers to access.

State initiatives were also often hindered by limits on revenue sources. General tax revenues are seldom a viable or reliable source, and initiatives are often dependent on a more limited potential revenue base of "sin taxes" (tobacco and alcohol excise taxes), earmarked sales taxes, or complicated provider "assessments." In addition, as the implications of recent federal budget reductions for welfare and Medicaid begin to be felt at the state level, state budget problems are likely to deteriorate.

The Balanced Budget Act of 1997, despite a legislative intent to reduce federal financial liabilities, sparked renewed interests among the states in expanding coverage. Beginning in the late 1990s, states focused on implementing their SCHIP programs, part of the Balanced Budget Act. Following delays in program implementation, most states have fully operational SCHIP initiatives, and the federal government has offered increased flexibility to states to use SCHIP as a platform for expanding coverage beyond children under 200% of poverty (www.state-coverage.net/schip.htm, February 9, 2001). As of the beginning of 2001, 38 states had extended SCHIP coverage to children to 200% or more of the federal poverty level (FPL), some through Section 1115 waivers and others by "disregarding" a portion of family income in determining SCHIP eligibility. Seven states extend eligibility to 300% of poverty or more, with New Jersey and Tennessee offering the most generous SCHIP eligibility limit at 350% and 400% FPL, respectively.

SCHIP addressed two major barriers to state policy to address the problem of the uninsured: lack of fiscal capacity and lack of technical competencies. SCHIP presented a new, long-term source of federal revenue to states for coverage expansions, with matching rates more favorable than Medicaid. Moreover, SCHIP pushed states to expand the capacity of their bureaucracies to implement broad new coverage mechanisms. For instance, many states focused for the first time on actively reaching out to nonwelfare populations and marketing state-subsidized coverage options. Many states also expanded their capacity to solicit and procure managed care contracts.

Some states have begun to use SCHIP as a platform for extending coverage to adults as well. As of January 2001, New Jersey, Rhode Island, and Wisconsin received federal approval to offer coverage to uninsured parents of some SCHIP recipients through Section 1115 waivers (www.state-coverage.net/schip-1115.htm, February 19, 2001). During the 2000 presidential campaign, then candidate George Bush voiced support for offering even greater flexibility to states to use federal SCHIP support to expand coverage further.

THE FUTURE: CONTINUING AND EMERGING ISSUES

Broad fundamental issues related to access are likely to continue in the short and medium term. Even with the SCHIP-sparked renewal of state action to cover the uninsured, large numbers of Americans remain without coverage, and patients and providers continue to struggle to cope with the consequences of this reality. As of 2001, three new sets of access issues are emerging that will become increasingly important.

First, within the next few years, virtually all Medicaid patients (except the elderly in long-term care and some special needs populations) will be enrolled in managed care, and state SCHIP expansions deliver coverage almost exclusively on managed care. Passage of the Balanced Budget Act of 1997 removes most restrictions on mandatory Medicaid managed care enrollment. While this transformation has the potential to help reduce some of the indirect barriers to care for public coverage program recipients, it also raises many new concerns and issues.

On the positive side, capitated payments create strong financial incentives for managed care plans to solve some noneconomic or quasi-economic barriers to care, for example, to the extent that preventable hospital admissions for conditions, such as asthma, can be reduced by more timely and effective outpatient management. (Better patient education on use of inhalers, improved medication regimens, and nurse hotlines for care management advice during acute flare-ups) or by development of a more accessible health care delivery system (longer clinic hours, shorter waits in clinics, child care services on site, and in-home visits). Managed care plans have an interest in solving these problems that have historically eluded the fee-for-service world. Research is needed to monitor how plans respond to develop new strategies to improve access as Medicaid and SCHIP managed care matures.

Publicly funded managed care also creates new enforcement mechanisms and opportunities for government agencies to assure better access for enrolled patients. For example, some states have instituted policies that plans must assure that patients with urgent care needs can obtain an appointment with their primary care provider within a specified period (e.g., 48 hours). Medicaid patients have historically adapted to long wait times for appointments at some clinics and outpatient departments (60 days or more in many cases) by using emergency rooms for routine care or by turning to Medicaid mills for much of their care. Medicaid agencies often had no effective means to compel providers to be more responsive because of the logistical problems of monitoring a huge number of care sites and the difficulties inherent in penalizing providers who were often already in financial distress and who were critical to assuring some access in low-income communities. Moreover, since patients often used multiple providers, it was not possible to hold any single provider responsible for patient care, for example, when a newborn failed to receive the requisite schedule of well-baby care visits or appropriate immunizations, it was not always clear who should be held accountable.

In a managed care environment, a single health plan is responsible for each patient. Regulators can more effectively monitor the performance of the smaller number of plans (e.g., using mock patients attempting to schedule appointments with the plan's providers by telephone; monitoring disenrollment rates; tracking performance indicators for immunizations, well-baby visits, or follow-up after hospitalization) and have a realistic enforcement mechanism to assure accountability: closing enrollment for new patients or denying reenrollment of current patients. Noncomplying plans can be forced to expand capacity or improve performance of their primary care providers, or face serious loss of revenue. Again the potential may exceed the reality. Accordingly, a critical issue for the future concerns the extent and effectiveness of government oversight of Medicaid managed care. The explosion of Medicaid managed care is happening at a time of overall government cutbacks, and it will be critical to examine whether and how public agencies will adapt to this new environment.

Medicaid managed care also presents a serious risk of creating a whole new set of barriers to care for low-income patients. The confusion associated with the enrollment process undoubtedly has negative consequences. For example, many patients may enroll in plans not realizing that they will be required to change providers, perhaps requiring unrealistic travel times to new care sites and certainly disrupting continuity of current utilization patterns. Other problems are likely to emerge, as well. Aggressive, entrepreneurial plans may enroll more patients than their primary care network can adequately serve. New providers brought in by managed care plans may underestimate the special needs of Medicaid populations. Requirements that patients use a gatekeeping primary care practitioner may discourage needed care among patients who have difficulty adapting to the new rules. And, of course, the most serious concern relates to the new set of incentives for providers: provision of less care can mean higher profits or a bigger margin. While barriers to care may ultimately lead to increased morbidity and costly hospitalization for some patients, in the short run, low or no utilization of primary care services may be highly profitable. As patients jump on and off Medicaid and from one plan to another, some plans may find no financial advantage in improving access for many of their patients. Therefore, it is critical that policymakers have a capacity to monitor these developments carefully and to learn more about how these new incentives are affecting utilization and outcomes.

There are new risks as states gain more flexibility to structure public coverage programs through managed care plans. Until the Balanced Budget Act, states were required to apply for waivers to mandate managed care enrollment of Medicaid beneficiaries. Waivers brought extra layers of scrutiny from the federal government through mandated program evaluations. But today, states may employ managed care plans to deliver care under Medicaid and SCHIP without waivers, and less scrutiny may put program beneficiaries at greater risk.

The second set of emerging issues relates to the consequences of the changing health care marketplace. With the growth of managed care (in commercial, Medicare, and Medicaid markets) and the strengthening of market forces in the health care sector, the ability of traditional safety-net providers to survive, as discussed previously, remains in some doubt. The consequences of their failure are likely to be most dire for the uninsured, especially among immigrant populations who will find it increasingly difficult to take advantage of public programs to provide health insurance coverage. While the market clearing effect of competition may help reduce system-wide overcapacity, the impact on patients dependent on these vulnerable providers may be serious. A critical issue in the next decade will be how well the imperative to reduce unneeded beds and services is balanced by efforts to assure the availability of resources to these vulnerable populations. Will we allow these safety-net providers to fail? What will be the consequences of such failures for other providers who begin to see more uninsured patients in their emergency rooms and outpatient departments?

Finally, as efforts to cope with access problems continue to devolve to states and localities, it will be become critical to more fully understand the impact and limits of incremental reforms at these levels. What are the most effective means of expanding coverage for children? How should insurance coverage be balanced with support/subsidies to providers for direct services to the uninsured? What about uninsured adults (who use substantially more health resources than children)? Will children, and adults, in similar economic circumstances but living in different states be treated equitably?

As other innovations are attempted at the state and local levels, sorting out the balance between what is politically feasible (programs for children and pregnant women) and where limited funds might be invested most effectively (adult immigrant populations, substance abuse programs, safe-ty-net providers) will undoubtedly be a major challenge. Disparities among states and localities will also emerge as some move forward while others remain intransigent, and it will be important to monitor the extent and effect of these differences.

Clearly, serious access problems will remain for many millions of Americans for the foreseeable future. The ultimate issue is when these problems will reemerge as a major national policy concern, at least regarding economic access, and whether national policymakers will yet again fail to find a politically viable and financially affordable strategy to assure universal access to needed care.

CASE STUDY

You are the governor of a midsize industrial state. You have just read this chapter and have decided you want to take on the "health reform/health care access" issue. How would your proceed? How would you staff the effort? Who are the stakeholders? How would you obtain input from stakeholders? How would you limit inappropriate influence by stakeholders? What is the likely nature of the problem in your state? What are the realistic range of solutions/reforms that might be considered? What is the likelihood of meaningful reform?

DISCUSSION QUESTIONS

1. Who are the uninsured and what does this tell us about the nature of the problem?
2. What are the implications of characteristics of the uninsured on efforts to expand coverage?
3. Who is responsible for reducing noneconomic and quasi-economic barriers to timely and effective health care?
4. What are the costs of barriers to access and how are these costs financed in the current health care delivery system?
5. What were the critical factors in the failure of the Clinton Health Plan? What are the prospects for meaningful reform in the immediate future?

REFERENCES

Allen, D., & Kamradt, J. (1991). Relationship of infant mortality to the availability of obstetrical care in Indiana. *Journal of Family Practice, 33*(6), 609.

Ayanian, J. Z., Kohlker, B. B., & Toshi, A. (1993). The relationship between health insurance coverage and clinical outcomes among women with breast cancer. *New England Journal of Medicine, 329*(5), 326.

Berk, M. L., Bernstein, A. B., & Taylor, A. K. (1983). The use and availability of medical care in health manpower shortage areas. *Inquiry, 20*(4), 369.

Billings, J., Anderson, G., & Newman, L. (1996). Recent findings on preventable hospitalizations. *Health Affairs,* 239.

Billings, J., Mijanovich T, & Blank, A. (1997). *Barriers to care for patients with preventable hospital admissions.* New York: United Hospital Fund.

Billings, J., & Teicholz, N. (1990). Uninsured patients in the District of Columbia. *Health Affairs,* 158.

Billings, J., Zeitel, L., & Lukomnik, J. (1993). Impact of socioeconomic status on hospital use in New York City. *Health Affairs,* 162.

Bindman, A., Grumbach, K., Osmond, D., Komaromy, M., Vranizan, K., Lurie, N., & Billings, J. (1995). Preventable hospitalizations and access to health care. *Journal of the American Medical Association, 274*(4), 305.

Blendon, R. J., Benson, J. M., & Brodie, M. (1997). Voters and health care in the 1996 election. *Journal of the American Medical Association, 277*(15), 1253.

Blendon, R. J., Benson, J. M., Brodie, M., Altman, D. E., & James, M. (2000). Health care in the upcoming 2000 election. *Health Affairs,* 210.

Blendon, R. J., Brodie, M., & Benson, J. (1995). What happened to Americans' support for the Clinton health plan. *Health Affairs,* 7.

Braveman, P. A., Egerter, S., Bennett, T., & Showstack, J. (1991). Differences in hospital resource allocation among sick newborns according to insurance coverage. *Journal of the American Medical Association, 266*(23), 3300.

Braveman, P. A., Oliva, G., & Miller, M. G. (1989). Adverse outcomes and lack of health insurance among newborns in an eight-county area of California, 1982–1986. *New England Journal of Medicine, 321*(8), 508.

Carlisle, D. M., Leake, B. D., Brook, R. H., & Shapiro, M. F. (1996). The effect of race and ethnicity on the use of selected health care procedures: A comparison of south central Los Angeles and the remainder of Los Angeles County. *Journal of Health Care for the Poor and Underserved, 7*(4), 308.

Cohen, J. W. (1989). Medicaid policy and the substitution of hospital outpatient care for physician care. *Health Services Research, 24*(1), 33.

Cooper, R. A. (1995). Perspectives on the physician workforce to the year 2020. *Journal of the American Medical Association, 274*(19), 1534.

Cotton, P. (1990a). Is there still too much extrapolation from data on middle-aged white men? *Journal of the American Medical Association, 263*(8), 1049.

Cotton, P. (1990b). Examples abound of gaps in medical knowledge because of groups excluded from scientific study. *Journal of the American Medical Association, 263*(8), 1051.

Council on Ethical and Judicial Affairs, American Medical Association. (1990). Black-white disparities in health care. *Journal of the American Medical Association, 263*(17), 2344.

Council on Scientific Affairs, American Medical Association. (1991). Hispanic health in the United States. *Journal of the American Medical Association, 265*(2), 248.

Fiscella, K., Franks, P., Gold, M. R., & Clancy, C. M. (2000). Inequality in quality, addressing socioeconomic, racial, and ethnic disparities in health care. *Journal of the American Medical Association, 283,* 2579.

Franks, P., Clancy, C. M., & Gold, M. R. (1993). Health insurance and mortality: Evidence from a national cohort. *Journal of the American Medical Association, 270*(6), 737.

Friedman, E. (1994). Money isn't everything: Nonfinancial barriers to access. *Journal of the American Medical Association, 271*(19), 1535.

Gaston, R. S., Ayres, I., Dooley, L. G., & Diethelm, A. G. (1993). Racial equity in renal transplantation: The disparate impact of HLA-based allocation. *Journal of the American Medical Association, 270*(11), 1352.

Gornick, M. E., Eggers, P. W., Reilly, T. W., Mentnech, R. M., Fitterman, L. K., Kucken, L. E., & Vladeck, B. C. (1996). Effects of race and income on mortality and use of services among Medicare beneficiaries. *New England Journal of Medicine, 335,* 791.

Grumbach, K. (1995). *The problems of shortages of physicians and other health professionals in urban areas.* Report prepared for the Council on Graduate Medical Education. San Francisco: University of California, San Francisco, Center for the Health Professions.

Hadley, J., Steinberg, E. P., & Feder, J. (1991). Comparison of uninsured and privately insured hospital patients: Conditions on admission, resource use, and outcome. *Journal of the American Medical Association, 265*(3), 374.

Held, P. J., Pauly, M. V., & Bovberg, R. R. (1988). Access to kidney transplantation. *Archives of Internal Medicine, 148,* 2594.

Henshaw, S. K. (1995). Factors hindering access to abortion services. *Family Planning Perspectives, 27*(2), 54.

Jacobson, P. D., Merritt, R., & Bartlett, L. (1994). California health care delivery: A competitive model? In *State health reform initiatives: Progress and promise.* Baltimore, MD: Health Care Financing Administration.

Johnson, P. A., Lee, T. H., & Cook, E. F. (1993). Effect of race on the presentation and management of patients with acute chest pain. *Annals of Internal Medicine, 118*(8), 593.

Kaiser Commission on Medicaid and the Uninsured. (2000). *Health insurance coverage in America—1999 data update.* Washington, DC: Author.

Kindig, D. A., & Ricketts, T. C. (1991). Determining adequacy of physicians and nurses for rural populations: Background and strategy. *Journal of Rural Health, 7*(Suppl.), 313.

Kirsch, I., Jungeblut, A., Jenkins, L., & Kolstad, A. (1993). *Adult literacy in America: A first look at the results of the National Adult Literacy Survey.* Washington, DC: National Center for Education Statistics, U.S. Department of Education.

Kjellstrand, C. M. (1988). Age, sex, and race inequality in renal transplantation. *Archives of Internal Medicine, 148,* 1305.

Lantz, P. M., Weigers, M. E., & House, J. S. (1997). Education and income differentials in breast cancer and cervical cancer screening. *Medical Care, 35*(3), 219.

Lieu, T. A., Newacheck, P. W., & McManus, M. A. (1993). Race, ethnicity, and access to ambulatory care among U.S. adolescents. *American Journal of Public Health, 83*(7), 960.

Lipson, D. J., & Schrodel, S. P. (1996). *State initiatives in health care reform: State-subsidized insurance programs for low-income people.* Washington, DC: Alpha Center.

Lurie, N., Slater, J., & McGovern, P. (1993). Preventive care for women: Does the sex of the physician matter? *New England Journal of Medicine, 329*(7), 478.

Lurie, N., Ward, N. B., Shapiro, M. F., Gallego, C., Vaghaiwall, R., & Brook, R. H. (1986). Special report: Termination of Medi-Cal benefits: A follow-up study one year later. *New England Journal of Medicine, 314*(19), 1266.

Mathews, S., Ribar, D., & Wilhelm, M. (1997). The effects of economic conditions and access to reproductive health services on state abortion rates and birthrates. *Family Planning Perspectives, 29*(2), 52.

Millman, M. (Ed.). (1993). *Access to health care in America.* Washington, DC: National Academy Press, Institute of Medicine.

Nesbitt, T., Connell, F. A., & Hart, L. G. (1990). Access to obstetric care in rural areas: Effect on birth outcomes. *American Journal of Public Health, 80*(7), 814.

Newacheck, P. W. (1992). Characteristics of children with high and low usage of physician services. *Medical Care, 30*(1), 30.

Phillips, K. A., Mayer, M. L., & Aday, L. (2000). Barriers to care among racial/ethnic groups under managed care. *Health Affairs,* 65.

Politzer, R. M, Harris, D. L., & Gaston, M. H. (1991). Primary care physician supply and the medically underserved. *Journal of the American Medical Association, 266*(1), 104.

Riley, A. W., Finney, J. W., & Mellits, E. D. (1993). Determinants of children's health care use. *Medical Care, 31*(9), 767.

Rosenblatt, R. A., Mattis, R., & Hart, L. G. (1995). Abortions in rural Idaho: Physicians' attitudes and practices. *American Journal of Public Health, 85*(10), 1423.

Schulman, K. A., Berlin, J. A., Harless, W., Kerner, J. F., Sistrunk, S., Gersh, B. J., Dubé, R., Taleghani, C. K., Burke, J. E., Williams, S., Eisenberg, J. M., & Escarce, J. J. (1999). The effect of race and sex on physicians' recommendations for cardiac catheterization. *New England Journal of Medicine, 340,* 618.

Short, P. F., & Banthin, J. S. (1995). New estimates of the underinsured younger than 65 years. *Journal of the American Medical Association, 274*(16), 1302.

Short, P. F., & Lefkowitz, D. C. (1992). Encouraging preventive services for low-income children: The effect of expanding Medicaid. *Medical Care, 30*(9), 766.

Solis, J. M., Marks, G., Garcia, M., & Shelton, D. (1990). Acculturation, access to care, and use of preventive services by Hispanics: Findings from HHANES 1982–1984. *American Journal of Public Health, 80*(Suppl.), 11.

Todd, K. H., Lee, T., & Hoffman, J. R. (1994). The effect of ethnicity of physician estimates of pain severity in patients with isolated extremity trauma. *Journal of the American Medical Association, 271*(12), 925.

Todd, K. H., Samaroo, N., & Hoffman, J. R. (1993). Ethnicity as a risk factor for inadequate emergency department analgesia. *Journal of the American Medical Association, 269*(12), 1537.

Udvarhelyi, I. S., Gatsonis, C., & Epstein, A. M. (1992). Acute myocardial infarction in the Medicare population. *Journal of the American Medical Association, 268*(18), 2530.

U.S. Census Bureau. (2000). *Health insurance coverage: 1999.*

Weiss, B. D. (1994). Illiteracy among Medicaid recipients and its relation to health care costs. *Journal of Health Care for the Poor and Underserved, 5*(2), 99.

Weissman, J., Gatsonis, C., & Epstein, A. (1992). Rates of avoidable hospitaliza-
    tions by insurance status in Massachusetts and Maryland. *Journal of the
    American Medical Association, 268,* 2388–2394.
Whittle, J., Conigliaro, J., & Good, C. (1993). Racial differences in the use of
    cardiovascular procedures in the department of Veterans Affairs Medical
    System. *New England Journal of Medicine, 329,* 627.
Williams, M. V., Parker, R. M., & Baker, D. W. (1995). Inadequate functional health
    literacy among patients at two public hospitals. *Journal of the American
    Medical Association, 274*(21), 1677.

16

Cost Containment

Kenneth E. Thorpe

LEARNING OBJECTIVES

☐ Understand the factors that contribute to the growth in health care costs.
☐ Describe the approaches employed by Medicare, Medicaid, and the private sector to control the growth in costs.
☐ Analyze the historic and recent performance of these cost-containment strategies.

TOPICAL OUTLINE

Factors accounting for health care expenditure growth
Efforts to control rising health care costs: The early experience
Efforts to control health care costs (1983–present)
Our Most Recent Experience—From 1999 On
Summary and conclusions

KEY WORDS

prospective payment, diagnosis-related group, managed care, point of service, preferred provider, hospital rate setting

Despite vigorous efforts to control health care costs, health care expenditures continue to rise at rates exceeding general inflation. In 2000, health care was 13.1% of our gross domestic product (GDP) (Heffler, Levit, Smith, Smith, Cowan, Lazenby, et al., 2001). Health care spending is expected to double this decade, rising from $1.3 trillion in 2000 to over $2.6 trillion by 2010. At the end of the decade, health care spending is expected to consume nearly 16% of the GDP. The most recent data reveal that health care spending is again on the rise. Between 1996 and 1999, national health care spending increased at a modest 5% per year. By 1999, however, the growth in spending increased, rising over 8%. The relatively low rates of growth in health spending over the past couple of years appear to be over.

Rising health care expenditures raise several issues. First, public expenditures for health care account for a substantial portion of the federal budget. Thus, past efforts to reduce the size of the federal budget deficit (estimated at approximately $50 billion in 1997) have focused attention on publicly financed health care programs. Other factors held constant, rising public health care spending could now reduce the size of our expected federal budget surplus. Second, though the growth in private health spending moderated through 1998, recent trends show a clear reversal. Lulled into 3 years of slow growth in insurance premiums, private insurance spending increased by 9.3% in 2000, with double digit increases expected in the near term (Heffler et al., 2001). The rising cost of health insurance will increase the number of uninsured, and slow the growth in take-home pay for workers with insurance.

The continued escalation in health care costs suggests that efforts by third-party payers to lower cost growth have achieved mixed results. Although some payers, in particular those with private insurance, have reduced the growth in expenditures for short periods of time, spending by others has remained stable or has increased, leaving the overall rate of growth in health care relatively unchanged. The factors accounting for the sustained increase in health care costs, the effects of recent public and private sector attempts to control this growth, and an assessment of the future direction of health care cost-containment serve as the focus of this chapter.

FACTORS ACCOUNTING FOR HEALTH CARE EXPENDITURE GROWTH

The United States spent $1.31 trillion on health care in the year 2000 (Heffler et al., 2001). This represents a 20% rise between 1997 and 2000 alone, a $217 billion increase. In its simplest construction, total spending equals price times the quantity of services. This reflects four major factors: general economy-wide inflation, inflation specific to the health care industry (over and above general rates of inflation), population growth, and changes in the nature and intensity of health care delivery. The relative contributions of these factors to yearly changes in health care costs are discussed below. It should be noted, however, that there is some debate over our ability to decompose the elements accounting for health spending growth. Aaron (1994), for instance, notes that we cannot directly measure the quantity of services produced. Moreover, Aaron, along with other economists, is quite skeptical about our ability to distinguish health-sector-specific increases in prices from overall inflation. The decomposition presented below should keep those important caveats in mind.

The most recent data suggest that after general inflation is taken into account, that medical care prices accounted for over two thirds of the most recent increase in spending (Heffler et al., 2001). The recent emergence of price in the spending equation largely reflects the growing role that pharmaceutical expenditures have assumed in the rise in health spending. Two factors commonly thought responsible for the rise in health care costs are the rapid spread of comprehensive health insurance (traced to demand-side distortions) and technological change (a supply-side issue). These factors and their interrelationships are explored below.

Demand-Side Distortions

Economists have traditionally identified the spread of health insurance as a primary cause for health care cost growth (Pauly, 1986). The rapid increase in availability of health insurance has generated continued increases in demand for health care, in terms of both volume and perceived quality. The rapid increase in the scope (type of health care insured) and comprehensiveness (the proportion of a health care bill paid by a third party) of health insurance during the 1960s and 1970s has been traced to the tax treatment of health benefits (Manning, Newhouse, Duan, Keeler, Leibowitz, & Marquis, 1987). In particular, employer contributions for health insurance benefits are exempt from federal and state income taxation. With employer health benefit contributions exceeding $200 billion in 1999, this exemption translated into a $76 billion loss in taxes (Office of Management and Budget, 1998). The tax treatment subsidizes the marginal dollar of fringe benefits that employees receive from employers relative to other forms of compensation (e.g., wages), thereby increasing the demand for health insurance relative to other goods.

The tax treatment of health insurance benefits has two consequences. First, individuals purchase more insurance than they would without the tax subsidy. Second, more extensive health insurance results in higher health care spending. With respect to insurance, the tax laws encourage individuals to purchase less preventive care and to insure against marginal risks. More comprehensive policies with few cost-sharing obligations also lead to higher spending. The magnitude of the additional expenditures is substantial. An experimental study, conducted by the Rand Corporation, examined the impact of insurance on health care spending. Their results indicate that the use of services responds to the level of cost sharing. In short, per capita expenditures in plans with no cost sharing were approximately 33% greater than in plans with a 95% coinsurance obligation (Manning et al., 1987). Moreover, relative to a free-care plan, per capita spending among those enrolled in plans with 25% coinsurance was approximately

15% lower. Lower expenditures did not result in measurable reductions in patient health status. For example, for an average individual enrolled in the plan, the Rand study did not detect significant differences in health status across insurance plans during the 3-year tracking period. These findings suggest that low coinsurance obligations result in higher rates of utilization with few measurable short-run health benefits.

Supply-Side Factors

Imperfect information and cost increasing technological changes represent two supply-side factors that distinguish the health care industry from more "competitive" markets. These factors, in conjunction with the demand-side distortions noted above, have also contributed to the real changes in medical care prices as well as intensity of medical care over time.

Imperfect Information

Potential consumers of medical care have imperfect information concerning its price and quality. High search costs and extensive health insurance coverage reduce the potential net benefits of searching for lower-cost providers. The importance of search costs and their impact on medical care prices have received much attention. The "increasing monopoly" thesis, outlined by Pauly and Satterwaite (1981), consists of two observations. First, consumer information concerning physicians and other providers decreases with higher numbers of providers. Second, if the search for providers is more difficult, consumers are less price sensitive, and physicians have more discretion in increasing fees. Thus, according to this thesis, growth in the per capita number of physicians would result in higher prices.

Even with extensive price shopping by consumers, comprehensive health insurance coverage reduces any potential savings resulting from identifying low-cost providers. Thus, both high search costs and extensive health insurance coverage dilute the incentives for consumers to engage in vigorous price shopping.

Further complicating the consumer's task is the lack of information concerning provider quality. Measuring the quality of care provided by individual physicians or hospitals has traditionally been very difficult. Although we have witnessed an explosion of medical outcomes research over the past 10 years, the development of outcome-based measures remains in its infancy. Instead, consumers have often used proxies such as the physician's board certification or a hospital's teaching affiliation as an indicator of higher quality. As a result, higher perceived quality is also associated with higher fees and costs. At issue is whether these higher fees and prices reflect unobserved quality differences. Thus, price competition among providers will continue to be limited until consumers are able to compare both price and quality differences accurately.

Despite the informational problems facing consumers, hospitals and physicians do compete. The features of the health care delivery system noted above, however, have encouraged competition in perceptions of quality rather than price. This includes both inadequate information on price and quality differences and the pervasiveness of first-dollar health insurance coverage. Thus, instead of competing on a price basis to attract patients, hospitals have competed to attract physicians (and through them patients). Hospitals in more concentrated (competitive) markets attempt to attract physicians through specific capital investments. These capital investments include the latest technologies, a broad range of clinical services, and other amenities. Because new technology increases service intensity, quality competition is quite costly. Whether the additional service intensity translates into better health outcomes remains at issue.

That hospitals have traditionally pursued competition in quality, rather than in price, has been the subject of numerous empirical investigations. The results generally lead to the conclusion that, other factors held constant, hospitals in more competitive markets produce more services and have significantly higher costs (Robinson & Luft, 1988). Although these results generally held through the mid-1980s, efforts by state governments and other payers to encourage price competition have altered the behavior of hospitals. The more recent roles of competition and market structure are discussed below.

Technological Change

The demand-side distortions noted above, combined with traditional "nonprice" competition among providers, have created an environment for rapid adoption and diffusion of new technologies. These technologies generally fall into three categories: replacing accepted medical practices (e.g., hip replacement techniques and coronary artery bypass surgery), new therapies (e.g., liver, heart, and other organ transplants; new classes of drugs), and new imaging devices (e.g., magnetic resonance imaging). Without question, many of these new technologies clearly extend years of active life to many who, even 25 years ago, would have died. The downside is that many of the new technologies have large price tags.

Although international comparisons of health care delivery systems often raise more questions than they answer, some studies have attempted to document the role of technology in increasing health care costs (Aaron & Schwartz, 1984). Based on their analysis of the U.S. and British health care systems, Aaron and Schwartz conclude that per capita health care costs would fall 10% if U.S. physicians used 10 key technologies (e.g., hip replacement, computed tomography, intensive care units) and intensive care at (population-adjusted) rates similar to those of their British counterparts. Their analysis did not detect significant differences in health status resulting from the less intensive use of these technologies.

The critical role assumed by technological change (discussed above as increased service intensity) in rising health care costs has generated a growing volume of research focused on practice patterns and the appropriateness of medical procedures. This research has been spurred by international comparisons as well as by large geographic variations in practice patterns documented domestically. One early pioneer of this type of study, John Wennberg, noted magnitude differences in rates of specific procedures completed by physicians. Fourfold differences in hysterectomy rates, prostatectomies, tonsillectomies, and other common surgical procedures were discovered within and between states (Wennberg, 1984). Subsequent research indicates that these variations are not related to underlying differences in patient characteristics but rather to physician's practice patterns. These large variations among common procedures have resulted in a significant body of research aimed at examining the "appropriateness" of these differences (Wennberg, 1996).

Researchers at the Rand Corporation have also been active in examining the appropriateness of various practice patterns. Their studies of four surgical procedures—coronary artery bypass surgery (CABG), carotid endarterectomy, coronary angioplasty, and upper gastrointestinal endoscopy—examined the magnitude of unnecessary procedures and hospitalizations. With respect to CABG, the Rand researchers judged that 44% of the procedures examined were performed for inappropriate reasons (Chassin, 1987). Some 17% of coronary angiographies, used to diagnose blockages in heart arteries, were deemed inappropriate, as were a similar volume of gastrointestinal endoscopies. Eliminating inappropriate surgery would result in continued savings of billions of dollars per year. Although the precise magnitude of the savings remains speculative, if the rates of inappropriate use found in these procedures are extrapolated, reducing unnecessary use could reduce health care spending by over $50 billion per year. More recent studies have reached similar conclusions. The landmark Harvard Medical Practice Study, whose findings were recently examined by an Institute of Medicine panel, found that inappropriate medical procedures were (if extrapolated nationally) associated with up to 100,000 patient deaths per year (Kohn, Corrigan, & Donaldson, 2000).

Private health plans, the federal government, drug makers, and large employers have attempted to further the work on "appropriateness." The federal government, under the sponsorship of the Agency for Healthcare Research and Quality (AHRQ) has examined several areas of medical practice and produced a number of specific guidelines designed to help physicians practice the best quality medicine. Moreover, the concept of appropriateness has generated a new nongovernmental industry that attempts to "manage" the process of care, known as "disease management." Here vendors have developed specific protocols for treating specific medical conditions such as asthma, diabetes, and cancer, among others. As disease management is in its formative stage, it is too early to detect its impact on practice.

Large employers, members of both the Washington Business Group on Health and the Business Roundtable (which formed the Leapfrog Group) have become more active in pushing for improvements in the quality of health care. The Leapfrog Group, comprised of several Fortune 500 companies, has recently published a series of recommendations focused on reducing provider errors (Leapfrog Group, 2001). A renewed call for evidence-based medicine, and computerized physician order entry (to reduce information errors, and prescribing errors) is among their recommendations. However, the introduction of new technologies (Internet-based for instance) into the physician's office remains a slow process.

Improvements in quality are likely to come at a cost, however. Recent analyses (Phamaceutical Research and Manufacturers Association of America, 2001; Schwartz, 1994) outline the flood of new technologies that will come on-line over the next 10–15 years. Much of the innovation is traced directly to the scientific findings from the Human Genome Project. Indeed, today there are approximately 500 distinct targets for drug intervention. Over the next decade or so, the number of therapeutic targets is expected to rise to 3,000–10,000—an explosion of new technologies converging on the market (Pharmaceutical Research and Manufacturers Association, 2001). These include new classes of pharmaceuticals that will treat persons with the acquired immune deficiency syndrome (AIDS) and a range of additional autoimmune diseases, treatment of Parkison's and dementia, advances in molecular and cell biology that could change clinical medicine fundamentally, and advances in genetics. These new technologies are, in the short run, likely to place persistent pressure on the growth in health care spending. It remains to be seen whether the "march of science" will result in slower or higher growth in spending in the longer run.

EFFORTS TO CONTROL RISING HEALTH CARE COSTS: THE EARLY EXPERIENCE

This section summarizes previous and current efforts by third-party payers to control health care costs. We focus specifically on hospital cost containment, the area that has attracted most of our cost-control efforts.

Limits on Hospital Inputs

Historically, efforts to control the use of inputs by hospitals have focused on capital expenditure decisions. Government has assumed a major role in initially financing and subsequently limiting hospital capital expansion for more than 40 years. The initial role of the government in health planning was to facilitate expansion of the hospital industry. In this capacity, the Hospital Survey and Construction (Hill-Burton) Act of 1946 supplied federal funds to underwrite new hospital construction. These funds were allocated to states according to population and state per capita income levels to redress a perceived shortage and maldistribution of hospital beds. Using some simple bed-to-population guidelines, local health planners allocated the funds to expand the nation's hospital bed supply.

In light of the rapid growth in the capacity of the hospital sector, health planning efforts have recently focused on limiting future hospital capital expansions. Although some voluntary efforts preceded it, the most comprehensive planning efforts commenced in 1974 with the National Health Planning and Resource Development Act. This act provided federal funding for local health systems agencies (HSA) and state health planning and development agencies. The health planning act developed because of growing concern over rising hospital costs increasingly linked to facility (both physical plant and technology) duplication. Thus, a primary role of the HSA's was to develop planning recommendations for specific hospital investments exceeding some dollar threshold (often $100,000). Based on the work of the local HSA, a certificate of need (CON) was usually issued at the state level granting permission to spend capital. Although health planning agencies reached their peak during the 1970s, HSA's were generally phased out during the mid-1980s.

Regulating the Utilization of Medical Care

This section focuses on public sector efforts to limit the utilization of hospital services. More recent attempts by the private sector to manage the course of a patient's treatment are addressed below. Efforts to prevent unnecessary and low-quality care delivered to publicly insured patients commenced in 1972 with the advent of professional standard review organizations (PSROs). The goals of the PSRO program, albeit quite broadly defined, were to "promote the effective, efficient, and economical delivery of health care services of proper quality." Thus, the language in the enacting legislation included both cost-containment and quality-enhancement goals. The lack of clear direction in the program's goals likely contributed to the inability of most PSROs to focus their efforts effectively. In practice, PSROs focused primarily on Medicare and Medicaid beneficiaries, although some anticipated a broader spillover to privately insured patients. Despite the broad range of goals articulated under the original act, most PSROs attempted to reduce the length of stay among the Medicare population.

Evaluations of the PSRO program showed that it produced mixed results. On average, the PSROs appeared to reduce total days of hospitalization among Medicare patients by 1.5% (Congressional Budget Office, 1981). PSROs appear to have reduced total days through reductions in length of stay rather than by preventing admissions. Although some studies suggest that the PSRO program produced some public sector savings, these costs appear to have been shifted to other payers (Congressional Budget Office, 1981). The impact of the program on the Medicaid population remains unknown. However, Medicare savings (through reduced utilization) were nearly offset by the administrative costs of the program. Viewed more broadly, the Congressional Budget Office researchers found that savings to the Medicare program were offset by increases in charges (and expenditures) by private payers. Hence, when administrative costs and charges in total health care expenditures were examined, the PSROs appeared less effective.

The PSROs were replaced with peer review organizations (PROs) in 1984. The PRO differs from its predecessor, the PSRO, in that PRO contracts are awarded in a competitive bidding process, based in part on the bidder's projected and/or demonstrated ability to achieve specific utilization goals. These goals are developed through negotiations with the Health Care Financing Administration (HCFA) and relate to five objectives (Office of Technology Assessment, 1981, Appendix G):

1. to reduce unnecessary hospital re-admissions;
2. to assure the provision of adequate care, that, if not given, would cause serious complications;
3. to reduce the risk of mortality associated with specific procedures and conditions;
4. to reduce unnecessary surgery; and
5. to reduce avoidable postoperative or other complications.

Negotiations between a PRO and the HCFA define specific performance markers (e.g., reducing readmissions resulting from substandard care by 20% could be used to evaluate the effectiveness of each PRO).

Starting in 1989, PROs assumed an extended set of responsibilities beyond hospital care, including review of outpatient procedures, home health care, and care provided to military personnel and their families. By 1993, however, the program's effectiveness was in question, especially given its $300 million annual price tag. Starting that year, PROs began adopting a new strategy called the Health Care Quality Improvement Initiative. Under this initiative, PROs shifted their focus from identifying individual clinical errors to helping providers improve the mainstream of medical care. The PROs use statistical quality controls to examine variations in both the processes and the outcomes of care. They then share this information with hospitals and physicians and work with them to interpret and apply the findings.

The Process of Cost Reductions

Effective rate-setting programs provide incentives for hospitals to adjust their "behavior" across many dimensions. Most notably, rate-setting programs provide incentives for hospitals to reduce the service intensity of medical care. In an earlier section, increased service intensity was identified as a major factor accounting for real increases in yearly health care costs. Reductions in service intensity are possible through lower staffing levels, a less expensive mix of personnel (e.g., the substitution of licensed practical nurses for registered nurses), slower adoption of new technology, or all of the above. The early literature on rate setting found evidence of adjustment across all dimensions (Cromwell & Kanak, 1982).

More effective rate-setting programs reduced costs by limiting the inputs (most notably technology) used to produce medical care. Hospitals in rate-setting states adopted new technologies at slower rates. Among the diffusion patterns examined were such major expense items as intensive care units, open heart surgery, coronary artery surgery, obesity surgery, and burn care units (Romeo, Wagner, & Lee, 1984). Moreover, other technologies, most notably imaging devices such as the computerized axial tomography (CAT) scanner, were adopted by hospitals at a slower pace in rate-setting states.

Rate setting also resulted in reduced hospital payroll expenses per patient day (Kidder & Sullivan, 1982). These "productivity" increases were achieved through both reductions in staff per adjusted day and changes in the mix of personnel. In some instances, particularly in teaching hospitals, administrators reduced their ancillary staff component, including intravenous and phlebotomy teams, messenger/transporters, and clerks, among others. Their tasks were generally absorbed by resident physicians, nurses, or both.

Although rate-setting programs during the 1970s achieved some of their goals, some dysfunctional side effects were evident. Rate-setting programs that focused solely on the day of care often led to increases in the average length of a hospital stay (Sloan & Becker, 1984). In some cases, average hospital occupancy rates also increased. As a result, per capita days of care remained relatively stable after the implementation of rate-setting programs, blunting the full cost-containment potential. The first rate-setting programs appeared less effective in reducing per capita health care spending. This led many observers to speculate that hospitals merely shifted their fixed costs to other, unregulated payers (often termed cost-shifting) or unregulated sources of revenue (e.g., outpatient care) (Eby & Cohodes, 1985). The ability of hospital administrators to escape the full regulatory potential of the rate-setting laws created increased demand for alternative cost-containment strategies. Sharp increases in charges to unregulated payers—who were largely commercial health insurers—created growing allegations that they bore the burden of any cost savings enjoyed by regulated (generally, government) payers (Sloan & Becker, 1984). The growing differential between "costs" reimbursed by regulated payers and "charges" to unregulated payers raised concerns about the overall effectiveness and equity of rate-setting programs. These concerns were largely responsible for the subsequent generation of rate-setting programs, competitive bidding schemes, and alternative delivery systems described below.

Efforts to Control Health Care Costs (1983–Present)

Informed by the early experience with hospital rate setting, attempts to control rising health care costs changed in four important aspects during the mid-1980s. First, private payers and employers increased their efforts to develop cost-containment programs. Second, state governments and Medicare experimented with new approaches to hospital rate setting. Third, both the public and private sectors created incentives for hospitals to compete on the basis of price, rather than other dimensions. Finally, the cost-containment debate was extended to physician payment in addition to institutional payment reforms.

Role of Private Payers

Perhaps the most important story trend the past 5 years with respect to health care spending has been the slower growth in private health insurance spending. During this time employers have become increasingly vigilant in their efforts to control their expenditures; the evidence indicates that these efforts have achieved some level of success.

Facing sharply rising health insurance premiums during the early 1980s, private payers extended their efforts to control health care costs (particularly hospital costs) in three important directions. First, private payers and employers increased efforts to "manage" the utilization of health care. Second, dissatisfied with the ability of private health insurance carriers to control costs, a growing number of employers decided to "self-insure." Third, using their purchasing power for leverage, private payers increasingly negotiated rates of payment with health care providers.

Growth in Managed Care

Managed care is a term applied to a wide variety of health plans (see also chapter 11). In its most general formulation, the managed care plans link patients with primary care physicians for care. Health plans providing care under this rubric may be entirely or partially capitated. Perhaps the best known form of managed care organization is the health maintenance organization (HMO).

The spectacular growth in HMO enrollment noted above was enhanced by their well-documented ability to reduce total health expenditures. Early, nonexperimental experience placed the magnitude of these cost savings between 20% and 40%, compared to those enrolled in more traditional health care plans (Luft, 1981). More recent studies have estimated that HMOs reduce the use of services by 20% compared to traditional health plans (Congressional Budget Office, 1995). As such plans also negotiate price discounts, the overall reduction in spending is even larger. Though these studies have used statistical methods that attempt to estimate spending in HMOs and traditional plans among populations "randomly" assigned to such plans, such selection in practice is not likely. Thus, there is residual concern that some portion of the estimated savings linked to HMOs may in fact simply reflect the enrollment of healthier patients in such plans.

Evidence from the Rand Health Insurance Experiment (HIE) provided insight into the selection issue. Using an experimentally controlled population, the HIE found that, compared to a free, fee-for-service plan, HMOs reduced total expenditures by 29% (Manning et al., 1987). The magnitude of these reductions was impressive, similar to those observed under a 95% coinsurance rate. Thus, the experimental results indicated that HMOs did not require favorable selection to achieve their large apparent cost savings. Remaining at issue, however, is whether these savings represent one-time or continued reductions in health care spending. One early comparison of premium growth among traditional plans with that of HMOs found little difference in rates of increase (Newhouse, Schwartz, Williams, & Witsberger, 1985). If these results are valid, they suggest that HMO savings, although substantial, may be transitory.

Spurred by the studies documenting their effectiveness, selected aspects of HMOs, such as a second surgical opinion, pre-authorization of selected hospital admissions, concurrent review, and outpatient surgery and testing requirements, assumed standard roles in many health plans (Jensen, Morrisey, & Marcus, 1987). In some cases, immediate reductions in health care spending resulted. Although evaluations of the cost savings traced to private sector utilization programs are rare, one study provided some early insight. For the large private health insurer examined, hospital utilization review (which included preadmission certification and on-site and concurrent review) reduced admissions by 12.3%, inpatient spending by 11.9%, and total per capita expenditures by 8.3% (Feldstein, Wickizer, & Wheeler, 1988). More recent studies have confirmed these earlier results (Zwanziger & Melnick, 1996).

In addition to avoiding state benefit mandates, there are other incentives for companies to self-insure. For instance, self-insured funds are not subject to state premium taxes or to laws governing capital and financial reserve requirements. Moreover, self-insured funds do not contribute to state "risk pools," designed to finance insurance for high-risk, low-income individuals through state taxes. Growth in the number of self-insured plans is also symptomatic of the longer-term trend away from "community"-rated plans and toward "experience" rating. Built into traditional group health insurance premiums are costs stemming from uncompensated care, insurance company profits, and cross-subsidies of high-cost policyholders. The rising number of uninsured individuals and uncompensated care has accounted for a portion of the yearly increases in health insurance premiums. Firms that self-insure avoid these additional costs, which are built into a typical group health insurance premium. In this sense, self-insuring eliminates any cross-subsidies included in health insurance premiums. However, the move to self-insuring also transfers all (or in some cases most) of the financial risk of catastrophic cases from private insurers to firms.

Despite the benefits accruing to firms that self-insure, the comparative ability of such plans to contain costs remains unproved. One study compared the level and rate of increase in costs among self-insured, commercial, and Blue Cross plans. The results found no significant differences in expenditures across plans between 1981 and 1985 (Jensen & Gabel, 1988). Moreover, firms self-insuring during this period actually experienced sharper increases in health care spending compared to commercial and Blue Cross plans. Although our experience with self-insured plans is relatively new, their ability to significantly reduce cost growth relative to more traditional payers appears questionable. Though few recent studies have directly compared health insurance premiums between insured and self-insured firms, one recent examination found few significant differences in premiums (Acs, Long, Marquis, & Short, 1996).

Point-of-Service Products

Another important trend is the growing popularity of point-of-service (POS) plans. These hybrid plans combine key features of HMO and traditional indemnity products. Enrollees are permitted to choose at the point of service whether to use the plan's provider network or seek care from nonnetwork physicians. Typically, in-panel physicians are paid on a capitated or discounted-fee basis, and out-of-panel physicians receive traditional fee-for-service reimbursement.

From the consumer's perspective, free choice of providers is a major selling point for POS plans. The reimbursement provisions of these plans, however, are designed to dissuade enrollees from exercising the out-of-network option. Most enrollees in open-ended products pay coinsurance in the 30% range and deductibles of up to $300 for use of out-of-network providers, whereas services provided in-network are subject to minimal co-payments (KPMG, 1996). These financial differentials effectively deter out-of-network care. Strongly encouraging, but not requiring, use of in-network physicians, POS plans aim to reap the benefits of tightly managed care while bypassing its least popular feature, that is, restricted consumer choice.

Growth in Preferred Provider Organizations

Finally, private payers and self-insured firms have increasingly used their purchasing power to negotiate payment rates with providers. Under a preferred provider organization (PPO) arrangement, private payers negotiate a discounted rate with selected physicians and hospitals, often guaranteeing the provider a specified volume of business. For hospitals suffering from low occupancy rate (generally in California, Colorado, and Florida), the arrangements are quite attractive.

Although the sponsorships, form, and incentives found in PPOs differ widely, today's PPOs share four common characteristics:

1. PPOs represent an organized network of providers (e.g., hospitals, physicians) available to provide care.
2. Patients enter the PPO network through financial incentives in their benefits, a physician gatekeeper, or both.
3. PPOs negotiate discounts from providers from prevailing market payment rates.
4. PPOs include a variety of managed care elements, usually including physician gatekeepers, utilization review, and second-opinion programs.

Early PPOs focused on negotiating reduced rates of payment to both hospitals and physicians. Little attention was directed toward including checks on utilization. As a result, early experience with PPOs provided mixed results. Although unit costs fell, the volume of services often increased, reducing the success of the ventures. More recently, insurers have developed hybrid programs incorporating utilization-control features along with negotiated payments. The utilization-control features in these hybrid plans are similar to those found in most HMOs. A central feature of these plans is the use of a gatekeeper primary care physician. The primary care physician in essence manages the patient referral process. Most hybrid plans include financial incentives for the gatekeeper to monitor utilization by setting specific targets for hospital admissions, total hospital days, and outpatient surgery. Because these hybrid plans are so new, few empirical analyses have assessed their impact on health care expenditures. One recent study reference, however, examined the impact of a PPO for a large western company. The study found no discernible difference in spending among those enrolled in the PPO compared to other employees. Whether these results will generalize to other settings remains unknown.

Innovations in Hospital Rate Setting—Growth in Diagnosis-Related Group Payment Systems

Perhaps the most important change in hospital rate setting during the 1980s was Medicare's shift from a retrospective cost-based program to a prospectively determined payment based on diagnosis-related groups (DRGs). Under this system, hospitals are paid a preestablished amount per case treated, with payment rates varying by type of case. The DRGs measure hospital output by originally classifying patients into 23 major diagnostic categories (MDCs), based on major body systems. The MDCs are divided further into more than 470 diagnostic groups based on the patient's diagnosis or surgical procedure used and on age, sex, and other clinical information. Three aspects of this approach differ from Medicare's previous payment methodology. First, the payments are determined in advance and are fixed. Second, the unit of payment changed from per day to per admission. Finally, payment rates were eventually divorced from each hospital's own cost experience.

The new payment scheme implemented by Medicare applies only to inpatient, operating costs. Excluded are payments for physicians' services (discussed below), capital (which Medicare continues to reimburse at levels slightly below interest and depreciation expenses), direct medical education (e.g., salaries for attending physicians and residents), and outpatient and emergency departments. Not all hospitals were included in Medicare's case payment system. Some specialty hospitals, such as children's, long-term care, rehabilitation, and psychiatric hospitals, were exempt. Also exempt were four states (New York, Massachusetts, Maryland, and New Jersey) receiving waivers from the HCFA to develop their own experimental payment programs. By 1993, however, only Maryland had retained its waiver.

Payment that an individual hospital receives for treating Medicare patients in a given DRG depends on the DRGs "cost" weight (i.e., its cost relative to an average Medicare admission) multiplied by a "standardized" average cost for all Medicare patients. The standardization process includes adjustments for inter-hospital differences in wages, teaching status, and amount of care provided to low-income patients. Different rates are also set for urban and rural hospitals. In addition, payment amounts to hospitals are adjusted each year by a "trend factor," consisting of a measure of the price of goods and services purchased by hospitals and a discretionary adjustment factor to account for changes in new technology and productivity. The original plans called for a gradual phase-in of the case payment system over 3 years. In the first year (1984), 75% of a hospital's per-case payments were to be based on its own cost experience. This level gradually declined over time; by 1988 payment rates (known as prices) to hospitals were based on national standardized average costs per admission. Movement to a pricing system divorced payment rates from each hospital's costs.

The Impact of the Medicare DRG Program

Medicare's experience with the DRG system has produced mixed results. Initially, hospitals responded quite dramatically to the altered incentives created by the DRG payment system. The payment of a fixed price per admission provided hospitals clear incentives to reduce costs. Any savings stemming from these reductions could be retained by the hospital. The new opportunity to earn short-term profits resulted in impressive changes during the early years of the program. In its first year (federal fiscal year 1984) inpatient expenditures declined as the number of full-time equivalent

(FTE) employees fell 2.3%, reversing the trend of earlier years. Although lengths of stay among the elderly had been falling for years, the DRG program accelerated the decline. Finally, total admissions fell 2.6% during the first year of the DRG program, again reversing a long trend toward increased admissions.

Falling lengths of stay, admissions, and employment levels resulted in slower hospital expenditure growth. Total Medicare inpatient operating costs decreased by 6% during the first year of the program. Inpatient cost per admission increased slightly, by approximately 1.3%, significantly below the 4.7% update in Medicare payments allowed during the first year. With cost growth slower than increases in revenue, hospital operating margins rose sharply. By 1984 it was 11.3%, the highest in nearly 2 decades (AHA, 1988).

The second decade of experience with the Medicare DRG program differs sharply from the experience in the 1980s (see Table 16.1). Starting in the late 1980s, both the nominal and real (here adjusted for the percent change in the consumer price index) growth in Medicare inpatient hospital payments and hospitals costs started to decline. By the early 1990s the inflation-adjusted growth in hospital costs had declined to approximately 4%. By 1994, the growth in inflation adjusted payments had declined to 2.6%.

The 1990s witnessed another major difference in the interaction between Medicare hospital payments and costs. Throughout the course of the DRG program, payments to hospitals had always increased at a slower rate than hospital costs. By 1993, however, Medicare payments to hospitals started to rise faster than the overall growth in hospital costs. The dramatic slowdown in costs is partially attributed to changes in Medicare payment policies, as well as to changes in medical technology that have redirected a substantial volume of cases to the outpatient setting. Although these trends are important, the most recent reduction in hospital costs appear primarily motivated by the substantial increase in cost-containment pressures applied by the private sector. The demand for cost containment among private payers has generated an overall reduction in the growth of hospital costs.

Although it appears that the growth in Medicare inpatient hospital spending has slowed dramatically, the growth in outpatient hospital spending continued to rise. Unlike payments for inpatient expenses, Medicare currently employs a variety of methods to pay for outpatient services (i.e., laboratory, ambulatory surgery, other diagnostic). Though some of Medicare's payments are prospective in nature (e.g., laboratory services), most are based in large part on reported hospital costs. Thus, Medicare payments for outpatient services generally rise as costs rise. This differs significantly from the inpatient methodology, where the growth in payments and costs is not directly linked.

In addition to the rapid growth in outpatient payments, Medicare faces additional issues with its outpatient payment methodology. Under current law, Medicare beneficiaries face a 20% coinsurance based on hospital outpatient charges, as opposed to payments. Over the past decade, outpatient

TABLE 16.1   Percentage of Change in Medicare-Related Hospital Costs and Payments, Federal Fiscal Years 1988–1998

Year	Cost per case	Payment per case	Consumer Price Index
1988	9.0%	6.0%	4.1%
1989	9.5%	6.8%	4.7%
1990	8.1%	6.1%	5.0%
1991	7.0%	6.1%	5.1%
1992	4.6%	6.2%	3.0%
1993	1.2%	3.5%	3.1%
1994	–1.1%	3.1%	2.6%
1995	–1.2%	4.9%	2.5%
1996	–1.1%	4.6%	3.3%
1997	.5%	1.7%	1.7%
1998	1.5%	–2.3%	1.6%

Source: Medicare Payment Advisory Commission. (2000). *Selected Medicare issues, report to Congress.* Washington, DC: MedPac.

charges have risen at a faster pace than Medicare payments, imposing an increasing amount of cost sharing on Medicare beneficiaries. For example, during federal fiscal year 1995 Medicare payments for hospital outpatient services totaled $19.4 billion, 37% of which was financed by beneficiary payments (Prospective Payment Assessment Commission, 1995, Table 2-21). Several proposals have been advanced to "fix" this beneficiary overpayment. One proposal seeks to have the Secretary of Health and Human Services establish a prospective payment program for outpatient care. The design of such a program has embraced the difficult issue of defining the clinically and financially relevant DRG equivalents.

The Managed Care Revolution: Impact on Private Health Care Spending

Perhaps the most notable change in the structure of health care payments and costs is the dramatic growth in managed care in both the public and private sectors. As interest among employers intensified after the demise of President Clinton's health care reform effort to control costs, they relied almost exclusively on managed care as the vehicle to deliver savings. The growth in the percentage of workers enrolled in such plans over 4 years has been impressive (see Table 16.2). As late as 1993, 42% of workers employed in firms with over 3 employees were enrolled in traditional fee-for-service plans. By 1996 only one quarter (26%) of all workers were enrolled in such plans. The most recent data for 1999 reveal that only 9% of all workers remain in a traditional fee-for-service plan. The demise of fee-for-service plans was accompanied by a rapid growth in enrollment in POS plans and HMOs.

**TABLE 16.2   Percentage of Workers Enrolled in Traditional
Fee-for-Service and Managed Care Plans, 1992-1999[1]**

Plan type	1992	1993	1994	1995	1996	1998	1999
Traditional Fee-for-Service	45	42	35	31	26	14	9
Point-of-Service	8	10	15	18	16	24	25
Preferred Provider	26	22	25	22	25	35	38
Health Maintenance Organization	22	26	25	29	33	27	28

[1] There is no available data for 1997.

Source: Kaiser Family Foundation. (2000). *Employer health benefits, 1999 annual survey.*
Menlo Park, CA: Author.

The growth in managed care has not been limited to the private sector. The growth in managed care within the Medicaid program has been the most impressive. As of July 1999, over 40% of Medicaid beneficiaries were enrolled in managed care plans. This compares to only 9.5% enrollment in Medicaid managed care in 1991 (www.hcfa.govoffice/managed care). By enrolling certain Medicaid beneficiaries into managed care, several states have generated savings that have, in part, been used to expand coverage to the previously uninsured. Though the growth in Medicare managed care has been slower, there is substantial interest by many policymakers to increase the use of managed care within the program to slow the growth in total Medicare spending. As of 2000, an estimated 7 million Medicare beneficiaries—approximately 18% of total enrollees—were enrolled in managed care plans (Congressional Budget Office, 2000). This compares to only 3.7% enrollment in managed care plans in 1991 (Health Care Financing Administration, 1996). Though the increased use of managed care appears to have generated substantial savings within the private sector and the Medicaid program, there is considerable debate surrounding the savings (if any) attributed to the use of managed care in the Medicare program. Some studies have suggested that Medicare saves money through managed care enrollment; other studies disagree. The lack of program savings relates, in part, to the formula used by the federal government in setting payment rates to HMOs. Under current law, Medicare pays each HMO 95% of the estimated (after adjusting for age, sex, disability status, and location) costs of providing services to beneficiaries in the fee-for-service sector. There remains substantial suspicion and some empirical documentation that even with these adjustments, healthier patients are enrolling in managed care. As a result, Medicare ends up paying more than they would have paid for the patients had they remained in the fee-for-service part of the program.

Employers have used several means to shift their workers into managed care plans. These include relying on "defined" contributions toward the price of insurance. In general, the premiums associated with managed care plans are lower than fee-for-service plans. Thus, this would increase enrollment in managed care plans relative to fee-for-service plans. Another method used by employers to direct enrollment into managed care plans is to limit their employees' choice of plan options. Among workers employed in firms with over 200 employees, 43% have a choice of only one plan, 17% have a choice of two plans, and the remaining 40% may select among three plans (Kaiser Family Foundation, 1999).

The movement of workers into managed care plans has generated impressive reductions in private-sector health care spending (see Table 16.3). For instance, spending by employers on health insurance increased at an average annual rate of 11.3% between 1985 and 1990 but declined to 6.8% during the 1990s. This includes spending growth on active workers (described in Table 16.2) as well as for retirees. The ability of employers to control the growth in spending among these two populations had differed. In general, the growth in spending among active workers has slowed dramatically, whereas the growth in retiree health spending provides few indications of any decline. The growth in household spending (both on health insurance premiums and out-of-pocket) decreased from 8.9% annually between 1985 and 1990 to 6% during the 1990s. More recent data reveal even sharper reductions in spending among active workers (see Table 16.2). Among such workers, the growth in health insurance premiums across all plans has declined steadily since 1991. By 1996 the growth in health insurance premiums decreased to a low of 0.5%.

A major issue in the managed care revolution is whether the impressive reductions in the growth in private health care spending represents a one-time savings as workers shift to managed care plans or whether the savings will be sustained over time. As the movement into lower-cost managed care plans is still in process, it is difficult to distinguish savings from migration into managed care plans from ongoing savings generated among those enrolled in such plans. As the managed care marketplace becomes more saturated in certain areas, it will become easier to isolate these two effects.

TABLE 16.3 Percentage of Change in Private Health Insurance Premiums, 1991-1999[1]

	1991	1992	1993	1994	1995	1996	1998	1999
Total	11.5	10.9	8	4.8	2.1	0.5	3.7	4.1
By number of employees								
200–999	—	10.6	8.8	4.6	2.8	1.1	3.5	4.7
1,000–4,999	—	10.3	7.3	5.4	2.2	0.5	4.4	3.1
5,000+	—	11	8	4.6	1.9	0.3	2.6	4.2

Sources: Kaiser Family Foundation. (1999). *Health Benefits of Small Employers in 1998.* Kaiser Family Foundation and Health Research and Educational Trust. (2000). Employer health benefits, 1999 annual survey. Menlo Park, CA: Author.

[1] There is no available data for 1997.

Reform of Physician Reimbursement

During much of the 1980s, efforts to reduce health care costs often focused on payments to institutions (especially hospitals), rather than payments for physician and outpatient services and hospital capital. After implementing the DRG system, however, policymakers turned their attention to reforming the way in which Medicare pays physicians. This attention was justified. Between 1975 and 1987, total Medicare expenditures for physicians increased by an average of 18% annually (Physician Payment Review Commission, 1988). More recent data show a slight reduction in the growth in nominal spending, but the growth remains high after adjusting for inflation. The Health Care Financing Administration projects that physician payments will rise 11% per year between 1993 and 2005 (1999).

Medicare's traditional method for reimbursing physicians was based on the "customary, prevailing and reasonable" (CPR) reimbursement system, a methodology that was typical of the fee-for-service methods used by most third-party payers. Under the CPR method, payments for each service performed were based on the lowest figure for the physician's historic charge, the billed charge, or an average charge of similar physicians in the area. Payment rates were also limited to yearly increases in the Medicare Economic Index (MEI). This system was roundly criticized as inflationary and complex. In addition, it provided higher payment rates (relative to costs) for specialists and those performing complex procedures (relative to those performing more cognitive tasks). This structure was frequently cited as influencing physicians' specialty choices. The apparent "surplus" of surgeons and subspecialists projected over the next 20 years has often been traced to this payment system.

Two options were frequently advanced to address both the cost growth and the specialty choice issues. The first payment option was to expand the number of physicians paid on a capitated basis. The role of capitation in addressing cost growth was addressed earlier. The second option was a new fee schedule for physicians.

In the 1989 Budget Act, Congress chose the second option. It mandated the implementation of a specific type of fee schedule, called a resource-based relative value scale (RBRVS), starting in 1992. This particular relative value scale has three components: a measure of total "work" by the physician, an allowance for practice costs, and an allowance for the cost of malpractice insurance. Each service is assigned a given number of relative value units (RVUs). These RVUs are then multiplied by a national conversion factor to determine a dollar amount of payment for that service. As of 1997, the federal government had created three conversion factors: one for surgical services, one for primary care, and the third for other services.

A major objective of the RBRVS was to develop a more equitable method of reimbursing physicians. In contrast to the CPR, two services that require the same amount of work, practice expense and malpractice expense, should be reimbursed at the same level (except for an adjustment to account for different price levels in different geographic areas). This was intended to eliminate the distortive effect that the CPR has on specialty choice and service mix.

In the 1989 Budget Act, Congress also made two other changes to the way that physicians are reimbursed for services they provide to Medicare patients. First, limits were placed on the amounts that physicians could charge patients above a Medicare-approved amount. In 1992 doctors were not allowed to charge more than 20% more than the Medicare-approved amount. From 1993 on, this percentage dropped to 15%.

The final reform was the creation of the Medicare volume performance standard (MVPS). The MVPS is a target rate that Congress sets annually to reflect its view of the appropriate growth rate in Medicare spending for physician services. It is intended to take into account both general cost inflation and acceptable increases in volume and intensity of services provided.

Under the CPR system, payment rates each year were updated by the amount of the MEI. The MVPS simply adds another layer to this process. After a year has ended, the MVPS rate of increase in spending and the actual rate are compared. If the MVPS is lower than the actual rate of increase (i.e., spending grew at a higher level than Congress considered appropriate), then the next year's increase (normally the MEI) is decreased by the amount of the excess. If the MVPS is higher than the actual rate of spending, then the annual update is increased by the amount of the shortfall.

OUR MOST RECENT EXPERIENCE—FROM 1999 ON

As the discussion above illustrates, the dramatic shift to managed care in the private sector generated a one-time reduction in private health spending. The most recent data show a substantial increase in private spending starting in 1999. What has accounted for this change? First, the growth in pharmaceutical spending has increased sharply. Pharmacy expenses account for approximately 15%–20% of the costs of a typical private insurance package. Drug spending has, since 1999, increased by 17% per year—accounting for 3–4 percentage points of the increase in private health insurance (Heffler et al., 2001). Much of the savings traced to managed care resulted in a one-time reduction in hospital days per capita. In addition, managed care plans successfully negotiated lower payments to hospitals and physicians. However, the shift to managed care also reduced the out-of-pocket co-payments and deductibles facing consumers for prescription drugs. At the same time, managed care plans did not achieve similar success in controlling the use and prices for pharmaceuticals. The combined effects of lower co-payments, and an explosion of new drugs hitting the market (fueled in part by a billion dollar plus direct-to-consumer advertising blitz to increase patient demand) have created double-digit increases in drug spending.

A second factor associated with the recent rise in private insurance spending is the changing nature of the managed care marketplace. Fueled in part by consumer voiced problems associated with closed-panel HMOs, and a variety of process of care initiatives developed by managed care plans to control costs, several states have enacted patients' bill of rights legislation. The new legislation has targeted the tools used by managed care plans to control utilization of health care. The state rules have resulted in congressional attentions as well. The pending passage of federal legislation will further weaken many of the tools used by the industry to control costs.

3) A third and related factor is the tightness of the labor market. Employers have competed, in part, for scarce labor using health benefits. To attract and retain labor, employers have changed the nature of their managed care plan offerings, by offering more open network plans. This has led to more choice, less utilization control, and somewhat higher spending. The demand by employers and employees for broader choice of providers combined with state-based interventions has changed the nature of managed care operations, creating looser networks of care, and less effective cost-control algorithms.

Given these changes in managed care, combined with the pending explosion of new technologies, the nature of future approaches for controlling health care costs, while improving the quality of care and providing incentives for the diffusion of cost-effective new technologies, is unknown. Clearly, the old approaches used by managed care plans—tight utilization controls directed by the plans—has met considerable resistance by physicians and the public. To be successful in the new century, it would indeed appear that the industry will have to reinvent itself and focus on new approaches for managing costs and quality.

SUMMARY AND CONCLUSIONS

Our earlier discussion indicated that the fundamental force driving up health care costs was the diffusion of new technologies. The results from the Human Genome Project, and the recent spike in spending on pharmaceuticals, represent our most recent example of technology-driven spending increases. Of the estimated sevenfold real increase in health care spending since 1950, new technologies and practice patterns account for up to 90% of the growth (Manning et al., 1987). Innovations in medicine have been nothing short of remarkable. Our capacity to increase average life expectancy and quality of life reflect these developments. The growth in transplant capacity, diagnostic imaging, and drugs represents a few of these medical innovations. If this increase in spending had generated commensurate increases in benefits, then the "problem" of health care cost growth would be illusory. In short, that we spend over 13% of our GDP in the health care sector may simply reflect societal preferences to direct limited resources to health rather than to other areas.

At the center of the debate over the growth of health care costs is whether the same level of health could be purchased for less. A growing body of research indicates that substantial savings could be achieved without significant changes in the health of our population. Critical examination of the appropriateness of various medical procedures indicates that health care spending could be reduced by several billion dollars without a deleterious impact on health. At issue is the appropriate intervention to address the underlying problem of health care cost growth in areas where problems remain. These problem areas include the Medicare program, the small group and individual insurance market, and spending in retiree health care services. Whether an expansion of managed care into these sectors can produce savings similar to those observed among workers in larger firms remains an important policy issue.

CASE STUDY

New York State recently adopted a new hospital payment system that relied on competitive bidding, rather than regulation, to determine hospital payments. New York also has over 2 million uninsured residents and the largest group of teaching hospitals in the country. Can competitive bidding and competition coexist with these other key health policy issues facing state policymakers? If so, how?

DISCUSSION QUESTIONS

1. Several states adopted rate setting that applied to all third-party payers, yet only Maryland's system has survived. What factors account for the demise in all-payer rate setting in the other states?
2. Compared to fee-for-service medicine, managed care appears to generate significant savings. How does managed care alter the delivery of medicine, and how are these savings achieved?
3. All-payer rate-setting systems were developed to contain the growth in hospital costs, but they also included a broader range of objectives. What were these additional goals, and how can these objectives be met with the demise of rate setting?

REFERENCES

Aaron, H. J. (1994). Thinking straight about medical costs. *Health Affairs, 13*(5), 7–13.

Aaron, H., & Schwartz, W. (1984). *The painful prescription: Rationing hospital care.* Washington, DC: The Brookings Institution.

Acs, G., Long, S., Marquis, S., & Short, P. (1996). Self-insured employer health plans: Prevalence, profile, provisions and premiums. *Health Affairs, 15*, 266–278.

Chassin, M. (1987). *Does inappropriate use explain geographic variation in the use of health care services? A study of three procedures* (N-2748). Santa Monica, CA: Rand Corporation.

Congressional Budget Office. (1981). *The impact of PSRO on health care costs: An update on the Congressional Budget Office's 1979 evaluation.* Washington, DC: U.S. Government Printing Office.

Congressional Budget Office. (1995). *The effects of managed care and managed competition.* Washington, DC: U.S. Government Printing Office.

Congressional Budget Office. (2000). Available: www.cbo.gov

Cromwell, J., & Kanak, J. (1982). The effects of hospital rate setting programs on volume of hospital services. *Health Care Financing Review, 4*(2), 67–88.

Eby, C. L., & Cohodes, D. R. (1985). What do we know about rate-setting? *Journal of Health Politics, Policy and Law, 10,* 299–327.

Feldstein, P., Wickizer, T., & Wheeler, J. (1988). The effects of utilization review programs on health care use and expenditures. *New England Journal of Medicine, 318,* 1310–1314.

Health Care Financing Administration, Office of the Actuary. (1999). *National health expenditures projections, 1998–2008* [On-line]. Available: www.ncfa.gov

Heffler, S., Levit, K., Smith, S., Smith, S., Cowan, C., Lazenby, H., & Freeland, M. (2001). Health spending growth up in 1999: Faster growth expected in the future. *Health Affairs, 20,* 193–203.

Jensen, G., & Gabel, J. (1988). The erosion of purchased health insurance. *Inquiry, 25,* 328–343.

Jensen, G., Morrissey, M., & Marcus, J. (1987). Cost sharing and the changing pattern of employer-sponsored health benefits. *Millbank Memorial Fund Quarterly, 65,* 521.

Kaiser Family Foundation and Health Research and Education Trust. (1999). *Health benefits of small employers in 1998.* Menlo Park, CA: Author.

Kaiser Family Foundation and Health Research and Education Trust. (2000). *Employer health benefits 1999 annual survey.* Menlo Park, CA: Author.

Kaiser Family Foundation and Health Education Research Trust. (2000). *Employer health benefits, 2000 annual survey.* Menlo Park, CA: Author.

Kidder, D., & Sullivan, D. (1982). Hospital payroll costs, productivity, and employment under prospective reimbursement. *Health Care Financing Review, 4*(2), 89–100.

Kohn, L., Corrigan, J., & Donaldson, M. (Eds.). (2000). *To err is human: Building a safer health system.* Washington, DC: Committee on the Quality of Health Care in America, Institute of Medicine.

KPMG Peat marwick. (1996). *Health benefits in 1996.* Newark, NJ: Author.

Leapfrog Group. (2001). *Patient safety* [On-line]. Available: www.leapfrog-group.com

Luft, H. (1978). How do health maintenance organizations achieve their savings? *New England Journal of Medicine, 298,* 1366.

Manning, W. G., Newhouse, J. P., Duan, N., Keeler, E. B., Leibowitz, A., & Marquis, W. D. (1987). Health insurance and the demand for medical care: Evidence from a randomized experiment. *American Economic Review, 77,* 251–277.

Medicare Advisory Payment Committee. (2000, June). *Report to Congress: Selected Medicare issues.* Washington, DC: MedPac.

Newhouse, J. P., Schwartz, W., Williams, A., & Witsberger, C. (1985). Are fee-for-service costs increasing faster than HMO costs? *Medical Care, 23,* 960.

Office of Management and Budget. (1998). *Federal budget* (p. 48). Washington, DC: U.S. Government Printing Office.

Office of Technology Assessment. (1981). *Policy implications of the CT scanner: An update.* Washington, DC: Author.

Pauly, M. (1986). Taxation, health insurance and market failure. *Journal of Economic Literature, 24,* 629–675.

Pauly, M., & Satterwaite, M. (1981). The pricing of primary care physicians' services: A test of the role of common intervention. *Bell Journal of Economics, 12,* 488–506.

Pharmaceutical Research and Manufacturers Association of America. (2001). *Industry profile, 2000.* Washington, DC: Author.

Prospective Payment Assessment Commission. (1995, June). *Medicare and the American health care system: Report to Congress.* Washington, DC: ProPac.

Physician Payment Review Commission. (1989). *Annual report to Congress, 1989.* Washington, DC: U.S. Government Printing Office.

Robinson, J. C., Luft, H. S., McPhee, S. J., & Hunt. S. S. (1988). Hospital competition and surgical length of stay. *Journal of the American Medical Association, 259,* 696–700.

Romeo, A., Wagner, J., & Lee, R. (1984). Prospective reimbursement and the diffusion of new technologies in hospitals. *Journal of Health Economics, 3,* 1–24.

Schwartz, W. (1994). In the pipeline: A wave of valuable technology. *Health Affairs, 13*(3), 70–80.

Sloan, F., & Becker, E. (1984). Cross-subsidies and payment for hospital care. *Journal of Health Politics, Policy and Law, 8,* 660–685.

Wennberg, J. (1984). Dealing with medical practice variations: A proposal for action. *Health Affairs, 3*(2), 6–32.

Wennberg, J. (1996). On the appropriateness of small-area analysis for cost containment. *Health Affairs, 18*(4), 164–167.

Zwanziger, J., & Melnick, G. (1996). Can managed care plans control health care costs? *Health Affairs, 15,* 185–199.

IV

Futures

Part IV, "Futures," is concerned with the futures of health care delivery in the United States. Knickman explains the importance of thinking about the future for health care management and policy. Next, he describes different approaches used to forecast the future. Then he analyzes what social factors drive change in the health care system. These factors include the preferences and ideology of various population groups, aging and ethnic changes in our population, and the growing importance of health behavior in determining health status.

Knickman concludes with a review of future changes that he sees as most significant: increased services for the elderly and chronically ill, advances in molecular genetics and associated technological change, changes in health system markets, the restructuring of Medicare, and the explosion of information technology.

Three appendixes and two indexes follow this section. The appendixes include a glossary, a guide to sources of data, and an essential guide to the World Wide Web in health care. Indexes are by author and by subject.

17

Futures

James R. Knickman

LEARNING OBJECTIVES

- ☐ Explain the importance of thinking about the future for management and policy.
- ☐ Describe different approaches to forecasting the future.
- ☐ Analyze what social factors drive change in the health care system.
- ☐ Predict what changes are likely to be most important to the future of health care.

TOPICAL OUTLINE

Forecasting: Definition and approaches
Key drivers of change in the new millennium
Areas where change may be most striking in coming years
Conclusions

KEY WORDS

forecasting, Delphi method, drivers of change, aging of the population, behavioral risk factors, molecular genetics, technological change, market change, fixed-benefit programs, information technology, health promotion

FORECASTING: DEFINITION AND APPROACHES

Imagine the future: I wake up, take a reading on my health monitor (connected to a health information system that tracks 300 aspects of my health status, including a list of specialized self-chosen health goals). I lean over to the monitor, make a few clicks, and quickly get key information on how my 105-year-old mother—who lives 800 miles away—did overnight and get a forecast about how she will feel during the coming day. As I get in my car to commute to work, I am comforted by its advanced anticollision system that makes life-threatening accidents a concern of the past. I do find the many billboards advertising health-enhancing services of every stripe a general nuisance and source of visual pollution. My grandchildren cannot believe my stories of how physicians used to work in small groups or by themselves and how there were thousands of hospitals, each one operating on its own rather than as a part of the four national chains of health plans that now compete vigorously in the health care market.

Will the future really look like this? Although it's tough to know what the specifics of tomorrow's health system will look like, it is an important exercise to think about the future and spend time forecasting what might be, what could be, and what forces will shape the future. The 16 chapters that precede this one look very closely at key parts of the health environment, explaining the current status of the health system and key issues currently facing the health system. Understanding the present and being knowledgeable about the past are the first steps in predicting the future, that is, forecasting, and shaping the future.

Many readers of this book are beginning careers in the health care field; they will play key roles in shaping the future and should recognize the importance of taking time periodically to think about where the health system is headed and what levers are available to make it head in a desired direction. The saying goes: "If you don't know where you're going, you might wind up somewhere else."[1]

Exercises in forecasting have many practical values. Most important, forecasting is a crucial step in strategic planning. In the public sector and the private sector, deciding where to focus attention depends on a sense of future trends and prospects. What new products must be designed? How large should a new hospital be? How many elderly will use Medicare services 20 years from now? Questions like these guide current actions, and some approach to forecasting is crucial to give tentative answers to these questions.

Forecasting also forces us to look at history. In essence, every approach to forecasting attempts to look at patterns of past trends to make predictions about future trends. In this sense, as Norman Cousins stated, "history is a vast early warning system" (Fitzhenry, 1993). Looking at and studying what caused what in the past is often the approach for devising innovations and new solutions to current problems. Epidemiologists, for example, use the natural patterns of past behavior and events to sort out what

---

[1] This famous quote is from Yogi Berra. Not all pundits agree with this logic, however; Albert Einstein said: "I never think of the future. It comes soon enough." And Euripides is quoted: "What we look for does not come to pass. God finds a way for what none foresaw." These quotes are all found in Fitzhenry (1993).

behaviors, environmental factors, and interventions seem to lead to good and bad health outcomes (McMahon & Pugh, 1970). This type of analysis then leads to ideas for how to improve health outcomes. Most social scientists use the same basic approach in studying how the health system works and how it can be improved.

Finally, a value of forecasting is that it gives us a reference point in the future to assess our past logic. Six years ago (in early 1994), Anthony Kovner prepared a chapter on "Futures" as the capstone to a previous edition of this volume (Kovner, 1995). Reading the chapter in 2000 provides useful information about how we thought about health care dynamics 6 years ago and about how our logic has evolved in just 6 years. Some of the events forecasted by Kovner in 1994 are happening and some are not, but one real value of his earlier paper when read today is that it allows us to sharpen our analytic abilities to pursue the always important task of linking causes to effects.

There are varied methods for making forecasts. Economists, for example, have developed highly quantitative approaches for analyzing data from the past to make forecasts of future economic events (Granger, 1989). This approach generally involves collecting time series data from the past on a set of economic variables, then developing theories about how each variable influences the others, then testing these theories with data from the past, and finally using statistical techniques to estimate how the variables will change in the future based on the estimated relationships of how they changed in the past. The economic approach works only when extensive empirical data are available, and even in these cases the approach is far from perfect as a forecasting technique and most useful for forecasts of the near future (Berndt, 1991).

The Delphi method, which is a more qualitative approach to forecasting, obtains expert opinion in a systematic manner with an end goal of achieving consensus. Delphi administrators poll experts about their forecasts of the future with a self-administered questionnaire. Participants complete three or four rounds of questionnaires, but after each round, results are tabulated and disseminated to the group. The group completes a Delphi when it reaches a convergence of opinion (Fink, Kosecoff, Chassin, & Brook, 1984).

The Delphi method overcomes geographic barriers that plague many consensus-building exercises. Flexibility represents another strength of the Delphi method as it easily applies to health and medicine, as well as to war and weapons systems and to all levels of decision making. The fact that reliability, as well as required work, increases as the number of rounds and experts increases sets limitations on the utility of the Delphi method. Problems of questionnaire design and expert identification also inhibit the Delphi method.

A third, and least scientific, approach to forecasting is to rely on nationally recognized leaders in a field to apply their experience about the past and the dynamics of the present to make predictions about the future. This is the approach used on Sunday morning television and the approach used by many magazines and trade journals. In addition, almost every article in a journal like *Health Affairs* ends with expert authors assessing what the analyses presented in their papers imply for the future. Thus, forecasting is a natural part of most analysis and comment by experts. It is often the ultimate reason for undertaking an analysis.

The approach to looking at the future employed in this paper is of the third variety. I hope to draw on the wide literature contributed by experts analyzing the present to predict the future and to present my interpretation and inferences of what current patterns in the health system suggest for the future. My analysis of "Futures" is shaped by my vantage point—working at a philanthropy that supports efforts to improve the health and health care of the American public. I have the privilege of interacting with many experts in the health field who use our foundation's resources to try to shape the future so that Americans can live in better health and have health care services as accessible and responsive to their needs as possible.

KEY DRIVERS OF CHANGE IN THE NEW MILLENNIUM

It is often difficult to know for sure that a given period—as it is happening—is one of rapid change, but the 1990s surely had a reputation of being a time of fundamental change in how we organize and deliver health care and how we think about "maintaining health." As change seems to occur all around us, it often is difficult to distinguish drivers of change (the topic of this section) and key aspects of change itself (the topic of the next section). At the core of the dynamics shaping change, however, there seem to be three fundamental forces:

1. the preferences of consumers (in economic-speak) or the ideology of the citizenry (in political science-speak);
2. the demographic change in the American population shaped both by aging and ethnic shifts in the general population; and
3. the growing understanding that individual and environmental behavior drives health outcomes more than health services.

Preferences and Ideology of People

We often talk in 2001 about market forces as a key driving influence right now in health care, but in fact, the current flurry of system change is derivative of the preferences and ideology of the public. Over the past few years, Americans have made clear the preferences and ideology that characterize the majority of the voting population.

Perhaps most striking is the ongoing distrust that Americans place in their governments, especially the federal government. The majority of

Americans remain convinced that the federal government cannot be trusted to sponsor or manage large social programs. In 1964, when the American National Election Study first asked about public trust, three fourths (76%) of Americans said they trusted the federal government to do the right thing always or most of the time. This figure declined through the 1970s to a low point of 25% in 1980. This low level of public trust in the government has increased only slightly through the year 2000 (to 30%) according to an *ABC News/Washington Post* survey. (*ABC News/Washington Post*, 2000). The closeness of the 2000 presidential election and the contentiousness of the process used to select the winner are not indicators that trust in the political system will improve in the near future.

Of course, not all Americans view the government the same way. Hispanic and African Americans, who look to the federal government to redress racial and ethnic inequalities, express higher than average trust. Those with lower incomes, as well as young adults, also view the government as more trustworthy than does the average American. Deviations remain small, however; according to the 1995 *Washington Post*/Kaiser/ Harvard survey, only about one third of each of these groups believed the federal government does the right thing always or most of the time (Blendon et al., 1998).

Although political scientists often cite reactions to the conduct of the Vietnam War and to the lack of success of the social programs of the 1960s as the core source of American distrust of government (Nye, Zelikow, & King, 1998), the impact of the high periods of inflation in the economy during the late 1970s and early 1980s and the large federal budget deficits also seem important in shaping Americans' attitudes about the role of government in key parts of the economy. Whether or not Americans' reactions to government efforts of the past are justified, their reactions sharply curtail health system interventions that involve large public sector roles.

Perhaps related to this economic history, as well as the slow economic growth during the 1985–1995 period, Americans were fundamentally price-conscious in the 1990s. This price consciousness partly drives the movement toward managed care in that Americans will choose lower priced insurance options as long as those options have acceptable quality standards (Knickman, Hughes, Taylor, Binns, & Lyons, 1996). In a recent survey of consumers in 15 communities around the country, concerns about the costs of health care consistently outranked concerns about the potential "evils" of managed care in each community (Blendon et al., 1998).

One other strong preference of Americans that will shape change over the next few years is the importance they place on "choice" in any health care system. Americans are accustomed to being able to pick and choose from various options when making purchases in almost every part of the economy. The ability to "exit" from service systems that they do not like will continue to be a strong preference among consumers, and market changes will have to take this into account.

Aging and Ethnic Changes in the Population

The continued aging of the American population will command significant attention among health care providers and policymakers over the next 30 years. Approximately 47% of all hospital admissions are currently made up of Americans over 65, who account for just 13% of the population. The number of people over 65 will double in the next 25 years, thus driving up demand for many types of health care, especially care focused on chronic illnesses and support services for the frail elderly. The population growth rates are most dramatic for the eldest of the old, who are among the very highest users of health and support services.

Even if managed care leads to dramatic decreases in the use of health care, person by person, the aging of the population should make health care and supportive services (e.g., home care and assisted living) an important growth industry in the United States. The style of health care and the sensitivity of the system to the special concerns of the elderly will have to evolve. All of this growth will take place while informal support systems continue to shrink. The number of adults aged 21–65—the main cadre of informal caregivers—will decrease from 12.5 per elderly person (over age 75) in 1980 to 6.5 per elder in 2025 (U.S. Census Bureau, 1992).

An interesting possibility, of course, is that we will find ways of diverting some personal energies and social resources away from children and toward elders. An important statistic, not often cited in relationship to the growing burdens of an aging society, is that the share of the population who need support services because they are young will shrink as the elderly share increases. In 2000 there were two children for each person over age 65, but this number will shrink to just 1.18 by 2030 (Francese, 1995).

A second key population shift whose effect is more difficult to predict is the growing ethnic diversity of Americans. By 2060 it is expected that a majority of Americans will be ethnic minorities. Although the nonHispanic Caucasian population will increase only moderately from 196 million in 2000 to 213 million in 2050, minority groups will see bigger increases. Between 2000 and 2050, the population of nonHispanic African Americans will increase from 36 million to 54 million, and the size of the Hispanic population will triple, from 32 million to 98 million. Asian groups will more than triple, from 11 million in 2000 to 36 million in 2050 (U.S. Census Bureau, 2000).

The impacts of this ethnic transformation of America on health care requirements depend crucially on how quickly the growing ethnic groups assimilate into the economic mainstream of American life. Currently, the African American population and Latino population have greater than average health care needs, principally related to lower incomes and the associated stresses on health-related behaviors. If population growth occurs mostly among the low-income part of the American population and if distribution of wealth continues to be as skewed as it was in the 1990s, we can expect growing demands for health care and public health services.

Even if ethnic America does better economically in the future and has health status patterns closer to overall averages, health care will have to respond to diversity in the style of medicine that will be demanded by growing ethnic populations. It is clear that ethnic minorities prefer services delivered by providers who understand their culture and preferably match their ethnicity. Creating a more diverse health care workforce will be a key challenge facing the health system of the 21st century.

A third population shift will be a significant change in the income and asset status of the elderly. As recently as the 1960s, more than one third of the elderly were poor. In 1999, although 17% of children were poor, less than 10% of the elderly were poor. In 1999, the median household income of the elderly was $22,812, almost double that of the median household income in 1967 ($12,677 in 1999 dollars).

Health and Behavior

Increasingly, Americans are understanding that the real determinants of health have little to do with the trillion dollars we currently invest in the health care system each year, but have more to do with the way we lead our lives and the environment we live in. It has been estimated that about half of all deaths in the United States could be attributed to both individual behavioral and environmental factors, including use of alcohol, tobacco, and other drugs; diet; activity patterns; microbial and toxic agents; firearms; sexual behavior; and motor vehicles (McGinnis & Foege, 1993). The most prominent contributors to these deaths include tobacco, diet, activity patterns, and alcohol (see Figure 17.1).

Despite the established linkages between behavioral risk factors and subsequent morbidity and mortality, only about 3% of total health care expenditures in the United States is spent on well care, including preventive care (Centers for Disease Control [CDC], 1994). This investment pales compared with the $425 billion in direct health care costs for persons with chronic conditions in the United States (Hoffman, Rice, & Sung, 1996).

An understanding that lifestyles and behavior must change in order to improve population health status should translate into growing demands for public health activities that attack environmental factors associated with health problems and for behavioral health care that attempts to improve the way individuals act to maintain their own health. The Robert Wood Johnson Foundation, for example, is investing in efforts to get managed care providers to institutionalize (or implement) state-of-the-art behavioral interventions to assist patients to stop smoking or reduce their risky drinking practices. Similarly, we recognize that improved health outcomes are much more likely to occur if cities can rethink how they intervene in the lives of low-income children than if we expand the number of cardiac catheterization laboratories in a city.

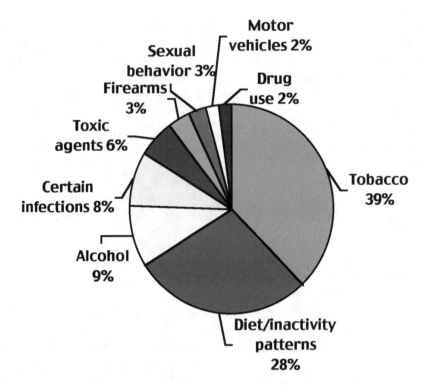

FIGURE 17.1   Actual causes of death (attributed to both individual behavioral and environmental factors) in the United States, 1990.

Source: McGinnis, J. M., & Foege, W. H. (1993). Actual Causes of Death in the United States. *Journal of the American Medical Association, 270,* 2207–2212.

A focus on behavior as a key determinant of health problems could lead to more attention for research to improve interventions aimed at helping individuals change behaviors that involve health threats. It also supports the idea that capitated payments should reward providers and health systems that head off the need for expensive health care interventions by intervening early enough in the onset of chronic health problems to prevent costly disease complications and flare-ups. A number of managed care organizations have successfully demonstrated cost-effective approaches to behavioral risk factor management, but it is clear that additional incentives that encourage investments in preventive care are needed (CDC, 1995). A 1999 article in *Journal of the American Medical Association* demonstrated that significant short-term health care costs result when health plans do nothing to influence modifiable health risks such as physical inactivity, obesity, or smoking. Over an 18-month period, costs associated with overweight and inactive smokers were almost 50% higher than for those beneficiaries who did not have these behavioral risk factors (Pronk, Goodman, O'Connor, & Martinson, 1999).

AREAS WHERE CHANGE MAY BE MOST STRIKING IN COMING YEARS

Serving the Elderly and the Chronically Ill

The aging of the population will refocus the health system so that its primary concerns revolve around chronic disease management, geriatrics as a medical specialty, and the general field of services for the frail. This transformation will occur slowly and steadily over the next 30–50 years, but the contrast in what preoccupies the medical and service fields now and in the future will be striking.

The prospects of positive change in this area are strong. On the medical care side, large analytic investments are well under way to experiment with two quite different but interrelated changes in the service system. First, more sophisticated ways of paying managed care organizations for the care they deliver to the chronically ill are being designed and tested. Second, physicians and other providers are testing new approaches to better manage the way clinical care is delivered to the chronically ill, with central emphasis on four components: evidence-based care protocols, data management systems that track the care of patients with chronic conditions, patient self-management and activation, and the use of coordinated teams of providers with different expertise (Wagner, Austin, & von Korff, 1996). When economic incentives embedded in payment systems change so that managed care plans are rewarded for enrolling and providing better care for the chronically ill, we should expect widespread implementation of some of the current experiments in chronic disease management.

To date, managed care plans have had perverse incentives relative to services for the chronically ill. Because plans tend to get paid much less than actual costs for the care of each chronically ill person enrolled (and reciprocally much more than actual costs for nonchronically ill enrollees), the natural incentive of a plan is to avoid enrolling the chronically ill through various selection strategies. And there are surely no strong incentives to provide innovative care for the chronically ill so that it will attract greater numbers from this population to a given health plan. The incentives will reverse if risk-adjusted payments can be made more sophisticated, and more closely match payments to the expected costs of a person with a chronic illness.

Increasingly, Americans are recognizing that the quality of a managed care plan should be judged by how well it takes care of life-threatening medical episodes (such as care after a heart attack or a serious malignancy) and how well it takes care of chronic diseases. It is the medical care that accompanies these serious health threats that is most valuable to Americans. Thus, in deciding whether to remain in a specific health plan, increasing numbers of people will judge not how well they are taken care of when basically in good health but in how well their friends and relatives who have chronic illnesses and life-threatening problems are cared for. This new mind-set will also help to refocus the attention of managed care plans on the care they provide to the chronically ill.

Many health providers are experimenting with new methods of organizing care for the chronically ill. Wagner and colleagues (1996) have developed principles that can guide such innovation:

- Information systems are needed to track the care the chronically ill receive from different medical care providers.
- Protocols are needed to make sure providers deliver evidence-based care.
- Multidisciplinary teams need to be involved in caring for the chronically ill.
- Patients need to be educated and activated so that through "self care" they become partners with medical providers in the management of the chronic illness.

There also are good prospects for better integration of services directed at both the medical problems of the chronically ill and the social support needs of this population. In the past, health insurance tended to pay only for acute medical services, and most individuals had to use out-of-pocket funds to pay for services such as home care, nursing home care, and assistance with chores. For the poor and for those who became poor because of the high costs of these support services, government would pay for many support services through the Medicaid program and other state and local initiatives. Unfortunately, the two very different financial approaches to covering medical versus support services ignore important interrelationships that jointly determine the needs for these services. Without coordinated planning and recognition that unmet needs in the support area can often lead to severe medical setbacks, the chronically ill have not received cost-effective care that maximizes health outcomes and functioning.

Prospects are changing for better integration of services, partly because of interests of state governments in better coordinating resources coming from Medicare (which focuses mostly on medical care) and Medicaid (which pays for many more support services). Arizona, Tennessee, Oregon, and Minnesota have taken early leads in experimenting with better integration of Medicare and Medicaid funds for the chronically ill (Bonnyman, 1996; McCall, Wrightson, Paringer, & Trapnell, 1994). Other states are moving in similar directions.

Ironically, integration of services is likely to happen more quickly for the poor and near poor than for the wealthy and middle class, who are less likely to be eligible for Medicaid services. With the steady but slow growth of private long-term care insurance and with an emerging new wave of public sector approaches to help people pay for long-term care needs, however, the experience that managed care plans gain on service integration for the population dually eligible for both Medicare and Medicaid can later be applied to the broader population.

The final aspect of change related to the chronically ill is the likely emergence of a new industry catering to the various needs of an aging population. The next Microsoft or McDonald's will likely be in the area of services for the elderly. New approaches to assisted living will be in great demand, new approaches for management of retirement resources will be in demand, and approaches for "one stop shopping" to get medical, support, and lifestyle services in a trusted, easy environment will be desired by the quickly aging population. It is difficult to predict exactly what a new service sector will look like, but it will involve large resources and will likely be led by private corporations.

Advances in Molecular Genetics and a Range of Technological Innovations

Currently, the federal government is funding one of the largest targeted research efforts since the project to create an atomic bomb (the Human Genome Project). This time, however, the investment is directed at health as opposed to defense, with a focus on mapping each of the human genes. This effort is one of basic science directed at a better understanding of our human genetic makeup, and the exact payoffs of this effort in terms of medical knowledge will not be known for some time, but the likely implications for health and medical care are immense.

Perhaps the most dramatic advance in the genetics field in terms of foreshadowing future possibilities is the successful cloning of a sheep in 1996 by a team of applied geneticists in Scotland (Kolata, 1997). The methods used are claimed to be applicable, eventually, for human cloning, which raises a host of ethical concerns that must be dealt with in the early part of the 21st century.

Genetics research, however, will lead to an even broader range of medical interventions and prevention possibilities for dealing with many medical problems. These advances will likely make us a healthier population—at least in terms of morbidity and mortality associated with many traditional diseases. The advances will also transform the methods of medical providers and the ways that medical providers spend their time. Many of the efforts that currently take time and energy will be avoided because of better prevention efforts, but new technology will make new medical interventions possible. Constant retraining of medical providers will be more important than it is currently.

Most predictions about the future of new technology and medical interventions suggest that they will add to our health care cost bill (Weisbrod & LaMay, 1999). Economists currently are studying exactly how and why different sectors of the technology industry invest in cost-increasing versus cost-reducing technologies. With the spread of managed care and capitated payments, there should be more investments in cost-reducing technologies than in the past 20 years (Weisbrod, 1991). An optimistic prediction is that there will be a better balance in the introduction of new technologies, with cost-decreasing inventions and strategies somewhat compensating for cost-increasing inventions. What will be essential are better social mechanisms for deciding which of the cost-increasing technologies that emerge in fact enhance quality of life and thus are worth investing in. Americans will continue to be willing to pay for quality-enhancing technologies even if they cost more.

One potential negative side effect of increased knowledge and knowhow will be the overuse of testing and medical interventions (Welch & Fisher, 1999). Few diagnostic tests are error free, and to the extent that new tests lead to a fair number of false positives (i.e., indicating a problem when none in fact exists), expensive, unnecessary treatments may be done and people's quality of life may be affected by unnecessary health concerns. An added fear is that some of the genetic testing will identify problems or the likelihood of future problems for which nothing can be done. Again, knowledge of this sort could actually have significant negative impacts on psychological well-being. We may be headed toward a world where we have too much information for our own good.

Health System Change

Perhaps the easiest change to predict is the continued transformation of the way our health care services are organized, financed and delivered. Narrowing in on the ultimate destination of this transformation is much more difficult. While the proposed government-led reforms debated vigorously during the early and mid-1990s never wound up taking hold, the threat of such reforms unleashed a rapid series of market driven changes that continue to unfold today.

To better understand these changes and what they mean for people, in 1995 The Robert Wood Johnson Foundation began supporting a large-scale initiative known as Health Tracking. Health Tracking is a longitudinal study that combines information from families, providers, employers and market leaders to explain health system changes and the implications of these changes for consumers in 60 different markets across the country. While "health system change" is still a work in progress, the initiative has helped provide objective information (some of which is outlined below) to counter anecdotes about the types of changes we are passing through and the effects of those changes on people.

Over the last decade, most Americans experienced some change in their health insurance. Fewer than 20 percent of employees of mid- and large-size firms were enrolled in HMOs in 1988, compared to more than half by 1998 (Gabel et al., 1998; Reschovsky & Kemper, 2000). The mid-1990s, in particular, saw rapid and dramatic shifts to all types of managed care. Between 1993 and 1997 alone, the number of employees in fee-for-service plans dropped by 60% from 46% to 18%, with nearly half of employees enrolled in point-of-service or preferred provider type plans and one third in HMOs by 1997 (Marquis & Long, 1999).

Accompanying these changes were remarkable slowdowns in premium increases as well as in underlying health care costs. Annual premium hikes dropped from 11% in 1992 to less than 1% in 1996, as many insurers priced products below cost to gain market share. Underlying cost increases also slowed from 7% in 1992 to 2% in 1996 (Ginsburg, 1999). Among health care providers, various organizational change strategies were pursued to help to navigate or mitigate the effects of these changes. Consolidation was rapid, with more than 700 mergers and acquisitions completed among hospitals between 1994 and 1997 (Lesser & Brewster, 2001).

Physicians experienced a unique set of pressures in the shift to managed care, stemming from dramatic changes to both their practice and their payment. By 1997, less than half of physicians were in solo or two-physician practices. Two years later, the number in solo practice had declined even further—accounting for fewer than one third of physicians in 1999 (Center for Studying Health System Change, 1996–1997). Managed care's emphasis on primary care and the coordination of specialty care left over 90% of primary care physicians acting as gatekeepers for their patients (St. Peter, 1997). Both primary care physicians and specialists agreed that the scope of care for primary care doctors increased over the period, with a sizeable minority believing this scope was greater than it should be (St. Peter, Reed, Kemper, & Blumenthal, 1999). Over half of doctors reported receiving capitated payments for at least some of their patients (Lake & St. Peter, 1997). While capitation by no means accounts for the bulk of physician revenue, even some can pose a conflict for physicians between care delivery and business decisions. For example, in 1997, one in four doctors didn't think they could make clinical decisions in the best interest of their patients without possibly reducing their income (St. Peter, 1999).

Consumers also felt some discomfort with these new arrangements as the shift to managed care became more pronounced. Over 40% of Americans feel that their doctors are strongly influenced by insurance company rules when making decisions about their care (Hargraves, 2000). One in six is concerned that their doctor might not refer them to a specialist when needed (St. Peter, 1997).

Although, early on, the public seemed enthusiastic about the possibility of cost savings from managed care—(in 1997, for example, almost 60% said that they would be willing to accept limits in choice of hospitals and physicians if it meant lower costs (Cunningham & Tu, 1997)—many lacked a choice of plans, forced by their employers to switch to managed care. Perhaps this lack of plan choice, combined with unprecedented economic growth and "a great ride" of moderate cost increases, shifted consumer priorities, setting the stage for what grew into a severe backlash against managed care and its restrictions. "HMO Hell" described (and often fueled by) the media evoked a broad movement away from HMO restrictions and narrow provider networks.

Interestingly, a series of research papers carefully examining differences in a whole set of services between HMOs vs. non-HMOs, shows no significant difference in use, even of expensive services, among HMO and non-HMO consumers, yet it indicates lower satisfaction and trust among HMO patients (Kemper, Reschovsky, & Tu, 1999). Separate research confirms that perceptions, rather than the reality of HMOs, often drives consumer ratings. In fact, after correctly controlling for insurance types, even differences in consumer ratings between HMO and non-HMO participants shrink or disappear (Reschovsky & Hargraves, 2000). Despite the evidence of HMOs not skimping on services, extremely tight labor markets left employers wary of resisting employee demands for broad networks and choice. The result? A scenario where managing care and costs is nearly impossible. Not surprisingly, the latest data show that premium increases are back up, topping 8% in 2000, about double the overall rate of inflation (Ginsburg, Hogan, Ginsburg, & Gabel, 2000).

Although the future direction of health system change is uncertain, continued change is certain, as our current system for managing care and costs is unsustainable. A softening of the economy combined with continued premium increases will likely drive corrections once again. Response to these corrections from employers, consumers and providers will determine whether the insured get more or less managed care and whether the ranks of the uninsured will continue to grow.

Medicare

In thinking about future directions of public policy in the health field, the Medicare program stands out as the area most liable to face sharp changes in structure. Medicare represents a huge public commitment to health care, with expenditures reaching $215 billion in 1997 and projected to grow—unless changes occur—to $403 billion by 2008 (Health Care Financing Administration, 2000).

Perhaps more relevant to prospects for change, Medicare represents a substantial share of federal government expenditures. Spending on the major health and retirement programs as a percentage of GDP is expected to more than double between now and 2040, from 7.5% of GDP to almost 17% (Congressional Budget Office [CBO], 2000). To the extent that current concerns about budget deficits continue, Medicare will eventually be subject to even greater cost cutting attention than it typically faces. This is not to say that making changes in this insurance program for the elderly and disabled will be easy. Any efforts to tamper with the current system will face huge political hurdles because the approach would cap Medicare commitments and allow the exact amount of the commitment to be determined by the political process over time, through debates about how fast the fixed dollar amount would increase.

Either of these paths toward change will escalate the trend toward at least two tiers of medical care access in America. The wealthy will be able to opt out of managed care arrangements or specific managed care restrictions through use of point-of-service options. These options increasingly will let people gain access to services at the best medical centers if the individual pays a significant share of the costs for the specific service. The importance of being able to afford the top tier of medicine could become increasingly significant as new technology allows for expensive but effective interventions.

My sense is that the multitiered approach to Medicare is inevitable because of the alternative: equal access to a lower amenity, less intensive health care system will be unacceptable to the growing cadre of middle-class and wealthy elderly who will want an ability to spend their accumulated wealth on health-enhancing interventions. This desire, coupled with the continuing reluctance of Americans in the late 20th century to redistribute more of our growing wealth to the needy, leads to a prediction of more striking tiers in Medicare coverage.

Other changes in Medicare are more difficult to predict. How many resources will ultimately be devoted to home health and home care services—many of which improve quality of life but are far removed from actual medical care? How active will the federal government be in regulating the quality of medicine associated with the health plans that manage the care of the elderly? How active will government be in refereeing the conflicts that will continue to grow between providers of care and health plans? How will approaches to care and caring at the end of life be reformed to better reflect the needs and wishes of the elderly? Change in all of these areas is needed, but future leadership at the federal level will shape these changes.

Information

The ability to collect, process, and categorize information is changing faster than any other technology in America. The final moments of the 2000 presidential election were full of references to instant email communication on handheld devices between candidates and their aides who monitored returns. By the time this book is published, wireless email will likely be available at a low cost.

The effects of new information technologies will be striking in the health care field although, again, the exact path of change is difficult to predict, and actual changes are likely to be more dramatic than any predictions one would make at the present time. Despite the potential for change, an important concern about confidentiality and privacy may inhibit some uses of new information technology. For example, it would be straightforward, with existing technology, to track the use of multiple providers by one individual so that each provider could better coordinate the care being considered. However, privacy concerns have slowed efforts to implement such tracking systems. Privacy concerns even hamper efforts to implement computerized systems to track immunization information for young children.

The privacy concerns are important, though, and more creativity is needed to meet the demands of consumers for privacy. Some solutions may come from technological advances. Perhaps data systems will be designed so that they are accessible only if a consumer provides a private code, or methods could be designed to limit access for specific providers only to certain information, depending on the need for that information.

Information technology, however, will go far beyond tracking health and health care patterns for individuals. Virtual imaging and related technologies will provide significant new information to help providers identify medical problems and potential solutions to the problems. This type of information may assist centrally located specialists in caring for individuals in remote areas of the country without face to face contact (Institute of Medicine, 1996).

Information technology will also provide more self-help information to consumers. Already, the Internet has increased the availability of health-related information dramatically. More than a third of Internet users spend time finding medical information on the Web (UCLA, 2000). With time, this type of information will become better cataloged and better designed to provide useful help for individuals concerned with their health.

Passive monitoring systems—perhaps like those described in this chapter's opening paragraph—could also provide "real time" information about emerging health problems with protocols for reacting to this information. The challenge will be to make sure that the deluge of new information improves the quality of our lives rather than complicating our lives and adding to the costs of medical care. As discussed earlier, if increased volumes of information about our health serves mostly to scare us about low-probability adverse events, we could end up worse-off rather than better-off. And if new information leads to more frequent interventions of questionable efficacy, again we could emerge worse-off after the information revolution. This inevitable revolution will call for creative management over the next 20 years.

Health Promotion

The growing awareness that healthy lifestyles have much more impact on long-range health than access to health care should translate into significant change in Americans' approach to health maintenance.[2] The key areas of focus will likely be on the five lifestyle factors that have been identified as most important to morbidity and mortality: smoking, unhealthy diets, sedentary lifestyle, alcohol and drug use, and risky sexual practices (McGinnis & Foege, 1993). The importance of noncompliance with medical regimens can also be added to this list. For example, Leventhal, Zimmerman,

---

[2] I want to acknowledge the strong influence of the work of Tracy Orleans, my colleague, in the arguments presented in section.

and Gutman (1984, p. 404) noted that "people are as likely to quit cigarettes or stick with their diets as they are to adhere to blood pressure treatment." Medical noncompliance has been estimated to result in $100 billion avoidable health care costs, and more than half of the elderly are reported to have compliance problems (Sullivan, Kreling, & Hazlet, 1990).

Why will change occur rapidly in lifestyle factors even though they have been so difficult to alter over the past 20 years? Koop and McDonald (1995) point to two "revolutions" to explain their optimism about improvements in behavioral health: "two revolutions—health system change and the building of the national information infrastructure—are transforming American health care . . . and give us some modest confidence that present-day concepts of what determines health and disease, and our methods of intervening, will be dramatically different in the not too distant future" (p. ix). Health system change creates better incentives of health systems to maintain a population's health through prevention approaches, and information technology, as discussed above, will expand the opportunity to get information about behavior change and self-help to consumers.

The payoffs from human genome research will also play a role in this area. Because few inherited diseases are likely to be candidates for drug or gene therapies in the near future, the identification of risk genotypes boosts the demand for more effective and better targeted prevention efforts. The next generation of behavior change strategies are likely to be strengthened by advances in understanding the bio-behavioral mechanisms linking behavioral risk factors and disease. For instance, advances in brain imagery have led to breakthroughs in understanding the neurological basis of drug addiction. Leshner (1997, p. 46), for example, notes that "drug addiction is not just 'a lot of drug use,' but a brain disease, that is expressed in behavioral ways and occurs in a social context." This awareness will spawn more effective combined pharmacological and behavior intervention approaches. Similarly, Glanz (1997) notes that research into the psychobiology of fat appetite and the role of metabolic factors as promoters of fat and protein intake, offers intriguing possibilities for new bio-behavioral models of food intake.

Besides advances resulting from the multidisciplinary bio-behavioral research into the mechanisms linking health behavior to health outcomes, new theories and models of the dynamics of health behavior change and population-based health improvement strategies will also increase our capabilities to address behavioral threats to health. Models such as the "stages of change" model continue to see enhancements in individualized and interactive interventions and the recruitment and retention of all members of an at-risk population (e.g., all smokers or sedentary members of a health plan), not just those who are motivated to change their behavior (Prochaska & Velicer, 1997).

In addition, advances in health behavior change have moved away from a strictly clinical behavior change model toward broader public health and public policy models of prevention. Accordingly, experts increasingly argue that strategies for improving healthy behaviors must focus on three very different intervention points: "downstream" interventions focused on the individual, "midstream" interventions focused on work sites and health providers, and "upstream" interventions that involve public health campaigns to change social perceptions about healthy behaviors and that include macro-level public policies to create incentives for health behavior (McKinlay, 1995). Predictions about how public policy will develop in this area is the most difficult to forecast, especially given America's traditional distrust of government.

CONCLUSIONS

In 1994, Kovner (1995, p. 552) concluded that it is important "to predict future directions in the American health care delivery system, not so much because of confidence that they will happen but rather to focus discussion on key issues, the constraints that surround them, and the opportunities for resolving them." This conclusion holds up, and it is hoped that the discussion of "futures" presented here provokes new ideas for improving our efforts to bring about better health for Americans.

CASE STUDY

Your governor appoints you executive director of a Commission on the Future of Health Care in your state. The commission has 1 year to develop a report outlining predicted changes in the health care field in your state. The purpose of this commission is to advise the governor on key changes in the state's health needs and resources so that he or she might develop public policies to make sure the health system evolves on a positive path.

1. How would you go about doing such a forecast? What methods and approaches would you use?
2. What types of people would you suggest that the governor appoint to the Commission? Explain how each could be helpful in the workings of the commission.
3. Outline what you would expect the final commission report to include.

DISCUSSION QUESTIONS

1. What are the reasons we spend time and energy trying to forecast what will happen in the future?
2. Discuss the advantages and disadvantages of different approaches for forecasting. When do you think it makes sense to be more technical in approach or less technical in approach?

3. What do you think are key drivers of change in the health care system at the turn of the century? Do you disagree with any of the items selected in this chapter? Would you add some other factors to the list?
4. What changes in health care do you think will be most significant?
5. Can you think of ways for public policy and private managers to shape some of these future changes in positive ways?
6. Take a specific topic covered in one of the previous chapters of this book. Forecast how that part of the health system is likely to change over the next 10 years and explain the drivers of these changes.

REFERENCES

Berndt, E. R. (1991). *The practice of econometrics: classic and contemporary.* Reading, MA: Addison-Wesley.

Blendon, R. J., Benson, J. M., Morin, R., Altman, D. E., Brodie, M., Brossard, M., & James, M. (1998). Changing attitudes in America. In J. S. Nye, Jr., P. D. Zelikow, & D. C. Kindig (Eds.), *Why Americans mistrust government.* Cambridge, MA: Harvard University Press.

Bonnyman, G., Jr. (1996). Stealth reform: Market-based Medicaid in Tennessee. *Health Affairs, 15*(2), 306–314.

Center for Studying Health System Change. (1996–1997). Community tracking study physician surveys. Unpublished raw data.

Centers for Disease Control. (1994). Medical care spending—United States. *Morbidity and Mortality Weekly, 43*(32), 581–586.

Centers for Disease Control. (1995). Prevention and managed care: Opportunities for managed care organizations, purchasers of health care, and public health agencies. *Morbidity and Mortality Weekly, 44*(RR4), 1–12.

Congressional Budget Office. (2000). *The long-term budget outlook.* Washington, DC: U.S. Government Printing Office.

Cunningham, P. J., & Tu, H. T. (1999). A changing picture of uncompensated care. *Health Affairs Special issue: The Safety Net versus the Market: Is the Safety Net in Crisis? 16*(4), 167–175.

Fink, A., Kosecoff, J., Chassin, M., & Brook, R. H. (1984). Consensus methods: Characteristics and guidelines for use. *American Journal of Public Health, 74*, 979–983.

Fitzhenry, R. L. (Ed.). (1993). *The Harper book of quotations.* New York: HarperCollins.

Francese, P. (1995, February). Americans at mid-decade. *American Demographics, 17*(2), 23–31.

Gabel, J., Hunt, K., Kim, J., Hurst, K., Hoover, S., & Hawkins, S. (1998). *Health benefits in 1998.* Arlington, VA: KPMG Peat Marwick, LLP.

Ginsburg, P. G. (1999). *Tracking health care costs: Long-predicted upturn appears* (Issue Brief 23). Washington, DC: Center for Studying Health System Change.

Glanz, K. (1997). Behavioral research contributions and needs in cancer prevention and control: Dietary change. *Preventive Medicine, 26*(5), S43–S55.

Hargraves, J. L. (2000). *Data Bulletin #17: Patients concerned about insurer influences.* Washington, DC: Center for Studying Health System Change.

Health Care Financing Administration. (2000). *National health expenditures projections 1998–2008* [On-line]. Available: http://www.hcfa.gov/stats/NHE-Proj/proj1998/proj1998.pdo

Hoffman, C., Rice, D., & Sung, H-Y. (1996). Persons with chronic conditions: Their prevalence and cost. *Journal of the American Medical Association, 276,* 1473–1479.

Hogan, C., Ginsburg, P. B., & Gabel, J. R. (2000). Tracking health care costs: Inflation returns. *Health Affairs, 19*(6), 217–223.

Institute of Medicine. (1996). *Telemedicine: A guide to assessing telecommunications in health care.* Washington, DC: National Academy Press.

Kemper, P., Reschovsky, & Tu, H. T. (1999). Do HMOs make a difference? Summary and implications. *Inquiry, 36,* 419–425.

Knickman, J. R., Hughes, R. G., Taylor, H., Binns, K., & Lyons, M. (1996). Tracking consumers reactions to the changing health care system: Early indicators. *Health Affairs, 15*(3), 21–32.

Kolata, G. (1997, February 26). Scientist reports first cloning ever of adult animal. *The New York Times, 1,* 22.

Koop, C. E., & McDonald, M. D. (1995). Foreword. In L. M. Harris (Ed.), *Health and the new media technologies transforming personal and public health.* Mahway, NJ: Erlbaum.

Kovner, A. (1995). Futures. In A. Kovner (Ed.), *Jonas's health care delivery in the United States* (5th ed., pp. 532–553). New York: Springer Publishing Co.

Lake, T. K., & St. Peter, R. F. (1997). *Payment arrangements and financial incentives for physicians* (Data Bulletin #8). Washington, DC: Center for Studying Health System Change.

Leshner, A. I. (1997). Addiction is a brain disease, and it matters. *Science, 278*(5335), 45–47.

Lesser, C. S., & Brewster, L. R. (2001). *Understanding health system change.* Chicago: Health Administration Press.

Leventhal, H., Zimmerman, R. A., & Gutmann, M. (1984). Compliance: A self-regulation perspective. In W. D. Gentry (Ed.), *Handbook of behavioral medicine* (pp. 369–434). New York: Guilford Press.

Marquis, M. S., & Long, S. H. (1999). Trends in managed care and managed competition 1993–1997. *Health Affairs, 18*(6), 75–87.

McCall, N., Wrightson, C. W., Paringer, L., & Trapnell, G. (1994). Managed Medicaid cost savings: The Arizona experience. *Health Affairs, 13*(2), 234–245.

McGinnis, J. M., & Foege, W. H. (1993). Actual causes of death in the United States. *Journal of the American Medical Association, 270,* 2207–2212.

McKinlay, J. P. (1995). The new public health approach to improving physical activity and autonomy in older population. In E. Heikkinen, J. Kuusinen, & I. Ruoppila (Eds.), *Preparation for aging: Proceedings of the Seventeenth International Congress of Aging* (pp. 87–104). London: Plenum Press.

McMahon, B., & Pugh, T. F. (1970). *Epidemiology: Principles and methods.* Boston: Little, Brown.

Nye, N. S., Jr., Zelikow, P. D., & King, D. C. (1998). *Why Americans mistrust government.* Cambridge, MA: Harvard University Press.

Prochaska, J. O., & Velicer, W. F. (1997). The transtheoretical model of health behavior change. *American Journal of Health Promotion, 12,* 38–48.

Pronk, N. P., Goodman, M. J., O'Connor, P. J., & Martinson, B. C. (1999). Relationship between modifiable health risks and short-term health care charges. *Journal of the American Medical Association, 282*(23), 2235–2239.

Reschovsky, J. D., & Hargraves, J. L. (2000). Health care perceptions and experiences: It's not whether you are in an HMO, it's whether you think you are. *Center for Studying Health System Change Issue* (Brief No. 30).

Reschovsky, J. D., & Kemper P. (2000). Do HMOs make a difference? *Inquiry, 36*(4), 364–377.

Sullivan, S. D., Kreling, D. H., & Hazlet, T. K. (1990). Noncompliance with medication regimens and subsequent hospitalizations: A literature analysis and cost of hospitalization estimate. *Journal of Research in Pharmaceutical Economics, 2*(2), 19–33.

St. Peter, R. F. (1997). *Gatekeeping arrangements in widespread use* (Data Bulletin #7). Washington, DC: Center for Studying Health System Change.

St. Peter, R. F., Reed, M. C., Kemper, P., & Blumenthal, D. (1999). Changes in the scope of care provide by primary care physicians. *New England Journal of Medicine, 341*(26), 1980–1985.

U.S. Census Bureau, Current Population Reports. (1992). *Population projections of the United States, by age, sex, race, and Hispanic origin: 1992–2050.* Washington, DC: U.S. Government Printing Office.

U.S Census Bureau, Population Division. (2000). *Projections of the resident population by race, Hispanic origin, and nativity: Middle series.* Washington, DC: U.S. Government Printing Office.

Wagner, E. H., Austin, B. T., & Von Korff, M. (1996). Organizing care for patients with chronic illness. *Milbank Quarterly, 74*(4), 511–544.

Weisbrod, B. (1991). The health care quadrilemma: An essay on technological change, insurance, quality of care, and cost containment. *Journal of Economic Literature, 29,* 523–552.

Weisbrod, B., & LaMay, C. L. (1999). Mixed signals: Public policy and the future of health care R&D. *Health Affairs, 18*(2), 112–125.

Welch, H. G., & Fisher, E. S. (1999). Avoiding the unintended consequences of growth in medical care: How might more me worse? *Journal of the American Medical Association, 281*(5), 446–453.

Appendix A

Glossary

---

access: An individual's ability to obtain medical services on a timely and financially acceptable basis. Factors determining ease of access also include availability of health care facilities and transportation to them, and reasonable hours of operation.

acute care: Medical care of a limited duration, provided in a hospital or outpatient setting, to treat an injury or short-term illness.

administrative costs: Nonmedical expenditures related to the delivery of health care services, including billing, claims processing, marketing, and overhead.

Advanced Practice Nurse: Registered nurse such as a Clinical Nurse Specialist, Nurse Practitioner, Nurse Anesthetist, and Nurse-Midwife with a master's or doctoral degree concentrating on a specific area of practice.

adverse selection: Occurs when some population characteristic such as age (e.g., a larger number of persons age 65 or older in proportion to younger persons), increases the potential for higher utilization than budgeted, and increases costs above those of the capitation rate.

average daily census: The average number of patients counted in a health care institution, usually over a 1-year period.

behavioral risk factor: An element of personal behavior, such as unbalanced nutrition, use of tobacco products, leading a secondary lifestyle, or the abuse of alcoholic beverages, that leads to an increased risk of developing one or more diseases or negative health conditions.

beneficiary: Any person, either a subscriber or a dependent, eligible for service under a health plan contract.

benefits: Specific areas of plan coverage or services provided, such as outpatient visits and hospitalization, that make up the range of medical services marketed under a health plan.

476

biotechnology: The application of a technology such as computer science, mechanical engineering, economics, or electronic imaging of one sort or another, to the prevention, diagnosis, evaluation, treatment, or management of a disease or negative health condition.

capitation: A payment method in which a physician or hospital is paid a fixed amount per patient, per year, regardless of the volume or cost of services each patient requires.

carrier: An insurer; an underwriter of risk that is engaged in providing, paying for, or reimbursing all or part of the cost of health services under group insurance policies or contracts, medical or hospital services agreements, membership or subscription contracts, or similar group arrangements, in exchange for premiums or other periodic charges.

case management: Often utilized as part of a managed care system; a practitioner known as a "gatekeeper" makes decisions regarding the type and volume of services to which the patient may have access.

case manager: An individual who coordinates and oversees other health care workers in finding the most effective methods of caring for specific patients.

catastrophic coverage: A type of insurance that pays for high-cost health care, usually associated with accidents and chronic illnesses and diseases, such as cancer and AIDS.

census: In the U.S., refers to counts of members of the national population and their demographic characteristics undertaken by the Bureau of the Census every 10 years on the 10th year, and in the health care delivery system specifically, the number of patients in a hospital or other health care institution at any one time.

Centers for Medicare and Medicaid Services (CMS): Administers Medicare, Medicaid, and the Child Health Insurance Programs. Formerly called Health Care Financing Administration (HCFA).

certificates of need: Franchises for new services and construction or renovation of hospitals or related facilities, as issued by states.

chronic care: Treatment or rehabilitative health services provided to individuals on a long-term basis (over 30 days), in both inpatient and ambulatory settings.

Clinical Nurse Practitioner: Nurse with extra training who accepts additional clinical responsibility for medical diagnosis or treatment.

clinical trials: The testing on patients in a clinical setting of a diagnostic, preventive, or therapeutic intervention, using a study design that will provide for a valid estimation of safety and efficiency.

closed panel: A managed care plan that contracts with physicians on an exclusive basis for services and does not allow those physicians to see patients for another managed care organization.

coinsurance: A provision in a member's coverage that limits the amount of coverage by the plan to a certain percentage, commonly 80%. Any additional costs are paid out-of-pocket by the member.

community hospital: A hospital offering short-term general and other special services, owned by a corporation or agency other than the federal government.

community rating: The rating system by which a plan or an indemnity carrier takes the total experience of the subscribers or members within a given geographic area or "community" and uses these data to determine a reimbursement rate that is common for all groups regardless of the individual claims experience of any one group.

complementary and alternative medicine: Refers to a series of diagnostic and treatment interventions that fall outside of the realm of state-licensed medical practice as it is defined by the privileges to use certain restricted diagnostic regimens, prescribe drugs from a restricted list, and practice surgery. Such disciplines include: chiropractic, acupuncture, homeopathy, herbal medicine, naturopathy, therapeutic touch, and the like.

Consolidated Omnibus Budget Reconciliation Act of 1985 (COBRA): A federal law (P.L. 99-272), that requires that all employer-sponsored health plans offer certain employees and their families the opportunity to continue, at their personal expense, health insurance coverage under the group plan for up to 18, 24, or 36 months, depending on the qualifying event, after their coverage normally would have ceased (e.g., due to the death or retirement of the employee, divorce or legal separation, resignation or termination of employment, or bankruptcy of the employer).

co-payment: A specified amount that the insured individual must pay for a specified service or procedure (e.g., $8 for an office visit).

comprehensive coverage: A health insurance system that pays for a broad range of services.

cost sharing: A provision that requires individuals to cover some part of their medical expenses (e.g., co-payments, coinsurance, deductibles).

cost-shifting: Refers to passing the cost of one group onto another group. For example, if the rate one group of health plan enrollees pays for services is less than the actual cost of those services, the difference can be made up based on charges higher than cost paid by another group.

credentialing: The most common use of the term refers to obtaining and reviewing the documentation of professional providers.

data: In health, an event, condition, or disease occurrence that is counted. In health services, an episode of care, costs of care, expenditures, quantification of manpower and facilities and their characteristics, and the like.

deductible: The amount a patient must pay out-of-pocket, usually annually on a calendar-year basis, before insurance will begin to cover costs.

demographic characteristics: Refers to such characteristics of an individual or a population group (averages in the latter case) as: age, sex, marital status, ethnicity, geographic location, occupation, and income.

denominator: For health care, the total number of people among whom numerator items are being counted (see "Numerator").

diagnosis-related groups (DRGs): Groups of inpatient discharges with final diagnoses that are similar clinically and in resource consumption; used as a basis of payment by the Medicare program, and as a result, widely accepted by others.

discharge planning: A part of the patient management guidelines and the nursing care plan that identifies the expected discharge date and coordinates the various services necessary to achieve the target.

disproportionate share hospital (DSH): A hospital that provides a large amount (or disproportionate share) of uncompensated care and/or care to Medicaid and low-income Medicare beneficiaries.

drug: A therapeutic drug is a chemical compound used in treating or managing a disease or negative health condition. A recreational drug is a chemical compound that alters the user's mood by providing diversion, relaxation, heightened sensation or other enjoyment or pleasure.

Employee Retirement Income Security Act (ERISA): A 1974 federal law (P.L. 93-406) that set the standards of disclosure for employee benefit plans to ensure workers the right to at least part of their pensions. The law governs most private pensions and other employee benefits, and overrides all state laws that concern employee benefits, including health benefits; therefore, ERISA preempts state laws in their application to self-funded, private employer-sponsored health insurance plans.

enrollment: The process by which an individual and family become a subscriber(s) for coverage in a health plan. This may be done either through an actual signing up of the individual or through a collective bargaining agreement on the employer's conditions of employment. A result, therefore, is that the health plan is aware of its entire population of beneficiary eligibles. As a usual practice, individuals must notify the health plan of any changes in family status that affect the enrollment of dependents.

entitlements: Government benefits (e.g., Medicare, Medicaid, Social Security, food stamps) that are provided automatically to all qualified individuals, and are therefore part of mandatory spending programs.

experience rating: A method used to determine the cost of health insurance premiums, whereby the cost is based on the previous amount a certain group (e.g., all the employees of a particular business) paid for medical services.

Federal Employee Health Benefits Program (FEHBP):   Also referred to as Federal Employee Plan or FEP. The health plans made available to federal employees as part of their employment benefits.

fee schedule: A listing of accepted fees or established allowances for specified medical procedures as used in health plans; it usually represents the maximum amounts the program will pay for the specified procedures.

fee-for-service: A billing system in which a health care provider charges a patient a set amount for a specific service.

fixed costs: Costs that do not change or vary with fluctuations in enrollment or in utilization of services.

for-profit hospitals: Those owned by private corporations that declare dividends or otherwise distribute profits to individuals. Also called "investor-owned," many are also community hospitals.

formulary: A listing of drugs prepared by, for example, a hospital or a managed care company, that a physician may prescribe. The physician is requested or required to use only formulary drugs unless there is a valid medical reason to use a nonformulary drug.

gatekeeper: A health care practitioner who makes decisions regarding the type and volume of services to which a patient may have access, generally used by health maintenance organizations (HMOs) to control unnecessary utilization of services.

generics: A therapeutic drug, originally protected by a patent, the chemical composition of which meets the standards for that drug set by the Food and Drug Administration, made by a company other than the company that originally developed and patented the drug. Generics are usually not manufactured and made available until after the original patent has expired.

governance: The activity of an organization that monitors the outside environment, selects appropriate alternatives, and negotiates the implementation of these alternatives with others inside and outside the organization.

governing board: A group of individuals, who under state law own an organization, whether or not they can obtain any financial advantage through such ownership.

graduate medical education: The education and training of physicians beyond the 4 years of medical school, in positions that may be termed internship, residency, fellowship, post-graduate year (PGY) 1, 2, 3, and so on. Although one can enter medical school only with an undergraduate degree of some sort at the baccalaureate level, in the United States, the 4 years of medical school leading to the MD or DO (Doctor of Osteopathy) degrees are customarily referred to as "undergraduate medical education."

group model: An HMO that contracts with a medical group for the provision of health care services. The relationship between the HMO and the medical group is generally very close, although there are wide variations in the relative independence of the group from the HMO. A form of closed panel health plan.

group practice: Three or more physicians who deliver patient care, make joint use of equipment and personnel, and divide income by a pre-arranged formula.

health care delivery: The provision of preventive treatment, or rehabilitative health services, from short-term to long-term, to individuals as well as groups of people, by individual practitioners, institutions, or public health agencies.

Health Care Financing Administration (HCFA): A part of the U.S. Department of Health and Human Services. In addition to its many other functions, HCFA is the contracting agency for HMOs that seek direct contract/provider status for provision of the Medicare benefits package. The name has recently been changed to Centers for Medicare and Medicaid Services (CMS).

health care providers: Usually refers to professional health service workers—physicians, dentists, psychologists—who are licensed to practice independently of any other health service worker.

health care workforce: All of the those people, professional and non-professional alike, who work in the health care services industry.

health maintenance organization (HMO): A managed care company that organizes and provides health care for its enrollees for a fixed pre-paid premium.

health promotion (personal): Personal health promotion is the science and art of helping people change their lifestyle to move toward a state of optimal health. Optimal health is defined as a balance of physical, emotional, social, spiritual, and intellectual health.

health systems: Organizations that work together in predictable ways because of contractual relationships. The systems may or may not be commonly owned.

hospitalization: The admission of a patient to a hospital.

hospitalization coverage: A type of insurance coverage that covers most inpatient hospital costs (e.g., room and board), diagnostic and therapeutic services, care for emergency illnesses or injuries, laboratory and X-ray services, and certain other specified procedures.

human genome: Projects to develop a draft of the human genetic code, involving billions of pairs of letters in the DNA sequence of 26,000–40,000 genes in the 23 human chromosomes.

incidence: The number of new events, disease cases, or conditions, counted in a defined population during a defined period of time.

indemnity insurance: Benefits paid in a predetermined amount in the event of a covered loss; differs with reimbursement, which provides benefits based upon actual expenses incurred. There are fewer restrictions on what a doctor may charge and what an insurer may pay for a treatment and generally there are also less restrictions on a patient's ability to access specialty services.

infant mortality: The death of a child born alive before he or she reaches 1 year of age.

information technology: Electronic systems for communicating information. Health care organizations want information technology that is accessible—with privacy safeguards—to multiple users within an organization.

integrated delivery system (IDS): A group of health care organizations that collectively provides a full range of health-related services in a coordinated fashion to those using the system.

integration, horizontal: Affiliations among providers of the same type e.g., a hospital forming relationships with other hospitals).

integration, vertical: Affiliations among providers of different types e.g., a hospital, clinic and nursing home forming an affiliation).

international medical school graduate: A U.S. or non-U.S. citizen physician who has graduated from a medical school not located in the United States that is also not accredited by the U.S. medical school accrediting body, the Liaison Committee on Medical Education.

investor-owned hospital: A hospital owned by one or more private parties or a corporation, for the purpose of generating a profitable return on investment.

Joint Commission on Accreditation of Healthcare Organizations (JCAHO): A national organization of representatives of health care providers: American College of Physicians, American College of Surgeons, American Hospital Association, American Medical Association, and consumer representatives. The JCAHO offers inspection and accreditation on quality of operations to hospitals and other health care organizations.

licensure: A system established by a given state recognizing the achievement of a defined level of education, experience, and examination performance as qualifying the person or organization meeting those standards to work or operate in a defined area of practice, prohibited to any person or organization that has not met those standards.

life expectancy: The predicted average number of years of life remaining for a person at a given age.

long-term care: A general term for a range of services provided to chronically ill, physically disabled, and mentally disabled patients in a nursing home or long-term home health care setting.

loss ratio: A term used to describe the amount of money spent on health care. A company with a loss ratio of .85, for instance, spends 85 cents of every premium dollar on health care and the remaining 15 cents on administrative costs, such as marketing and profits.

major medical: A precursor of "catastrophic coverage," it is coverage characterized by larger maximum limits, which is intended to cover the cost associated with a major illness or injury.

managed care: A system of health care delivery that influences or controls utilization of services and costs of services. The degree of influence depends on the model used. For example, a preferred provider organization charges the patients lower rates if they use the providers in the preferred network. HMOs, on the other hand, may choose not to reimburse for health services received from providers with whom the HMO does not contract.

mandated benefits: Benefits that a health plan are required to provide by law. This is generally used to refer to benefits above and beyond routine insurance-type benefits, and it generally applies at the state level (where there is high variability from state to state). Common examples include in vitro fertilization, defined days of inpatient mental health or substance abuse treatment, and other special condition treatments. Self-funded plans are exempt from mandated benefits under ERISA.

Medicaid: A joint federal/state/local program of health care for individuals whose income and resources are insufficient to pay for their care, governed by Title XIX of the federal Social Security Act, and administered by the states. Medicaid is the major source of payment for nursing home care of the elderly.

medical savings account: Accounts similar to individual retirement accounts (IRAs) into which employers and employees can make tax-deferred contributions and from which employees may withdraw funds to pay covered health care expenses.

Medicare: A federal entitlement program of medical and health care coverage for the elderly and disabled, and persons with end-stage renal disease, governed by Title XVIII of the federal Social Security Act, and consisting of two parts: Part A—For institutional and home care, and Part B—For medical care.

Medi-Gap: Also known as Medicare Supplement Insurance, a type of private insurance coverage that may be purchased by an individual enrolled in Medicare to cover certain needed services that are not covered by Medicare Parts A and B (i.e., "gaps").

morbidity: An episode of sickness, as defined by a health professional. A morbidity rate is the number of such episodes occurring in a given population during a given period of time.

mortality: A death. A mortality rate is the number of deaths (either the "crude rate," which is all deaths, or a "specific rate," which is by, for example, specific cause, specific location, or specific age group) occurring during a given period of time.

natality: A live birth. The natality rate is the number of live births occurring in a given population during a given period of time.

national health insurance: A system for paying for one or more categories of health care service, that is organized on a nationwide basis, established by law and usually operated by a government agency.

National Health Service: In the United States and Great Britain refers specifically to the comprehensive, government funded and operated system such as that found in Great Britain.

network: An arrangement of several delivery points (i.e., medical group practices affiliated with a managed care organization; an arrangement of HMOs, either autonomous and separate legal entities, or subsidiaries of a larger corporation) using one common insuring mechanism such as Blue Cross/Blue Shield; a broker organization (health plan) that arranges with physician group, carriers, payer agencies, consumer groups, and others for services to be provided to enrollees.

nonprofit or not-for-profit plan: A term applied to a prepaid health plan under which no part of the net earnings accrues, or may lawfully accrue, to the benefit of any private shareholder or individual. An organization that has received 501-C-3 or 501-C-4 designation by the Internal Revenue Service.

numerator: For health care, a number of events, disease occurrences, or conditions that are counted, over some defined period of time.

office visit: A formal, face-to-face contact between the physician and the patient in a health center, office, or hospital outpatient department.

open enrollment period: A requirement that all possible customers for a particular health insurance policy be accepted at all times for coverage and, once accepted, not to be terminated by the insurer due to claims experience.

outlier: Under a DRG system of payment, additional per diem payments are made to the hospital for cases requiring a patient to stay in the hospital beyond a threshold length of stay. Such cases are referred to as "long-stay outliers."

per diem payment: Reimbursement rates that are paid to providers for each day of services provided to a patient, based on the patient's illness or condition.

perspective, provider and patient: The two different vantage points from which the same health services event can be counted, over time. For example, visits by patients to physician offices can be counted as the number of patient visits a physician sees in a year (provider perspective) or the number of visits to the physicians office a patient makes in a year (patient perspective).

point-of-service plan (POS): A managed care plan that offers enrollees the option of receiving services from participating or nonparticipating providers. The benefits package is designed to encourage the use of participating providers, through higher deductibles and/or partial reimbursement for services provided by nonparticipating providers.

preexisting condition: A physical and/or mental condition of an insured that first manifests itself prior to issuance of a policy or that exists prior to issuance and for which treatment was received.

preferred provider organization (PPO and PPA): A limited grouping (panel) of providers (doctors and/or hospitals) who agree to provide health care to subscribers for a negotiated and usually discounted fee and who agree to utilization review. The arrangement created among the providers and others (employers, unions, commercial insurers, HMOs, etc.) is called the PPA or preferred provider arrangement.

premium: A periodic payment required to keep an insurance policy force.

prepayment: A method of providing, in advance, for the cost of predetermined benefits for a population group through regular periodic payments in the form of premiums, dues, or contributions, including those contributions that are made to a health and welfare fund by employers on behalf of their employees, and payments to HMOs and CMPs made by federal agencies for Medicare eligibles.

prescription: An order, usually made in writing, from a licensed physician or his or her authorized designee, to a pharmacy, directing the latter to dispense a given drug, with written orders for its use.

prevalence: The total number of events, disease cases, or conditions existing in a defined population, counted during a defined period of time, or at a given point in time (known as "point-prevalence").

primary care: The general health care that people receive on a routine basis, that is not associated with an acute or chronic illness or disability, and may be provided by a physician, nurse practitioner, or physician's assistant. Definitions of primary care physicians usually include those who practice family medicine, pediatrics, and internal medicine; other physicians often included in this definition are obstetricians and gynecologists, as well as practitioners of preventive and emergency medicine.

primary care practitioners: Doctors in family practice, general internal medicine, or pediatrics; nurse practitioners and midwives; and may also include psychiatrists and emergency care physicians.

privileges: Rights granted annually to physicians and affiliate staff members to perform specified kinds of care in the hospital.

public hospital: A hospital operated by a government agency. In the United States, the most common are the federal government's Department of Veterans Affairs; state governments' mental hospitals; and local governments' general hospitals for the care of the poor and otherwise uninsured.

public psychiatric hospital: A hospital devoted to the treatment and management of mental illness and disorders, owned and operated by a government agency (in the United States, most commonly at the state level).

quality assurance: A formal set of activities to measure the quality of services provided; these may also include corrective measures.

quality of care: Referring to the measurement of the quality of health care provided to individuals or groups of patients, against a previously defined standard.

rates, crude and specific: A rate is a measure of some event, disease, or condition occurring in members of a defined population, divided by the total number in that population. For crude rates, the whole population is the denominator. A specific rate defines the denominator by one or more demographic characteristics.

registered nurse: A nurse who is a graduate of an approved education program leading to diploma, an associate degree, or a bachelor's degree, who has also met the requirements of experience and exam passage to be licensed in a given state.

reinsurance: Insurance purchased by a health plan to protect it against extremely high cost cases.

relative value system (RVS):   A method of valuing medical services, especially physician services. The federal government changed to an RBRVS (resource-based relative value scale) physician payment system in early 1992, an RVS payment system for physician services to Medicare recipients. Each service is assigned a given number of relative value units based on, for example, how long it takes to do a procedure, which is multiplied by a national conversion factor to determine a dollar amount for payment of that service.

reserves: A fiscal method of withholding a certain percentage of premiums to provide a fund for committed but undelivered health care and such uncertainties as higher hospital utilization levels than expected, overutilization of referrals and accidental catastrophes.

resource-based relative value scale (RBRVS): On January 1, 1992, Medicare payments are based on a resource-based relative value scale, replacing the customary and prevailing charge mechanism for fee-for-service providers participating in the Medicare program. The objective is that physician fees should reflect the relative value of work performed, their practice expense, and malpractice insurance costs.

risk: Any chance of loss, or the possibility that revenues of the health plan will not be sufficient to cover expenditures incurred in the delivery of contractual services.

risk contract: A contract to provide services to beneficiaries under which the health plan receives a fixed monthly payment for enrolled members, and then must provide all services on an at-risk basis.

self-insurance: A program for providing group insurance with benefits financed entirely through the internal means of the policyholder, in place of purchasing coverage from commercial carriers. By self-insuring, firms avoid paying state taxes on premiums and are largely exempt from state-imposed mandates.

socialized health service: Usually an epithet used by opponents of any type of national government involvement in either the financing or operation of a health care delivery system on a nationwide basis, to describe any such system, regardless of whether such a government could itself be defined as "socialist" or not.

solo practice: Individual practice of medicine by a physician who does not practice in a group or does not share personnel, facilities, or equipment with three or more physicians.

staff model: An HMO that employs providers directly, and those provider see members in the HMO's own facilities. A form of closed panel HMO.

stakeholders: Persons with an interest in the performance of an organization. Examples of hospital stakeholders are: physicians and nurses, payers, managers, patients, and government.

strategic planning: A process reviewing the mission, environmental surveillance, and previous planning decisions used to establish major goals and nonrecurring resource allocation decisions.

surveillance: Ongoing observation of a population for rapid and accurate detection of events, conditions, or diseases.

teaching hospital: A hospital in which undergraduate and/or graduate medical education takes place.

underwriting: This refers to bearing the risk for something (i.e., a policy is underwritten by an insurance company), also the analysis that is done for a group to determine rates or to determine whether the group should be offered coverage at all.

uninsured: In the United States, a person who is not the beneficiary of any third-party source of payment for health care services.

universal health insurance: Usually refers to a national health insurance system that provides for comprehensive coverage for all permanent residents of a country.

utilization review: A system for measuring and evaluating the utilization by physicians for their patients of various health services ranging from diagnostic tests to admission to hospital, against a preestablished standard of "good" or "appropriate" utilization of such services.

vertical integration: The affiliation of organizations providing different kinds of service, such as hospital care, ambulatory care, long-term care, and social services.

vital statistics: Numbers and rates for births, deaths, abortions, fetal deaths, fertility, life expectancy, marriages, and divorces.

volunteers: People who are not paid for giving their time to the health care organization, their only compensation being the satisfaction they achieve from their work.

wraparound plan: Commonly used to refer to insurance or health plan coverage for co-payments and deductibles that are not covered under a member's base plan, such as Medicare.

Appendix B

A Guide to Sources of Data[1]

Jennifer A. Nelson and Mary Ann Chiasson

This appendix is a guide to the principal sources of health and health services data for the United States as of 2001. It contains descriptions of those sources, indicates how frequently each is published, lists the categories of data and other information they contain, and gives the address of the publisher and other ordering information as indicated, all as of 2001.

Almost all federal sources of data are available for purchase through the U.S. Government Printing Office (USGPO or GPO, for short), Superintendent of Documents, P.O. Box 371954, Pittsburgh, PA 15250-7954; http://bookstore.gpo.gov; tel. (202) 512-1800, FAX (202) 512-2250. There are local USGPO bookstores and phone ordering centers located in major cities around the United States. They are listed in the federal government section of the blue pages of local telephone directories under "Government Printing Office." These listings are also available at the above Internet address.

Not only are health data available in print form, but they are also available on the Internet. Many of the publications indicated in this appendix are available in whole or in part via the Internet; others may be ordered using the Internet. Basic statistical tables are often included on government and organization websites, sometimes via an interactive database that allows the user to design tables with variables of interest. In addition, many data sets are available for public use and can be downloaded from the Internet or ordered on CD-ROM.

---

[1] Much of the information about sources of health and health care data for the United States was adapted from the previous edition of this appendix, compiled by Steven Jonas and Christine T. Kovner.

Comprehensive Guides to Sources Published Annually

There are two comprehensive guides to sources of data that are published annually. The first appears in the *Statistical Abstract of the United States* (see item 1, below). The most recent edition as of this writing was for 2000, published in February 2001. Its Appendix I contains an extensive listing of sources of health data (as well as the sources of all other data appearing in the *Statistical Abstract*). Appendix III presents brief descriptions and analyses of the limitations of the major sources of data listed in Appendix I.

The second regularly published comprehensive guide to sources appears in *Health, United States* (see item 8, below). The most recent edition as of this writing was for 2000 (DHHS Publication No. [PHS] 2000-1232). Its Appendix I contains very useful, detailed descriptions of all the common health data sources published by the several branches of the federal government, the United Nations, and certain private agencies, ranging from the American Medical Association to the National League for Nursing.

Also, the *AHA Guide*, published annually by the American Hospital Association (see item 12, below), lists in its Part C the major national, international, U.S. government, state and local government, and private "Health Organizations, Agencies, and Providers" with addresses and telephone numbers. Health and health care data can be obtained from any of them.

Using the Internet to Access Data

The Internet is changing the way that we seek and retrieve data. Information and statistics on almost any topic can be easily obtained with a few clicks of the mouse. The volume of information available, however, can be overwhelming and it can be difficult to know where to begin to look for that particular bit of information that you need. The following are a few places to begin your search for health and health services data. Specific Internet addresses relating to the principal sources listed in the following sections are noted in those sections.

The federal government is a major source of health data. Each department of the U.S. government has an Internet address; some of them are listed in the sections below. All federal government department and agency websites can be accessed through http://www.firstgov.gov. In addition, access to federal data produced by more than 70 agencies in the U.S. government can be obtained via http://www.fedstats.gov. Two agencies that are responsible for a large amount of population, health, and health services data are the Census Bureau (http://www.census.gov) and the Centers for Disease Control and Prevention (http://www.cdc.gov). Exploring their websites is a good way to become familiar with the data available.

Most states and professional organizations have websites as well. Links to state sites, which can be excellent sources of state and local data, are available at http://www.piperinfo.com/state/index.cfm or http://www.loc.gov/global/state/stategov.html; the websites of state departments of health and other agencies can be reached via state homepages.

The National Association of Health Data Organizations website (http://www.nahdo.org) includes a Health Website Search Module, that includes links to the sites of federal and state agencies as well as numerous health care associations and nonprofit organizations that have health information and data. It provides an overview of health information sources available via the Internet as well as access to those sources. Internet search engines such as Yahoo, Google, Metacrawler, or Excite can be used to locate the sites of other organizations.

PRINCIPAL SOURCES OF HEALTH AND HEALTH CARE DATA

1. *Statistical Abstract of the United States.* Published annually by the Bureau of the Census, U.S. Department of Commerce, Washington, DC 20233, the *Statistical Abstract* contains a vast collection of tables reporting information and data collected by many different government (and in certain cases nongovernment) agencies. They are accumulated under the following headings: Population; Vital Statistics; Health and Nutrition; Education; Law Enforcement, Courts, and Prisons; Geography and Environment; Parks, Recreation, and Travel; Elections; State and Local Government Finances and Employment; Federal Government Finances and Employment; National Defense and Veterans' Affairs; Social Insurance and Human Services; Labor Force, Employment, and Earnings; Income, Expenditures, and Wealth; Prices; Banking, Finance, and Insurance; Business Enterprise; Communications; Energy; Science; Transportation—Land; Transportation—Air and Water; Agriculture; Natural Resources; Construction and Housing; Manufactures; Domestic Trade and Services, Foreign Commerce and Aid; Outlying Areas (under the jurisdiction of the United States); Comparative International Statistics; and Industrial Outlook. There are health and health services data of varying kinds reported in many of these categories, although the principal ones are of course found under the headings Population, Vital Statistics, and Health and Nutrition. This publication can be ordered via http://www.ntis.gov/product/statistical-abstract.htm or http://www.census.gov/statab/www/ or through the USGPO. It is also available to be downloaded as portable document format (pdf) files from the Census home page.

2. *U.S. Census of Population.* The U.S. Constitution requires that a census be taken every 10 years, at the beginning of each decade. The original purpose of the census was to apportion seats in the House of Representatives. Since it was first taken, the census and the voluminous amount of data it produces—going well beyond a simple count—have come to serve many other purposes as well. Many reports on the decennial censuses, as well as interim special counts and analyses known as "Current Population Reports"

(see item 3, below), are published by the Census Bureau (a part of the U.S. Department of Commerce). A good place to begin is in Section 1 of the *Statistical Abstract*. A good deal of highly detailed information drawn from the decennial national census data is published periodically in hardcover compendia. Also available are special analyses for a wide variety of geographical subdivisions of the country.

Census Bureau publications may be ordered from the USGPO through their comprehensive Census Catalog and Guide (itself available for purchase from the USGPO). Many Census Bureau products can be accessed and/or ordered via the Internet, either from the USGPO (orders only) or from the Census Bureau (http://www.census.gov). Product orders may also be sent to the U.S. Department of Commerce, Bureau of the Census, P.O. Box 277943, Atlanta, GA 30384-7943, tel. (301) 457-4100, FAX (310) 457-3842.

3. *Current Population Reports.* In addition to reports from the decennial censuses, the Census Bureau regularly publishes "Current Population Reports" (CPRs). They present estimates, projections, sample counts, and special studies of selected segments of the population. There are seven series of CPRs: P-20, Population Characteristics; P-23, Special Studies; P-25, Population Estimates and Projections; P-26, Local Population Estimates; P-28, Special Censuses; P-60, Consumer Income; and P-70, Household Economic Studies. Catalogs and information on the content of each series are available directly from the Bureau of the Census, U.S. Department of Commerce, Washington, DC 20233. Publications may be ordered through the USGPO. The data are also available in microdata files. The data files can be accessed and publications can be downloaded from the Census Bureau's Current Population Survey web page (www.bls.census.gov/cps/cpsmain.htm).

4. *National Center for Health Statistics.* Part of the Centers for Disease Control and Prevention, U.S. Department of Health and Human Services, the national Center for Health Statistics (NCHS) is the federal government's primary agency for vital and health statistics. Through its data systems, the NCHS collects data on health status, health behavior, and the use of health care; it also serves as the repository for data from the nation's vital statistics systems. Data is collected through national population surveys such as the National Health and Nutrition Examination Survey, the National Health Interview Survey, and the National Survey of Family Growth, and also through surveys of health care providers, such as the National Health Care Survey, which includes the National Hospital Discharge Survey and the National Ambulatory Medical Care Survey.

Data from the Vital Statistics System and the health surveys are published in a series of regular and periodic reports (see items 5–7, below). The center's website (http://www.cdc.gov/nchs/) serves as an entry to a great deal of information about these data systems and to data in tabular form, as well as publication lists and downloadable versions of many publications. In addition, many of these data sets are available for public use and can be downloaded from the website.

5. *National Vital Statistics report (NVSR).* NVSR is published by the National Center for Health Statistics (NCHS), Center for Disease Control and Prevention (CDC), U.S. Department of Health and Human Services, 6525 Belcrest Road, Hyattsville, MD 20782-2003, tel. (310) 458-4636. The NCHS periodically publishes catalogs of its various publications and electronic data products. The *NVSR* appears in several sections. "Provisional Data," published monthly, contains the most recent figures for the traditional "vital statistics"—births, marriages, divorces, and deaths. There is a series of NVSR supplements that appear on a semiregular basis, containing "Advance Reports" of the "Final Data" for the annually collected vital statistics. There are also reports titled "Advance Data." They present what are called "Vital and Health Statistics" for the health care delivery system, including, for example, results of the "National Home and Hospice Care Survey," the "National Hospital Ambulatory Medical Care Survey," and the "National Hospital Discharge Survey," as well as the results of special studies and technical information on methodology. All NVSR reports may be obtained by annual subscription, through the USGPO. Data and reports are also available via the Internet (http://www.cdc.gov/nchs/).

6. *Vital Statistics of the United States.* These are the full, highly detailed annual reports on vital statistics from the NCHS, the summary versions of which are published in the supplements of the NVSR.

7. *Vital and Health Statistics.* These publications of the NCHS, distinct from the "Vital Statistics" reports described in items 4 and 5 above, appear at irregular intervals. As of 1997, there were 14 series, not numbered consecutively. Most of them report data from ongoing studies and surveys that the NCHS carries out. The publication of some data shifts periodically between *Vital and Health Statistics* and *National Vital Statistics Report.* The 14 series of Vital and Health Statistics are as follows: Series 1, programs and collection procedures; Series 2, data evaluation and methods research; Series 3, analytical and epidemiological studies; Series 4, documents and committee reports; Series 5, international vital and health statistics reports; Series 6, cognition and survey measurement; Series 10, data from the National Health Interview Survey; Series 11, data from the National Health Examination Survey, the National Health and Nutrition Examination Surveys, and the Hispanic Health and Nutrition Examination Survey; Series 13, data on health resources utilization; Series 16, compilations of advance data from vital and health statistics; Series 20, data on mortality; Series 21, data on natality, marriage, and divorce; Series 23, data From the National Survey of Family Growth; Series 24, compilation of data on natality, mortality, marriage, divorce, and induced terminations of pregnancy.

8. *Health, United States.* Health, United States is published annually by the NCHS/CDC and is available for purchase from the USGPO. It may also be downloaded from http://www.cdc.gov/nchs/products/pubs/pubd/hus/hus.htm. A wide variety of health and health care delivery systems data are presented, under the following categories: population, fertility and natality, mortality, determinants of health, utilization of health

resources, health care resources, and health care expenditures. *Health, United States* also contains a useful appendix, "Sources and Limitations of Data" (described above), as well as a glossary. It is a boon to students and researchers in health care delivery systems analysis because it provides one-stop shopping for the most important health and health care data.

9. *Behavioral Risk Factor Surveillance System.* The Behavioral Risk Factor Surveillance System (BRFSS) is an ongoing data collection program that resides in the national Center for Chronic Disease Prevention and Health Promotion of the Centers for Disease Control and Prevention. It was designed to serve a dual purpose: to meet the need for behavioral health data, necessary for designing preventive programs to reduce mor-bidity and mortality, and to meet the need for that data at the state level where the activities and targeting of resources generally occur. States use a CDC-developed standard core questionnaire to conduct telephone sur-veys collecting data on health risks and behaviors. BRFSS data files are available free on CD-ROM or can be downloaded from the BRFSS web site (http://www.cdc.gov/hccdphp/brfss/). The 1999 CD-ROM is avail-able to order at http://www.cdc.gov/nccdphp/brfss/ordercdrom.htm; CD-ROMs with data from previous years may be ordered from the USGPO. In addition, "BRFSS Summary Prevalence Reports" are pub-lished annually; the most recent available is the 1999 report. Topics cov-ered include general health status, quality of life, health insurance, smoking status, alcohol consumption, immunization, HIV/AIDS, over-weight/obesity, and screening for diabetes, cholesterol, hypertension, and colorectal, breast, and cervical cancer. These reports are available to down-load from the BRFSS website. Prevalence and trends data are also available directly from the website.

10. *Morbidity and Mortality Weekly Report (MMWR).* This is a regu-lar publication of the Centers for Disease Control and Prevention. It is available by annual subscription from the USGPO. Following a large sub-scription price increase in 1982, however, *MMWR,* in the public domain, has been photocopied and circulated at cost by several organizations, including the Massachusetts Medical Society, P.O. Box 9120, Waltham, MA 02254-9120. It is now also available free via the Internet or email subscrip-tion (www.cdc.gov/mmwr/). In the past, *MMWR* has been concerned pri-marily with communicable disease reporting. As of 2001, the numbers by state of reported cases of the following diseases are published weekly: AIDS, chlamydia, cryptosporidiosis *Escherichia coli,* gonorrhea, viral hep-atitis, Legionellosis, Listeriosis, Lyme disease, malaria, *H. influensae* (inva-sive), salmonellosis shigellosis, measles, meningococcal disease, mumps, pertussis, rubella (German measles), primary and secondary syphilis, tuberculosis, and animal rabies. *MMWR* also reports deaths in 122 U.S. cities on a weekly basis. In the late 1990s, equally or perhaps more impor-tant, each week *MMWR* presented brief reports on special studies of such diverse health topics as alcohol consumption among pregnant and child-bearing-age women, human rabies, progress toward global poliomyelitis

eradication, rubella syndrome in the United States, adult blood lead epidemiology and surveillance, Clean Air Month, urban community intervention to prevent Halloween arson, sports-related recurrent brain injuries, a tobacco tax initiative in Oregon, and prevalence of cigarette smoking among secondary school students in Budapest, Hungary. *MMWR* also periodically publishes "Recommendations and Reports" of various governmental and nongovernmental health agencies and organizations, and the results of "CDC Surveillance Summaries."

11. *Health Care Financing Review.* The *Health Care Financing Review* is a quarterly publication of the Health Care Financing Administration (HCFA), USDHHS, Office of Strategic Planning, 1-A-9 Oak Meadows Building, 7500 Security Boulevard, C3-11-07, Baltimore, MD 21244-1850, tel. (410) 786-6572. It is available by subscription through the USGPO. It annually publishes the official HCFA reports, "National Health Expenditures" and "Health Care Indicators." It also publishes an extensive and wide-ranging series of academic articles, reports, and studies. The emphasis is on Medicare/Medicaid (for which HCFA is directly responsible), but "a broad range of health care financing and delivery issues" are also covered. Abstracts and information about the publication are available at http://www.hcfa.gov/pubforms/ordpub.htm. HCFA data and statistics, including data tables and data files from the Medicaid and Medicare systems, can be accessed at http://www.hcfa.gov/stats/stats.htm.

12. *American Hospital Association Guide to the Health Care Field and Hospital Statistics.* These are annual publications of the American Hospital Association (AHA) (http://www.aha.org), One North Franklin, Chicago, IL 60606-3401, http://www.ahaonlinestore.com. Publication ordering tel. (800) AHA-2626. The *AHA Guide* contains a listing of almost every hospital in the United States by location and gives basic data on size, type, ownership, and services of each one; a listing and brief description of the integrated health care delivery networks; a listing of the multihospital health care systems, and information on the AHA itself. It also contains the comprehensive lists of health and health care organizations referred to in the introductory section of this appendix, above. AHA also publishes *Hospital Statistics* annually. It contains a great deal of summary descriptive, utilization, and financial data on U.S. hospitals, presented in many different cross-tabulations. The two publications together contain the most detailed data available on hospitals in the United States. Other AHA data products and services are available for purchase at http://www.healthforum.com.

13. *Center for Health Policy Research of the American Medical Association.* The Center, located in AMA National Headquarters, 515 North State Street, Chicago, IL 60610, ordering tel. (800) 621-8335, http://www.ama-assn.org, produces a variety of useful data on the physician workforce and related subjects. Titles appearing on a regular basis include: "Physician Socioeconomic Statistics," "Physician Marketplace Statistics," "U.S. Medical Licensure Statistics and Current Licensure Requirements," "Physician Characteristics and Distribution in the U.S." and "Medical Groups in the U.S."

14. *National League for Nursing and National Council of State Boards of Nursing.* The National League for Nursing (http://www.NLN.org) provides information on Nursing Education Programs including enrollments. Information about their publications is available from the National League for Nursing, 350 Hudson Street, New York 10014, ordering tel. (800) 669-1656, publication information at http://www.nlnpress.jbpub. com. Titles appearing on a regular basis, incorporating results from an annual survey of nursing programs, are *State Approved Schools of Nursing* and *Nursing Data Source.*

The National Council of State Boards of Nursing (http://www. ncsbn.org) is a source of data about the licensing and employment of nurses. The Council annually compiles "Licensure and Examination Statistics" and publishes a series of reports on findings from the Job Analysis Study. Information, abstracts, and demographic data tables are available on line, while these and other publications may be ordered from National Council of State Boards of Nursing, Dept. 77-3953, Chicago, IL 60678-3953, tel. (312) 787-6555 ext. 177, http://www.ncsbn.org/publications/publist.asp. Links to other nursing and nursing statistics sites are available as well.

Another source for information about nursing data and data sources is the Interagency Conference on Nursing Statistics (ICONS) (http://www. ncsbn.org/icons.html). ICONS does not collect data itself, but rather serves as a coordinating association comprised of researchers from organizations that do collect and analyze nursing data.

INTERNATIONAL HEALTH AND HEALTH SERVICES DATA

What follows is not a comprehensive guide to sources of international population and health data, but an accounting of several major sources, that, along with the international sections of publications noted above, are good places to begin.

1. *United States Census Bureau International Programs Center.* The International Programs Center (IPC) of the U.S. Census Bureau (http:// www.census.gov/ipc/www/) produces a publication entitled *World Population Profile* (the most recent edition is for 1998). It includes data on population growth, fertility, mortality, migration, population aging, and contraceptive use for the world, regions, development categories, and some specific countries. It can be downloaded from the IPC website or ordered from the USGPO. The International Programs Center also produces other reports on various related topics. In addition, it administers an on-line International Database that has statistical tables of demographic and socioeconomic data for all countries of the world.

2. *United Nations.* The United Nations system is comprised of a host of agencies and organizations devoted to a wide variety of topics of international relevance; many of these collect and compile population and

health data. Most UN publications can be ordered through the UN Publications Department (United Nations Publications, Room DC2-853, 2 UN Plaza, New York, NY 10017, tel. (212) 963-8302 or (800) 253-9646, FAX (212) 963-3489; email publications@un.org or on-line at http://www.un.org/Pubs/, which also serves as an on-line catalog of UN publications. Specific ordering information for some publications can be found on individual agency websites. Links to the websites of all UN agencies can be found at http://www.unsystem.org. Some UN offices and agencies to consider when looking for international health data are World Health Organization (WHO), United Nations Population Fund (UNFPA), United Nations Statistics Division (UNSD), United Nations Children's Fund (UNICEF), Joint United Nations Program on HIV/AIDS (UNAIDS), and the Population Division of the United Nations Department of Economic and Social Affairs (UNPD).

The World Health Organization is the principal UN source for health and health care data. WHO publishes an annual *World Health Report* that includes a number of population health indicators as well as a narrative discussion of world health, each year examining one additional topic in more depth. For example, the 2000 *Report* includes a section on health systems with accompanying data on health systems. The report can be downloaded from the WHO website (http://www.who.int) or ordered from the WHO Publications Center USA, 49 Sheridan Ave., Albany, NY 12210, tel. (518) 436-9686, FAX (518) 436-7433. WHO also periodically produces the *World Health Statistics Annual* (most recent edition, 1996). The WHO Statistical Information System (http://www.who.int/whosis/) includes data from these two reports as well as links to a variety of other information and data, to other world health sites, and to Department of Health or Statistical Bureau websites for many countries.

The United Nations Statistics Division (http://www.un.org/Depts/unsd/) provides statistics on numerous topics including demographics and vital statistics. It publishes a quarterly journal, *Population and Vital Statistics Report,* that reports population estimates, and birth and mortality statistics for the world, regions, and 218 countries. It also publishes two general statistical compendiums: *Statistical Yearbook and World Statistics Pocketbook.* All of these publications can be ordered from the UN Publications Department. Many data files can also be downloaded or ordered.

UNFPA (http://www.unfpa.org) produces an annual report entitled *The State of the World Population,* which includes statistics. It can be downloaded from UNFPA or ordered through the UN Publications Department. Basic indicators related to child health can be accessed on-line via the UNICEF website (http://www.unicef.org). UNICEF also produces an annual report, *The State of the World's Children,* which includes many child health statistics. Portions of the current document are available on-line, as are the entirety of previous years' reports. The report can be ordered from the UN Publications Department.

The United Nations Population Information Network (POPIN) is supported by the Population Division and UNFPA. Via the POPIN website (http://www.undp.org/popin/) population-related data such as statistics on fertility, mortality, and migration can be accessed. Publications and other information on these and related topics are also available through this site.

3. *Demographic and Health Surveys.* The Demographic and Health Survey program, also known as MEASURE DHS+ (http://www.measuredhs.com) is administered by Macro International, Inc. and is a source of population and health data for developing countries. MEASURE DHS+ provides developing countries with assistance in undertaking surveys to collect data on population, family planning, maternal and child health, child survival, sexually transmitted infections, and reproductive health. This data is available for public use in a number of formats. Publications with comprehensive survey results for individual countries can be ordered on-line or by calling (301) 572-0958. Other publications available include comparative, analytic, and trend reports. Some of these reports can be downloaded. Data sets are also available to be downloaded. The DHS STATcompiler is an on-line database, that allows users to create custom tables drawing on hundreds of surveys from numerous countries and including hundreds of indicators. Tables of preset basic indicators can also be accessed through this database.

4. *Links to other sources of international data on the Internet.* Many of the sites listed above include links to other sites where international health data may be found. For links to other statistical sites including statistical agencies in countries around the world try http://www.census.gov/main/www/stat_int.html or http://www.bls.gov/oreother.htm. Links to an array of foreign government websites can be found at http://www.lib.umich.edu/libhome/Documents.center/foreignnew.html and http://www.lib.uiowa.edu/govpubs/forintl.html. Links to other sources of international data including individual country sites are available at http://www.un.org/Depts/unsd/sd_nat_data.htm.

INTERNET GUIDES

PBS Understanding and Using the Internet
http://www.pbs.org/uti/

Learn the Net
http://www.learnthenet.com

The Net: User Guidelines and Netiquette
http://www.fau.edu/rinaldi/netiquette.html

FOLDOC-Free On-Line Dictionary of Computing
http://www:foldoc.org

Appendix C

An Essential Guide to the World Wide Web in Health Care

Lesley Reis

OUTLINE OF RESOURCES

WEBSITE FINDERS AND LINKS

www.achoo.com

Achoo Internet health care directory; search engines and links

www.aha.org/resource/	American Hospital Association Resource Center; links to other health care related websites
www.auburn.edu/~burnsma/ha.html	Auburn University's directory ofhealth administration and policy links
http://www.healthfinder.gov	Health Finder; search engine and links to other health sites
http://neuro-www.mgh.Harvard.edu/hospitalweb.shtml	Hospital Web; listing of hospital and health system websites
http://epn.org/ideacentral/health.html www.looksmart.com	Idea Central; health policy links LookSmart; generic Internet directory with over 16,000 different subject categories and 250,000 reviewed site listings
http://medworld.Stanford.edu/medworld/medbot/	Medbot; Stanford University's medical and health web page search engine
www.medweb.emory.edu/medweb	MedWeb; Emory University's medical and health information search engine
www.mwsearch.com	Medical World Search; search full text of over 100,000 web pages from thousands of prescreened medical sites
www.health.gov/NHIC	National Health Information Center; links to websites of 1,200 health organizations
www.yahoo.com/Health/Health_Administration	Yahoo directory; health administration websites

GOVERNMENT WEBSITE FINDERS AND LINKS

www.fedworld.gov	FedWorld; links and information search engine for the federal government
www.firstgov.gov	FirstGov; links to all federal government department and agency websites
www.piperinfo.com/state/index.cfm	Piper Resources; links to state and local government websites, federal resources, national organizations, and other government links

www.loc.gov/global/state/stategov.html	State and local governments; index for state and local government information
www.hhs.gov/agencies/	U.S. Department of Health and Human Services; links to all HHS Agencies
www.statelocal.gov	U.S. State and Local Gateway; access to federal information
www.nttc.edu/gov_res.html	World Wide Web Virtual Library; U.S. government information sources

BIBLIOGRAPHICAL SEARCH

www.ahsr.org/search.htm	Association for Health Services Research; abstract search engine
http://igm.nlm.nih.gov	Grateful Med; health care bibliographical search engine
www.ipl.org	Internet Public Library
http://lcweb.loc.gov	Library of Congress
www.medmatrix.org	Medical Matrix; medical literature search engine
www.medscape.com	Medscape; medical search engine; access to on-line journals and current news
www.nichsa.org	National Information Center for Health Services Administration; focused on health administration and policy
www2.ari.net/chrc/oldchrc/nhirc/home_newlogsky.html	National Health Information Resources Center; clearinghouse and communications hub for health information
www.nlm.nih.gov/pubs/resources.html	National Library of Medicine; resource lists and current bibliographies in medicine
www.ncbi.nlm.nih.gov/PubMed/	Pub Med; National Library of Medicine's search engine that accesses citations in MedLine and Pre-MedLine and other related databases

http://www.lib.uiowa.edu/ hardin-www/hslibs.html	University of Iowa; links to medical libraries on the Web
www.webmedlit.com	WebMedLit; access to medical journals and literature search by subject

STATISTICS AND DATABASES

www.ahcpr.gov/data	Agency for Health Care Policy Research; access to the Healthcare Cost and Utilization Project, the National Medical Expenditure Survey, and other governmental data and studies
www.ahd.com	American Hospital Directory; on-line data for most U.S. hospitals constructed from claims data, cost reports, and other public use files obtained from HCFA; includes hospital characteristics, financial data, inpatient utilization, outpatient utilization, and links to the hospital's website
http://stats.bls.gov/oshhome.htm	Bureau of Labor Statistics; safety and health statistics
http://oshpd.cahwnet.gov	California Office of Statewide Health Planning and Development; utilization and financial data for California hospitals and long-term care facilities
http://chid.nih.gov	Combined Health Information Data Base; produced by Federal government health-related departments and agencies; links to most governmental health data sites
www.fedstats.gov	FedStats; links to federal data and statistics produced by government agencies

www.hcfa.gov/stats/stats.htm (HCFA has recently changed its name to CMS)	Health Care Financing Administration; HCFA data and statistics, including data tables and data files from the Medicaid and Medicare systems
www.hcfa.gov/medicaid/mcaidsad.htm (HCFA has recently changed its name to CMS)	Health Care Financing Administration; Medicaid utilization and financial data files from HCFA
www.hcfa.gov/stats/monthly.htm (HCFA has recently changed its name to CMS)	Health Care Financing Administration; Medicare Coordinated Care Health Plans; monthly reports from HCFA
www.hsls.pitt.edu/intres/guides/ statcbw.html	Health Sciences Library System; guide to locating health statistics on the Web
www.health.gov/healthypeople/	Healthy People; access to Healthy People 2010 prevention agenda and national health objectives information
www.hospitalselect.com	HospitalSelect; provides basic information on all hospitals in the United States
www.nahdo.org	National Association of Health Data Organizations; links to the sites of federal and state agencies, other health care associations, and nonprofit organizations that have health information and data
www.cdc.gov/nchs/	National Center for Health Statistics; basic source of data in the health care field
www.nlm.nih.gov/databases/ databases.html	National Library of Medicine; databases and electronic information sources
www.census.gov/prod/www/ statistical-abstract-us.html	*Statistical Abstract of the United States/Healthcare;* complete publications with over 1,500 tables and charts for years 1995–2000
http://www.census.gov/dmd/ www/2khome.htm	U.S. Census Bureau; Census 2000 data

GOVERNMENT AGENCIES

www.ahcpr.gov	Agency for Health Care Policy and Research
http://stats.bls.gov	Bureau of Labor Statistics
www.census.gov	Census Bureau
www.cdc.gov	Centers for Disease Control and Prevention
www.cms.hhs.gov	Centers for Medicare and Medicaid, formerly HCFA
www.cbo.gov	Congressional Budget Office
www.ha.osd.mil	Department of Defense, Health Affairs
www.ed.gov	Department of Education
www.dhhs.gov	Department of Health and Human Services
www.usdoj.gov	Department of Justice
www.dol.gov	Department of Labor
www.va.gov	Department of Veterans Affairs
www.epa.gov	Environmental Protection Agency
www.uscourts.gov	Federal Judiciary
www.ftc.gov	Federal Trade Commission
www.fda.gov	Food and Drug Administration
www.gao.gov	Government Accounting Office
www.gpo.gov	Government Printing Office
www.hrsa.gov	Health Resources and Services Administration
www.house.gov	House of Representatives
www.ihs.gov	Indian Health Service
www.medpac.gov	Medicare Payment Advisory Commission
www.nih.gov	National Institutes of Health
www.nlm.nih.gov	National Library of Medicine
www.surgeongeneral.gov/ophs/	Office of Public Health and Science
www.senate.gov	Senate
www.ssa.gov	Social Security Administration
www.whitehouse.gov	White House

TRADE ASSOCIATIONS

www.himanet.com	Advanced Medical Technology Association; organizations that manufacture health care products and equipment
www.aahp.org	American Association of Health Plans; information and statistics regarding managed health care plan enrollment, benefits, utilization, and prices
www.aahc.net	American Association of Healthcare Consultants; consulting firms focusing on the health care industry
www.aaihds.org	American Association of Integrated Healthcare Delivery Systems; PHOs, PSOs, PSNs, MSOs, IPAs, and other emerging forms of integrated delivery systems
www.abms.org	American Board of Medical Specialties; medical specialty and subspecialty societies
www.his.com/~afhha/usa.html	American Federation of Home Health Agencies; home health organizations
www.ahca.org	American Health Care Association; assisted living, nursing facility, and subacute care providers
www.aha.org	American Hospital Association; hospital and health systems
www.ambha.org	American Managed Behavioral Healthcare Association; health plans focused exclusively on behavioral (mental) health
www.amia.org	American Medical Informatics Association; dedicated to the development and application of medical informatics in support of patient care, teaching, research, and health care administration

www.aphanet.org	American Pharmaceutical Association; drug manufacturers and pharmacists
www.aslme.org	American Society of Law, Medicine and Ethics; provides information for professionals working with law, health care, policy and ethics; access to journals, newsletters, and research projects
www.ahcnet.org	Association of Academic Health Centers; medical and other health sciences schools in addition to their teaching hospitals
www.aamc.org	Association of American Medical Colleges; medical schools, academic societies, and teaching hospitals
www.aupha.org	Association of University Programs in Health Administration; graduate and undergraduate programs in health administration
www.chausa.org	Catholic Health Association; Catholic hospitals and health systems
www.fahs.com	Federation of American Health Systems; investor-owned hospitals and health systems
www.hiaa.org	Health Insurance Association of America; health insurance companies and managed care organizations
www.nahc.org	National Association for Home Care; home health providers
www.nacds.org	National Association of Chain Drug Stores; represents views and policy positions of member chain drug companies
www.naph.org	National Association of Public Hospitals and Health Systems; provides legislative and public policy information and publications

www.ncsbn.org	National Council of State Boards of Nursing; source of data about the licensing and employment of nurses; annual statistics and publications
www.nhpco.org	National Hospice and Palliative Care Organization; represents organizations that provide hospice and palliative care

PROFESSIONAL ASSOCIATIONS

www.aameda.org	American Academy of Medical Adminstrators; chief medical officers in hospitals and health systems
www.achca.org	American College of Health Care Administrators; managers of long-term care, assisted living, and subacute care facilities
www.ache.org	American College of Health Care Executives; executives/managers in all types of health care organizations
www.acpe.org	American College of Physician Executives; physician executives in all segments of the health care industry
www.healthlawyers.org	American Health Lawyers Association; attorneys specializing in the practice of health law
www.ama-assn.org	American Medical Association; physicians
www.ana.org	American Nurses' Association; registered nurses
www.am-osteo-assn.org	American Osteopathic Association; osteopathic physicians
www.apha.org	American Public Health Association; public health professionals
www.aone.org	Association of Nurse Executives; nurse managers

www.cmsa.org	Case Management Society of America; case managers
www.hfma.org	Healthcare Financial Management Association; financial management professionals in health care organizations
www.mgma.com	Medical Group Management Association; physician practice and medical group managers
www.nahq.org	National Association for Healthcare Quality; quality management professionals
www.nashe.org	National Association of Health Services Executives; African American health care executives
www.NLN.org	National League for Nursing; provides information on nursing education programs and publications
www.phrma.org	Pharmaceutical Researchers and Manufacturers of America; research-based pharmaceutical and biotechnology companies

OTHER HEALTH-RELATED ORGANIZATIONS: ASSOCIATIONS, ACCREDITING BODIES, CENTERS, INSTITUTES, AND FOUNDATIONS

www.aarp.org	American Association of Retired Persons
www.ahsr.org	Association for Health Services Research; membership organization of individuals involved in policy and management research
www.astho.org	Association of State and Territorial Health Officials; links to public health agencies in all states; state initiatives and publications
www.bluecares.com	Blue Cross/Blue Shield Association; represents Blue Cross and Blue Shield associations throughout the country

www.chcs.org	Center for Health Care Strategies; a health policy research and resource center affiliated with the Woodrow Wilson School of Public and International Affairs at Princeton University
www.futurehealth.ucsf.edu	Center for the Health Professions; University of California, San Francisco health manpower policy research center sponsored by the Pew Foundation
www.hschange.com	Center for Studying Health System Change; Washington-based research organization dedicated to studying how the country's health care system is changing and how these changes are affecting communities
www.tcf.org	The Century Foundation; research foundation undertaking analyses of major economic, political, and social institutions and issues
www.cmwf.org	The Commonwealth Fund; a nonprofit foundation engaged in independent research on health and social policy issues
www.ebri.org	Employee Benefit Research Institute; conducts research on employee benefits provided by commercial corporations
www.iom.edu	Institute of Medicine; a component of the National Academy of Sciences that studies health policy issues
www.iha.org	Integrated Health Association; California-based group of health plans, physician groups, and health systems, plus academic, purchaser, and consumer representatives involved in policy development and special projects focused on integrated health care and managed care

www.jcaho.org	Joint Commission on the Accreditation of Healthcare Organizations; accrediting body for health systems, hospitals, and other providers
www.kff.org	Kaiser Family Foundation; foundation supporting health services research and demonstration projects
www.mathematica-mpr.com	Mathematica Policy Research; conducts health and social policy research
www.nashp.org	National Academy for State Health Policy; disseminates information designed to assist states in the development of practical, innovative solutions to complex health policy issues
www.nchc.org	National Coalition on Health Care; the nation's largest and most broadly representative alliance working to improve America's health care; research and education about emerging health trends and policy studies
www.ncsl.org/programs/health/forum	National Conference of State Legislatures; Forum for State Health Policy Leadership
www.ncqa.org	National Committee for Quality Assurance; accrediting body for managed health care plans and designers of HEDIS
www.projecthope.org	Project Hope; nonprofit organization that conducts research and policy analysis on both United States and foreign health care systems
www.rand.org	RAND Corporation; nonprofit institution that helps improve policy and decision making through research and analysis
www.rwjf.org	Robert Wood Johnson Foundation; foundation that funds health services research and demonstration projects

www.uhfnyc.org	United Hospital Fund; health services research and philanthropic organization that addresses issues affecting hospitals and health care in New York City
www.urban.org	Urban Institute; nonprofit policy and research organization
www.wbgh.com	Washington Business Group on Health; national nonprofit organization devoted to the analysis of health policy and related worksite issues from the perspective of large public sector employers
www.wkkf.org	W. K. Kellogg Foundation; a foundation that funds health services research and demonstration projects

INTERNATIONAL HEALTH AND HEALTH SERVICES DATA

www.bls.gov/oreother.htm	Bureau of Labor Statistics; national and international statistical agencies
www.census.gov/ipc/www	International Programs Center of the U.S. Census Bureau; *World Population Profile* last published in 1998; on-line International Database
www.unsystem.org	United Nations; links to the websites of all UN agencies
www.unicef.org	United Nations Children's Fund; basic indicators related to child health; *The State of the World's Children* published annually
www.un.org/Depts/unsd/	United Nations Statistics Division; *Population and Vital Statistics Report* published quarterly
www.census.gov/main/www/ stat_int.html	U.S. Census Bureau; international statistical agencies

www.who.int   World Health Organization
www.who.int/whosis/   World Health Organization
                                          Statistical Information System

CONSULTING FIRMS

www.aahc.net   American Association of
                                          Healthcare Consultants

www.arthurandersen.com   Arthur Andersen, LLP
www.chpsconsulting.com   Center for Health Policy Studies
www.ey.com   Ernst and Young, LLP
www.kpmg.com   KPMG Consulting
www.lewin.com   The Lewin Group; health and
                                          human service consulting firm

www.pwc.global.com   Pricewaterhouse Coopers

ON-LINE INDUSTRY NEWS:
HEALTH INDUSTRY NEWS UPDATED DAILY OR WEEKLY

www.ahanews.com   AHA News; daily reports for
                                          health care executives

www.cnn.com/HEALTH   CNN; health news updated
                                          daily

www.hhnmag.com   Health and Hospitals Network;
                                          health industry news updated
                                          daily

www.individual.com/browse/   News Page for Healthcare; index
industry.shtml?level1=46610   of on-line news stories on a vari-
                                          ety of topics; updated weekly

www.newsrx.net   News Rx Network; current
                                          news stories; reports on
                                          bioscience, biotech/pharma,
                                          health, and medicine

MAGAZINES AND JOURNALS ON-LINE

www.apha.org/journal   *American Journal of Public
                                          Health and The Nation's
                                          Health;* published by the
                                          American Public Health
                                          Association; article archives

www.healthaffairs.org	*Health Affairs;* health policy articles and abstracts
www.hcfa.gov/pubforms/ordpub.htm	*Health Care Financing Review;* source of Medicare and Medicaid data and national health statistics and expenditures
www.healthforum.com	*Health Forum Journal;* selected articles available for the past 5 years
http://jama.ama-assn.org	*Journal of the American Medical Association*
www.trusteemag.com	*Magazine for Health Care Governance;* article archive
www.managedcaremag.com	*Managed Care Magazine;* access to current articles and analyses
www.Milbank.org/quarterly.html	*The Milbank Quarterly: Journal of Public Health and Health Care Policy;* access to current articles and archives
www.modernhealthcare.com	*Modern Healthcare;* weekly news journal for health care management professionals
www.cdc.gov/mmwr	*Morbidity and Mortality Weekly Report;* weekly publication of the Centers for Disease Control and Prevention
www.nejm.org	*New England Journal of Medicine*

JOB SEARCH

www.ache.org/career.html	American College of Healthcare Executives; career page; employment opportunities listing
www.futurestep.com	Future Step from Korn/Ferry; web-based job search/finding site for jobs in health administration
www.h-s.com	Heidrick and Struggles; executive search firm

www.kornferry.com   Korn/Ferry International;
                                     executive search firm

www.mcol.com/emp.htm   Managed Care On Line;
                                     employment opportunities
                                     listing

www.tylerandco.com   Tyler and Company; executive
                                     search firm

GENERAL INFORMATION RESOURCES: REPOSITORIES OF GUIDES, STUDIES, PAPERS, INFORMATION, AND MUCH MORE

http://hippo.findlaw.com   Health Hippo
www.healthonline.com   HealthOnLine
www.healthweb.org   HealthWeb
www.medconnect.com   MedConnect; on-line resource
                                     for medical professionals

www.refdesk.com/health.html   Refdesk; virtual encyclopedia for
                                     health and medicine

www.vh.org   The Virtual Hospital; University
                                     of Iowa Hospitals and Clinics

GLOSSARIES

www.medterms.com   Medicine Net; on-line medical
                                     dictionary

www.who.ch/pll/ter/dicfair.html   World Health Organization;
                                     medical terminology search
                                     engine and dictionary

Compiled from:

Pointer, D. D. (1999). *The essential health services WWW guide.* Unpublished
    manuscript. San Diego, CA.
Nelson, J. A., & Chiasson, M. A. *A guide to sources of data.* (Appendix II,
    this volume).
Volesko, M. M. (1998). *The RWJF Internet handbook: Basic, specialized,
    health care and grant seeking resources on the World Wide Web.*
    Princton, NJ: The Robert Wood Johnson Foundation.

Index

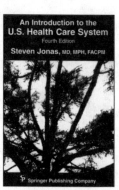